HOLY
intimacy

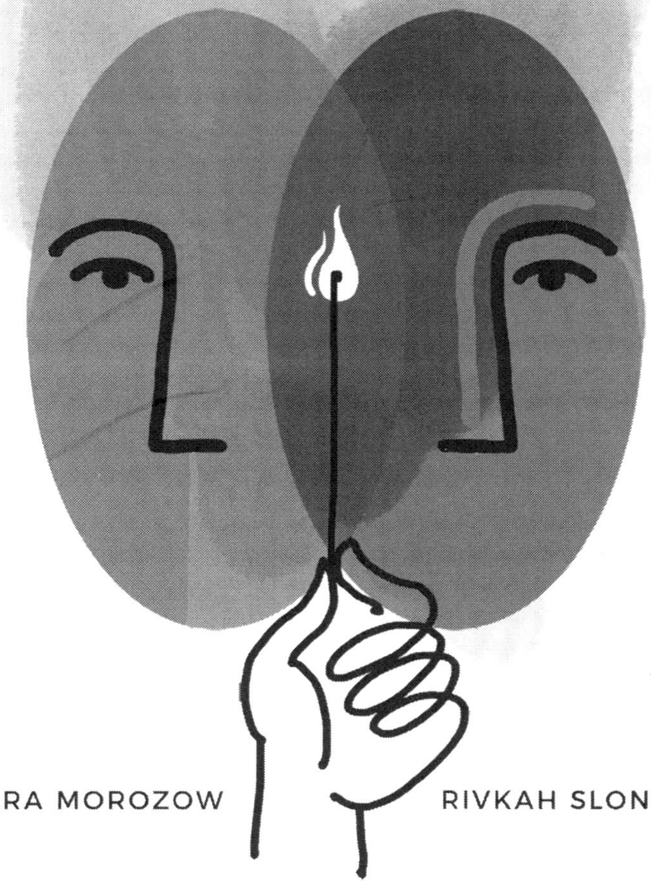

SARA MOROZOW   RIVKAH SLONIM

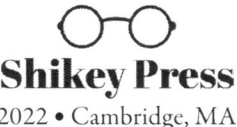

Shikey Press
2022 • Cambridge, MA

Holy Intimacy

Sara Morozow, Rivkah Slonim

© 2022, All Rights Reserved

ISBN: 978-1-958542-11-8

Published by Shikey Press

Cambridge, MA

www.ShikeyPress.com

info@ShikeyPress.com

Twitter @ShikeyPress

Readers can address questions and comments to the authors at:

Holyintimacybook@gmail.com

Cover and book illustrations by Annita Soble.

Design by David Shabtai and Annita Soble.

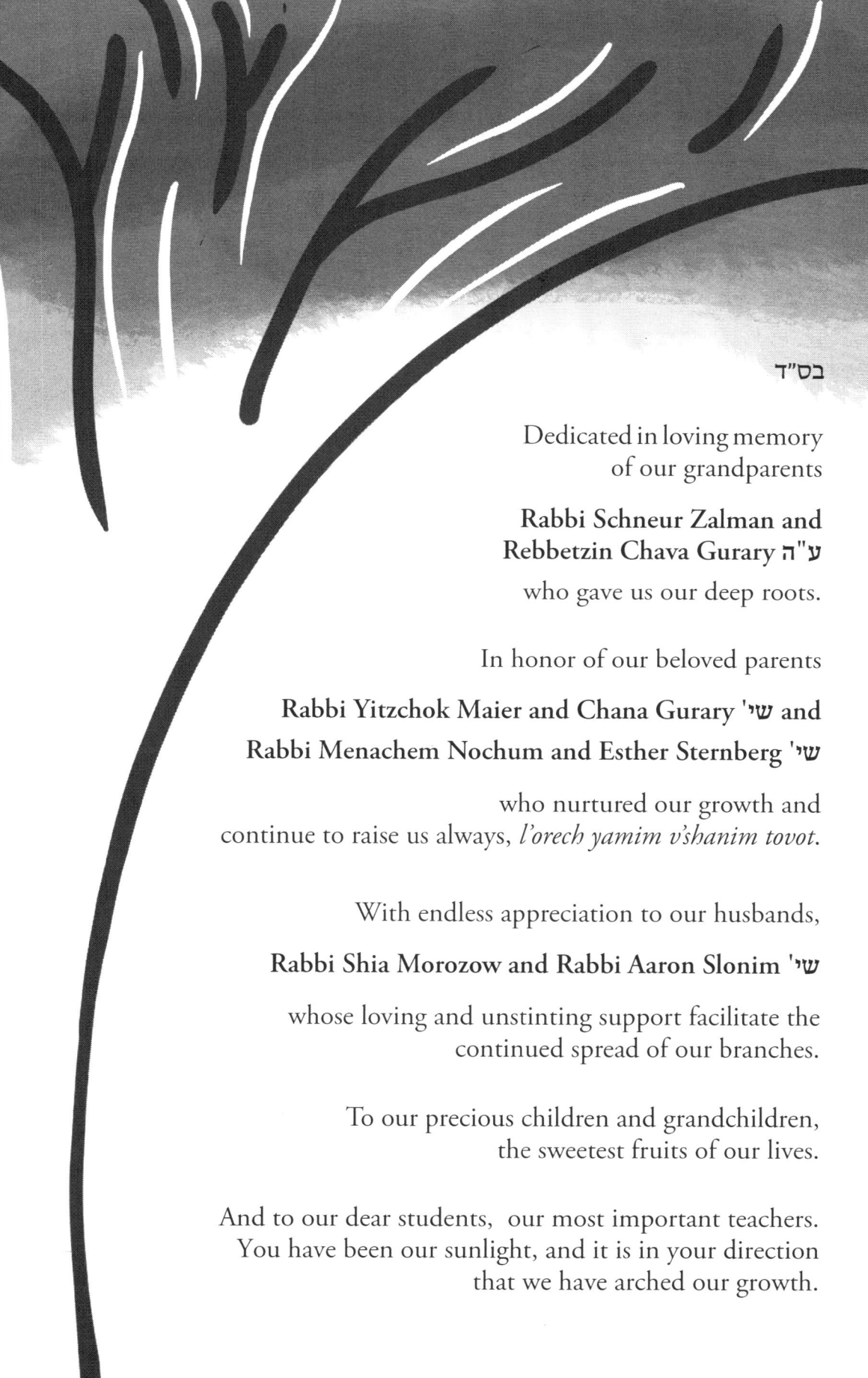

בס"ד

Dedicated in loving memory
of our grandparents

**Rabbi Schneur Zalman and
Rebbetzin Chava Gurary** ע"ה

who gave us our deep roots.

In honor of our beloved parents

Rabbi Yitzchok Maier and Chana Gurary 'שי and
Rabbi Menachem Nochum and Esther Sternberg 'שי

who nurtured our growth and
continue to raise us always, *l'orech yamim v'shanim tovot.*

With endless appreciation to our husbands,

Rabbi Shia Morozow and Rabbi Aaron Slonim 'שי

whose loving and unstinting support facilitate the
continued spread of our branches.

To our precious children and grandchildren,
the sweetest fruits of our lives.

And to our dear students, our most important teachers.
You have been our sunlight, and it is in your direction
that we have arched our growth.

ADVANCE PRAISE

What an important book. Rivkah Slonim and Sara Morozow tackle head-on the often avoided topic of sexual intimacy in a clear but respectful manner that demonstrates the comfort level for which they are advocating. While the framing of much of the discussion is on the Chabad outlook, the discussion of intimacy around familiar Jewish themes will speak to Jewish women of all backgrounds.

By interspersing their work with narratives of a large variety of women and readings by professionals, they have created a book that imparts crucial information in an eminently readable fashion. As a physician and Nishmat trained *yoetzet halacha* who has answered thousands of questions surrounding all of the topics discussed in the book, I know how important it is for women to have such information and how much accurate knowledge prevents suffering. I highly recommend this book for all, both lay and professional, to whom these topics are relevant.

Deena Zimmerman, MD, MPH, IBCLC

Dr. Deena Zimmerman is a pediatrician for Maccabi Health Services and TEREM-Immediate Medical Care in Israel, and Medical Advisor to the Jerusalem Breastfeeding Center. She is also a lactation consultant, *yoetzet halacha,* and medical advisor of Nishmat's Women's Health and Halacha websites.

Morozow and Slonim carry their balancing act through with panache, delicacy and realism, all shot through with holiness, practicality and even humor.

They take the most popular topic in the world, and project an inspirational view of the marriage relationship. This book suggests how to inspire respect, warmth, love, spirituality, dedication and other virtues into this relationship – which for most of us, is the most important relationship of our lives.

The focus is on Orthodox Jewish marriage, but there is much to inspire any reader. Whether you come from an environment which bombards readers with endless details about intimate relationships, or from an environment which shelters people completely, here is a beautifully described handbook enlightening the reader on ways to instill vital qualities into marriage – vital, but seldom or never explicitly discussed.

Kate Miriam Loewenthal, PhD

Kate Miriam Loewenthal, PhD, is emeritus Professor of Psychology in London University – Royal Holloway College and Professor of Abnormal Psychology at New York University in London, and editor of the journal Mental Health, Religion and Culture. Her research focuses on mental health, religion and culture, particularly mental health in the Jewish community.

Table of Contents

Acknowledgments i

Preface

    A Note From the Authors: Why You Are Holding This Book iii

Introduction ix

Part One

Marital Intimacy: A Play in Three Acts 1

    Chapter One

        Rupture in Gan Eden: Our Banishment 3

    Chapter Two

        Restore and Recalibrate: Our Life's Mission 11

    Chapter Three

        Gan Eden 2.0: Our Return 85

Part Two

Marriage: A Study in Three Parts 89

    Chapter Four

        When Does Kiddushin Begin? Your Choices Matter 91

    Chapter Five

        An Open Letter to the Kallah (or aspiring *kallah*) 113

    Chapter Six

        The First Night: Be'ilat Mitzvah 117

Part Three

My Home: Three Guideposts 131

    My Home: Hashem's Dwelling Place 133

  Chapter Seven
    Dinei Harchakah: Pulling Apart; Staying Together 137

  Chapter Eight
    Hide and Seek: The Mitzvah of Kisui Rosh 149

  Chapter Nine
    Fruitful: The Mitzvah of Pru U'rvu 177

Frequently Asked Questions Addressed in this Book 217

Part Four

Readings

  Appreciating Our Bodies: Inside and Out 223
    Rivky Boyarsky, APRN, CNM

  The Bodeket 249
    Channie Gurkov Akerman, RN

  A Jewish Mother and Midwife's Guide to Pregnancy and Childbirth 261
    Shayna Eliav, CNM

  Mother's Milk: A Lactation Primer 291
    Sarah Eichler, IBCLC

  Pru U'rvu: Understanding Fertility and Infertility 305
    Eliana Fine, MD, Bat-Sheva Lerner Maslow, MD, MSCTR, FACOG

  The Dream That Was: Understanding Pregnancy Loss 311
    Aimee Baron, MD

  Understanding Sexual Dysfunction: An Overview 323
    Pamela Klein, LCSW, AASECT

I'm So Confused, Am I Being Abused?
Guidance for the Orthodox Jewish Spouse & Those Who Are Trying to Help 337
    Lisa G Twerski, LCSW

Everything Sheitel Untangled 357
    Zlata Gitlin

Yakar Mikol Yakar: The Most Precious Time of Our Lives 367
    Esther Piekarski

The Holiness of the Wedding Day
Chabad Minhagim for the Yom HaChatuna 387
    Sara Morozow

Glossary 399

About the Authors 413

Acknowledgments

We are deeply grateful to Hashem for allowing us to work on and complete this book, and we offer a *tefillah* that it serves the purpose of guiding its readers towards achieving holy intimacy with their spouses and with *Hakadosh Baruch Hu*. We are grateful to the Lubavitcher Rebbe, זי"ע, for the inspiration and guidance he gave in speaking publicly – and encouraging others to speak openly – on this important topic, and for his vast Torah which saturates our work. The Rebbe's vision of a world perfected and redeemed – on the microcosmic and macrocosmic levels – is practical and tangible. He highlights the inherent greatness of each person and their ability to change the world by first changing themselves and their home. His passion for actualizing that potential, is *"ner leragleinu,"* the driving force of this project. We are humbled and filled with gratitude for the *zechut* to share so many of his ideas with our esteemed readers.

This book might have remained a dream without the integral assistance of the following individuals to whom we are deeply grateful:

Yehoshua November and Rachel Benaim-Abudarham for their masterful editing of the manuscript, and for their tremendous dedication to and support of – above and beyond anything we could have asked for – this project. The version of the book you hold is a profoundly improved version of what they were given.

Acknowledgments

Special thanks to Rabbis Yosef Y. Shusterman and Pesach Schmerling for their wise counsel, readiness to assist, and scrupulous review of many portions of this book. Rabbis Yitzchak Breitowitz, Tuvia Kasimov, and Mendel Lipskier, also answered our many questions and provided important guidance. Our gratitude goes to Mrs. Pamela Klein, LCSW for her counsel. Suffice it to say, all shortcomings and mistakes are the responsibility of the authors alone and we welcome feedback from our readers and most certainly, corrections.

Rabbi Yehuda Altein for the research, footnoting, and annotation.

Liz Rosenberg for her tutelage and counsel always, and specifically her editing of chapter one.

Miriam Lipskier, Hannah Siegel Mitrani, and Yehudah Slonim for reviewing the manuscript and providing invaluable critique and feedback. Special mention must be made of Chanie Diskin's review of multiple iterations of the manuscript and her constant and astute guidance.

Dr. Rhonda Levine's assistance with organizing an early version of this book, and Sara Raizel Wagner's expert review and wonderful suggestions regarding the chapter on *kisui rosh*.

All of our first readers challenged us to keep working and growing, revising, and perfecting. We are exceedingly grateful to them all.

Tobey Lass Karpel for introducing us to our publishers, Menachem Butler and Rabbi David Shabtai, MD of Shikey Press who embraced our project and shepherded it through the publication process.

Annita Soble for her brilliant artistic talent that graces our cover and so enhances each page of the book you hold.

Rabbi Motti Seligson for his sage counsel. Rabbis Tzvi Hirsh Gurary, Elkanah Shmotkin, and Avrohom YH Sternberg for their help with researching sources.

All of the contributors to the Readings section of the book for generously sharing their expertise with our readers.

And always, always to our husbands and children who supported our work and took our preoccupation with its gestation in stride.

Preface

A Note From the Authors:
WHY YOU ARE HOLDING THIS BOOK

Sara Morozow:

I was seventeen, in seminary, and still very naïve about all matters related to intimacy. Actually, I was rather clueless. I remember standing in my grandparents' home; I think I was looking at a *sefer,* holy book. My grandfather, a respected scholar and chassid, a Jew who relates to soul and identifies with chassidut, broke my reverie and, in a loving and direct way, said to me in Yiddish: "*Az a man un froi kushen zich nisht, zeinen zei nisht kein man un froi.*" *(If a man and woman do not kiss, they are not husband and wife.)* I was shocked, flabbergasted. I knew my grandparents to be deeply devoted to each other, even loving and tender...but kiss? And why was he talking to me about this? I looked at my grandfather. His piercing, slate-colored eyes didn't blink. He was not joking. To this day, I do not know what prompted this comment, but he must have understood that I needed to hear it.

Entering my own marriage a few years later, I was only slightly less naive and innocent than I had been, which definitely helped us create our private space. Back then, there was no comparing to anything or anyone. Perhaps my initiation into married life was slower, but, *boruch Hashem,* thank G-d, with patience, love, and understanding, we developed our unique, satisfying, and healthy intimate life.

Rivkah Slonim:

I was not yet twenty-one and had just arrived on *shlichut* to Binghamton, NY, with my husband and our five-month-old son, Levi. That was how I met Brenda, who lived across the hall from us. We were both mothers of young babies. Other than that, we were as different as two people could be. But even women from different planets can bond, and that's what we did when we ran into each other in the basement laundry room we both frequented. One day she casually asked for my opinion: "Hey, Rivkah, what do you think about John [her husband] having a vasectomy?"

I had learned of the procedure only months earlier but it was more than the term that threw me for a loop. I was flummoxed and shaken to my core. I think I managed to mutter something about how that seemed like an awfully radical form of birth control. Given their young age, I pressed on, they might try something more easily reversible even if they did not want more children at this time.

It's been close to forty years, but I still remember the encounter like it was yesterday. I went back into my apartment and consciously closed the door as if to put distance between me and what had just occurred. When I sat down on our couch to sort out my swirling feelings, I soon realized the source of my disorientation. I had come from a world where it was inherently understood that a master bedroom was a private place. No one ever told me that. Our parents' room was by no means off-limits to me and my siblings– we often hung out there. But I would never dream of going into someone else's master bedroom. In fact, to this day, even when enthusiastically invited to enter, even in the homes of my siblings or my children, I pause. And this woman I hardly knew was asking me to weigh in on a highly sensitive, private procedure her husband was contemplating?

• • • • •

Flash forward a few decades, and the two of us (Rivkah and Sara, close friends and first cousins), are talking. In addition to teaching in *Beis Rivkah,* a renowned Chabad school in Crown Heights, Brooklyn, and lecturing to diverse audiences, Sara has taught *kallot* in Crown Heights for over twenty-five years and is widely recognized as one of today's most experienced *kallah* teachers. Rivkah, as a *shluchah* at Binghamton University, has shared her life with thousands of college students across a number of generations and has been writing and lecturing across the globe for many years.

We compared notes about our respective experiences with preparing young women for marriage. Rivkah shared her fond memories of Sara's grandmother, Rebbetzin Rachel Altein *a"h*, who was her *kallah* teacher and a well-known Chabad *kallah* teacher at that time:

A Note From the Authors: Why You Are Holding This Book

> Rebbetzin Altein had one and only one thing to say about intimacy to our cohort, which she conveyed in her high-pitched voice and unflappable style: "It's natural girls, completely natural!" For me that was oddly reassuring and bolstering enough, Rivkah reflected. If it's natural, I thought, I will figure it out.
>
> We shared a laugh, and then we sobered up.

Today's *kallah* teacher could never get away with that, nor should she dream of it. Our globalized era necessitates that she elaborate far more on the subject. For most, it's not the neighbors across the hall who will unsettle you when you leave the proverbial bubble. It's the culture of social media, whose cloak of anonymity encourages sharing of information once considered deeply private, that may unnerve you. Online, anyone can appoint themselves an expert. Many do.

To be sure, digital spaces include a plethora of wonderful resources that offer information and advice in consonance with our *mesorah*. But there is so much more misinformation liberally sprinkled with the salacious and sensational.

Too many present information that is only pseudo-authoritative and in a manner that leaves little room for nuance, let alone context. When it comes to the basic facts of married life, it is unlikely today's seventeen-year-old needs to be set right by her grandfather. And yet, this generation's easy access to intimacy's most basic facts should not be equated with ease of access to clarity concerning intimacy's place in Jewish life. And certainly not guidance on how to approach the basic facts in a way that unleashes intimacy's profound spiritual and emotional possibilities.

Living in the twenty-first century means a tidal wave of information and imagery comes at you every minute of every day. The seemingly endless array of bloggers, podcast hosts, and influencers join the ever-expanding number of websites. The knowledge that an Instagram story will disappear within twenty-four hours unleashes a feeding frenzy of saving and forwarding. The ever-evolving social media scene stokes the increasingly urgent need for yet another dopamine hit.

This has left many to scramble for information often gleaned from a combination of informal conversations with friends and relatives and written materials rooted in secular values and perspectives. The result has been less than satisfying.

Over and over, women of all ages and stages, from highschoolers to those on the cusp of grandmotherhood, have asked the same question: Where in this sea of knowledge is the young woman serious about her relationship with *Hashem* supposed to find the wisdom and direction she seeks? Where in this barrage of images will she find the portrait of her life?

We have heard these questions over and over again. We feel for women of all ages, and especially for new brides. Engagement is such an exciting time; a couple's future lies ahead of them, filled with promise. But as the couple seeks to gain an understanding of the new life rapidly approaching, they may find themselves beset by anxiety, especially when it comes to the area of physical intimacy. The lack of accessible instruction that is down to earth but rooted in heaven has led to significant confusion. This vacuum has spawned both overly stringent and overly lax behaviors and attitudes, both of which can erode a couple's *shalom bayit,* domestic harmony.

So, together, we decided to write something just for you: our students, daughters, younger sisters, nieces, all of our friends, and all of your friends.

The contemporary *kallah,* as well as those young women not quite at that junction but curious and thinking, along with their mothers and grandmothers, should not have to guess, worry, or feel anxious. She should never feel deprived of important information. Most significantly, she should not have to scrounge for morsels of the Torah's truth and beauty; these are her birthright.

We live in exciting times. The sea of information that sometimes seems to engulf us serves as the precursor to the era when ומלאה הארץ דעה את ה' כמים לים מכסים, *the world will be filled with knowledge of Hashem as the waters cover the seabed.*[1] Humankind has not only the promise that *Yemot HaMashiach,* the days of the Messiah, are near, but we were handed a specific charge to hasten that day. Quoting the Arizal, the Lubavitcher Rebbe taught that the Jewish women of our generation are the *gilgulim,* the reincarnation, of the Jewish women who left *Mitzrayim,* Biblical Egypt.[2] Just as *Bnei Yisrael,* the nation of Israel, were redeemed in the merit of the righteous women of that day, so too, will today's women bring the present *geulah,* redemption.

In these final centuries before the *geulah,* Hashem has opened His treasure chest and gifted Jews with the teachings of chassidut. A couple hundred years ago, there were those who believed that these holy teachings should remain hidden and safeguarded, shared only with a select few. The first Chabad Rebbe, Rabbi Shneur Zalman of Liadi, on the other hand, insisted that chassidut must be revealed and serve as a powerful light in confusing times. To underscore the potency and necessity of chassidut in our era, he evoked the metaphoric image of a king's precious crown Jewel that, when ground up and mixed with water, could serve as the elixir that would heal the king's ailing son, *Bnei Yisrael,* and usher in *Yemot HaMashiach.*[3] True, Rabbi Shneur Zalman acknowledged,

---

1 *Yeshayahu* 11:9.

2 *Likkutei Sichot,* vol. 23, p. 240.

3 *Igrot Kodesh* by the Frierdiker Rebbe, vol. 3, pp. 326-328.

A Note From the Authors: Why You Are Holding This Book

we run the risk of diluting the preciousness of the stone and even squandering the droplets that fall from the mouth of the prince as he is fed. But what choice is there?

In a similar vein, for too long, discussions concerning sexual intimacy were compartmentalized; thought to be beyond the pale of *frum* life. We believe it is time to do away with this perceived division. This book addresses intimacy through the prism of Torah and chassidut.

Many of the ideas set forth in this book are predicated on Chabad Chassidut. Our aim is to present this content to Jewish women of all stripes, whether or not they have ever delved into Chabad Chassidut. We believe these ideas are foundational and enriching, regardless of background and *hashkafah,* religious outlook. Naturally, each reader can choose if and to what degree she incorporates the practices within her specific pathway in Torah and *mitzvot*.

We present this book with some degree of trepidation, as, historically, matters concerning intimacy have been imparted privately from mother to daughter, or via *kallah* teacher to her students.

The modern-day necessitates a different approach. During a *farbrengen* in 1968 the Lubavitcher Rebbe said:[4]

> **"Is this modest conduct?" you might ask, "Can one talk publicly about such things [intimacy]?" Today, intimate subjects are written about openly in the newspapers and are being taught to ten-year-old children in school. There is a rationalization for such practices. For a child's education to be complete, people explain, it is necessary to teach him about all the dimensions of married life. But they are being taught an immoral conception of married life. [In such an environment,] one should not be ashamed to speak about taharat hamishpachah. The listeners will know more than the teachers, but the listeners' knowledge will not have come from a holy source. So teach taharat hamishpachah. Don't be embarrassed. You will not reveal any secrets that your listeners do not know. Speak openly!**

---

[4] 12 Tammuz, 5728.

In 1974 the Rebbe similarly reiterated:[5]

> **I once asked a Rav why he doesn't speak about taharat hamishpachah. He responded that it isn't tzniut [to discuss matters related to physical intimacy], therefore he cannot speak about taharat hamishpachah. I told him that in years gone by, people were unaware; there wasn't widespread knowledge about these matters. Now, unfortunately, we live in an era when however many details the Rav knows, the individuals he must influence know even more!**
>
> **It is only that since Jewish daughters are proper, they know about this because they study it as a subject, whether it is called biology or something else. But they know all the details, and he does not need to disclose anything to them; they can teach him. What they don't know, however, is the importance of taharat hamishpachah…**

We have taken the Rebbe's charge to heart.

If you are reading this, you are, in all likelihood, already committed to a marriage and family built on a firm bedrock of foundational ideas. You understand intuitively that the strength of *Am Yisrael* depends on the *kedushah,* holiness, *taharah,* purity, and the emotional health of each *bayit ne'eman b'yisrael,* a faithful home among the Jewish people. Consider this read as a conversation between sisters, in the spirit of what our rabbis have taught: דברים היוצאים מן הלב נכנסים אל הלב, words that come from the heart enter the heart.[6]

---

[5] 19 Kislev, 5735.

[6] *Sefer Hayashar* (Rabbeinu Tam), ch. 13.

Introduction

No one is indifferent to the term sex. It evokes strong, often antithetical feelings: excitement, fear, anticipation, dread, curiosity, and often enough, confusion and anxiety. That is no wonder. More than any other aspect of life, this subject cries out for both detailed examination and larger context, without which sexuality is hardly understood.

Linking sex with intimacy, as in the term sexual intimacy, is a huge stride forward in the search for context, but it's just the beginning. We hope you find this book an enriching and inspiring read. This is the kind of book that will resonate in accordance with your age and stage in life. If you are reading it as a *kallah* or before you are engaged to be married, keep in mind that many life experiences still lie ahead of you. While we hope you will gain much from this book at the present time, we also invite you to revisit its pages again and at that later juncture, perhaps relate to its content in a whole new way. There may be paragraphs and chapters that don't speak to you at the present moment, and that's okay. This is a book to grow with.

While each reader of this book will choose how she wants to use it, we strongly suggest reading the book in its totality and optimally reading the sections in order. If at all possible, resist the urge to go straight to the practical questions and answers. To get the most out of this book, you will want to be familiar with the lofty and beautiful spiritual context that frames and informs the act of physical intimacy.

On style:

There are books that present ideas, philosophy, theology, mysticism etc.

There are books that offer assistance; the self-help genre.

This book is a hybrid. Its sections move in a zig-zag motion, presenting ideas and ideals rooted in *halacha*, chassidut, and Kabbalah, followed by practical analysis as well as commonly asked questions and answers. In explaining our thought process and goal, we offer the following analogy:

Not very far from Buckingham Palace sits an underrated tourist site known as the Royal Mews. There, in addition to seeing a working stable, curious tourists can view the royal family's collection of historic horse-drawn carriages, as well as the Royal Sleighs and the State Limousines; Bentleys, Daimlers, and a rare 1948 Rolls Royce Phantom IV.

There is a lot to take in, but, without a doubt, the most impressive item in the exhibit is the Golden State Coach replete with rich artistic intricacies. Aiming to own the most elegant coach ever seen, George III commissioned this piece in 1762. The Golden State Coach has been used at every coronation since that of George IV in 1821 and was employed as recently as 2002, on the occasion of Queen Elizabeth's Golden Jubilee year. The carriage is made of four tons - or 128,000 ounces - of gold, worth about $38,960,754.00 at today's price. Because of its weight, the coach requires eight horses to draw it and, even then, cannot move faster than walking speed. The body of the coach is slung by braces covered with Moroccan leather and decorated with gilt buckles. The interior is lined with velvet and satin.

A priceless piece of art, the coach screams royalty. And yet, all the luxury notwithstanding, for many years, the Golden State Coach provided an intensely uncomfortable ride. In the words of King William IV, a former naval officer, being driven in the Gold State Coach was like being on board a ship tossing in a rough sea. Queen Victoria complained of the distressing oscillation of the cabin and would often refuse to ride the Coach. A later monarch, King George VI, said that his journey in the coach on the day of his coronation was "one of the most uncomfortable rides I have ever had in my life." Clearly, more thought should have been invested in providing the occupants of the coach with a comfortable experience.

Every Jewish woman is a *bas Melech*, a daughter of the King. In His kindness and mercy, our Father, the King of all kings, has lovingly fashioned and presented us with a golden state coach, the Torah. Unlike the golden state coach designed for the English monarchy, Hashem conveyed the loftiest ideals of the Torah through a system of *halacha* designed with comfort in mind. Described as *darchei noam,* ways of pleasantness, our metaphoric carriage offers not only bare-bones practicality but also a smooth ride.

As believing Jews, we accept that our limited intelligence cannot grasp Hashem's *chochmah*; by definition, there will be much we cannot understand. We accept that, at times, fulfillment of *mitzvos* will necessitate a measure of *mesirat nefesh*, self sacrifice of the bodily sort, and a modicum of *mesirat haratzon,* abnegating our will before our Creator. Still, we recognize that the Ultimate Designer would not construct a coach bereft of basic amenities, a coach that fails to facilitate its riders' comfort.

On the contrary, our coach holds the promise of a smoother ride through life, of more peace of mind and harmony than any other vehicle might provide. It is simply a matter of making sure we recognize the ways in which the coach is properly outfitted to provide for our creature comforts. (Indeed, we will revisit, on various fronts, the notion that physical intimacy, one of our central creature comforts, proves most luxurious and smooth when guided by love and holy intent.)

While the Golden State Coach remains regal and splendid, unparalleled in its beauty, it is now fitted with modern amenities to provide greater comfort. In the analogy, our coach has no rival and boasts all of the bells and whistles built into the original mechanism. It is up to each generation to share this truth, and make it well known.

Throughout this book, we hope for you to be swept up in the majesty, the grandeur, and the privilege inherent in Jewish marriage, but no less important, we want you to revel in the ride.

On terminology:

In this work, we have chosen to use the term sexual intimacy, rather than euphemisms like "being together" or "the mitzvah," in the belief that when we speak of *halacha*, clarity is integral. Sexual intimacy is the best English term we can find to encapsulate the terms used in Torah sources such as *tashmish hamitah*, literally translated as the using of the bed, *chibbur*, connection, *zivug*, coupling, and *biah*, coming.

Furthermore, it is important that we nourish a positive, healthy attitude towards this important aspect of our lives. Like the words eating, sleeping, and breathing, the word sex describes a natural function. Lamentably, the term has come to be associated with a behavior that too often occurs outside of a meaningful relationship. But by studiously avoiding the term altogether, we further cement the erroneous but pervasive assumption that, for Torah Jews, there is something shameful about this subject. This is decidedly untrue.

There is nothing more holy in our lives than our marital relations. Surely, no physical relationship can ensue without the fusing of the couple's minds, hearts, and souls. We use the specific expression sexual intimacy to underscore this truth.

Enjoy the read!

Part One
Marital Intimacy:
A Play in Three Acts

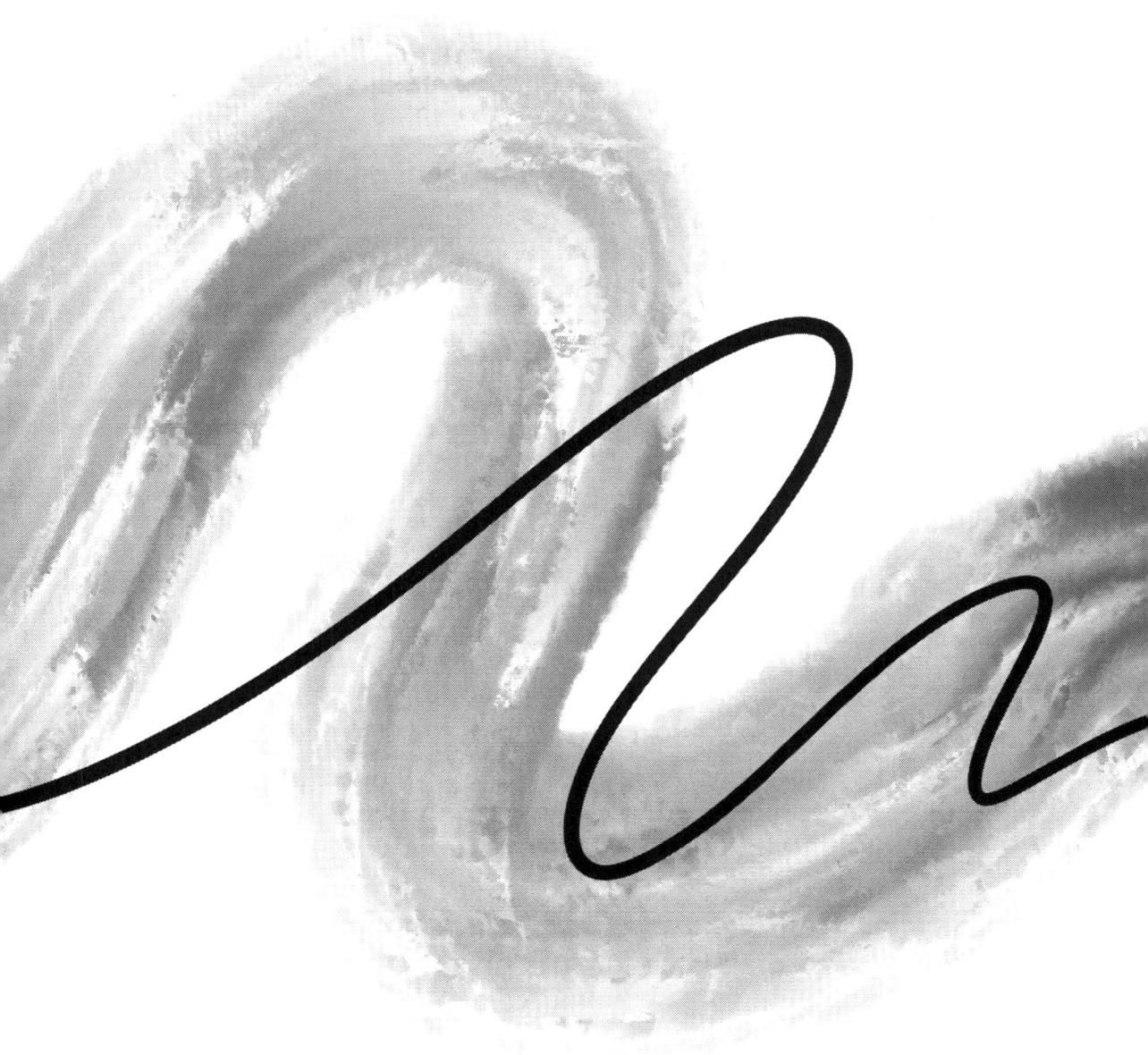

chapter one

Rupture in Gan Eden:
OUR BANISHMENT

To delve into the Torah's first few chapters is to understand sexual intimacy in its ideal state, its descent from that state, and the emergent possibility of intimacy that surpasses even the initial ideal. This book aims to help you achieve the latter form of intimacy. The first step is to go back to the very beginning, to revisit sexual intimacy's origins.

The story of humanity, and therefore that of human sexuality begins in Gan Eden. After placing Adam in Gan Eden, Hashem commanded him:

מכל עץ הגן אכל תאכל, ומעץ הדעת טוב ורע לא תאכל ממנו

> From every tree of the garden you may indeed eat, but from the Tree of Knowledge of Good and Evil you must not eat…[1]

History takes a very different turn. A surface reading of the Gan Eden narrative suggests Chava defaulted in eating from the tree. A chassidic teaching explains that something more profound was at play: Chava perceived that eating from the tree was the key to unlocking humanity's mission in the universe. (As we will see, it ushered free

---

[1] *Bereishit* 2:16-17.

will and, therefore, meaningful service of Hashem into the world.) And so she ate and invited Adam to as well.

Looking at a picture of human existence pre and post the *chet*, sin, helps bear out the ultimate Divine plan Chava had intuited. The Torah relates that just before Adam and Chava partook of the tree,

ויהיו שניהם ערומים האדם ואשתו ולא יתבששו

They were both naked, the man and his wife, and they were not ashamed.[2]

Immediately after they ate from the Tree, however, the Torah says:

ותפקחנה עיני שניהם וידעו כי עירֻמם הם, ויתפרו עלה תאנה ויעשו להם חגרת. וישמעו את קול ה' אלקים מתהלך בגן לרוח היום, ויתחבא האדם ואשתו מפני ה' אלקים בתוך עץ הגן. ויקרא ה' אלקים אל האדם, ויאמר לו איכה. ויאמר את קלך שמעתי בגן, ואירא כי עירֹם אנכי ואחבא.

The eyes of both of them were opened and they realized that they were naked. They sewed together fig leaves and made aprons for themselves.

They heard G-d's voice moving about in the garden with the wind of the day. The man and his wife hid themselves from G-d among the trees of the garden.

G-d called to the man and said, "Where are you?"

"I heard your voice in the garden," replied the man, "and I was afraid because I was naked, so I hid."

Hashem rejoins the conversation in the text with an illuminating question:

ויאמר מי הגיד לך כי עירֹם אתה, המן העץ אשר צויתיך לבלתי אכל ממנו אכלת?

Who told you that you were naked? Have you eaten from the tree from which I commanded you not to eat?[3]

The story of *chet etz hadaat tov v'ra*, the sin of [eating from] the Tree of Knowledge of Good and Evil, is bracketed by references to Adam and Chava in a state of undress. However, the way Adam and Chava experienced nakedness pre-*chet* could not be

---

2   *Bereishit* 2:25.

3   *Bereishit* 3:7-11.

more different from the way they experienced it post-*chet*, highlighting how the event drastically altered humanity's understanding of and relationship with the body. The episode of the *chet* is also key to deciphering our complex relationship with modesty and sexuality. More profoundly, the account of the *chet* underscores a rupture in our relationship with Hashem that led to our expulsion from Gan Eden. This estrangement precipitated many other shifts that still affect humanity today, including paramount changes in our experience of intimacy.

Synonymous with this breach initiated by the *chet* is a shift in human perception, or an awakening of *daat*. Conventionally, *daat* is defined as knowledge. Chassidut teaches that the term *daat* speaks more fundamentally about a dawning; a realization and consciousness, specifically, of the self. It is the way in which what we know affects us and becomes integrated into our psyches. As the *pessukim* spell out vis-a-vis Adam's and Chava's sudden realization of their nakedness, it was the *chet* that introduced this new dynamic of self-awareness.

The Rambam explains that before the *chet*, human intelligence functioned in black and white.[4] Man could differentiate between truth and falsehood from a state of emotional distance. Unencumbered by emotion, human perception was clear, unclouded, and unbiased.

After the *chet*, humans became יודעי טוב ורע, knowers of good and bad.[5] The terms good and bad describe our relationship with particular constructs. Things that attract us or resonate with us are labeled "good" while that which repulses us is labeled "bad." These terms represent subjective conventions, unlike the objective difference between right and wrong, truth and falsehood. And naturally, these repulsions and attractions extend out of the sense of self that dawned on Adam and Chava (and all of humanity after that), as a consequence of the *chet*.

In other words, the *chet* introduced an era of confusion in which good and bad could mix.[6] Endless criteria for assigning value, coupled with the new sensation of selfhood and a drive for self gratification, replaced the distinct sense of wrong or right that prevailed in the selfless and objective Gan Eden era.

Possessing absolute moral clarity before the *chet*, Adam and Chava experienced only a purposeful yearning for sexual relations as a means to fulfill the divine commandments

---

[4] *Moreh Nevuchim* 1:2.

[5] *Bereishit* 3:5.

[6] *Shaarei Kedusha*. 1:1; Rabbi Chaim Vital. *Sefer Hamamorim* 5725 p. 344.

to "become one flesh"[7] and to "be fruitful and multiply."[8] They engaged in sexual relations just as they did everything else: in service of Hashem.[9] The same applied to all the body's functions during this epoch. Just as there was no raging appetite for nor emotional attachment to sexual pleasures pre-*chet*, so too, Adam and Chava merely registered a healthy desire to eat rooted in acknowledging the body's nutritional needs.[10] In fact, their very bodies radiated an intense light of *kedusha*.[11] As chassidut teaches, not only did the first couple lack self-awareness, but, as will be further developed, they were subsumed, body and soul, in the Divine reality, wedded to G-d consciousness.[12]

Eating from the *etz hadaat* changed everything. It introduced consciousness of the self, *daat*, as distinct and apart from Hashem.[13] It heralded the possibility of disjunction between man and Creator; the eclipse of G-d consciousness by self-consciousness. It became the root of all spiritual ills and misalignments. Hence, suddenly, Adam and Chava felt shame in their nakedness. Shame is the emotion that wells up when a discrepancy exists between who you are and who you know you ought to be. Indeed, this first case of shame in world history came as a result of the couple's newfound possibility, even passion, for self-indulgence, an extension of their newfound sense of self navigating the mixed-up world they now inhabited. This new arrangement often put them at odds with the impulses of their souls, which continued to crave transcendence of self, to be swallowed in the Divine reality.

With our bodies and souls no longer automatically synchronized, human life simultaneously gained a new fragility and a new power. Humanity was stricken with mortality. Working and birthing now required exertion and pain. Human sexuality, eating, and drinking became complicated and subject to potential abuse. Simultaneously, humanity gained freedom of choice. Unique among all creations, and mirroring the Creator, human beings were vested with volition. The power to soar, achieve, and even transcend was matched only by the potential to stumble and fall. While expulsion from the Garden seemed to mark a demotion, in truth, it was Hashem saying, *Now you have choice. From now on, you will operate outside of the safe zone. I am graduating you to the sphere in which your actions will make all the difference.*

---

[7] *Bereishit* 2:24.

[8] *Bereishit* 9:7.

[9] *Reishit Chochmah, Shaar Hakedushah* 16:9.

[10] *Ramban Bereishit* 2:9.

[11] *Vayikra Rabbah* 20:2.

[12] *Torah Or, Bereishit* 5d.

[13] *Torah Or, Bereishit* 5c-d.

Rupture in Gan Eden: Our Banishment

This was also the beginning of reciprocity between Hashem and humanity. Just as humanity was banished from the Garden, so was Hashem's presence, the *Shechinah*, Divine presence, banished from the Earth, retreating upwards into the heavenly realms.[14] Indeed, this retreat created a vacuum that contributed to the new sense of self-awareness on the part of humanity noted earlier; it left space for humanity to view the world as independent of the Creator.

• • • • •

Chava intuited the ultimate secret of the universe in partaking of the tree: Hashem desired a splitting off of humanity from Himself that would subsequently enable a more profound reunion. In the pre-schism, Adam and Chava were "one flesh" with Hashem; their sole preoccupation was with the Divine, and they were completely subservient to His will. And yet, Chava sensed that humanity was meant to accomplish something greater.[15] While the serpent's intention was to create two opposing teams, pitting man against G-d, Chava knew that like herself and Adam, all of creation had been created as one with G-d, and commanded to become unified again.[16]

This model of separation for a deeper subsequent reunification was the true will of Hashem in His relationship with the larger world. In the beginning, the world was perfectly aligned with the *Ratzon Ha'Elyon*, the Supernal Will. Humanity was "one flesh" with Hashem, as it were; immersed body and soul, in the Divine reality. This arrangement left no room for humanity's contribution. If individuals could not rebel against Hashem, then they could not choose to embrace Hashem either.

This same dynamic is reflected in Adam and Chava's union. Originally, Hashem created Chava and Adam as one dimorphous being. Shortly thereafter, He declared: לא טוב היות האדם לבדו, It is not good for man to be alone, and severed them from each other.[17] They were separated, however, not to cause divisiveness but so, as two distinct individuals, they could consciously *choose* to unite.

---

14 *Midrash Tanchuma, Parshat Naso*, sec. 16.

15 *Torat Moshe* (Alshich) on *Bereishit* 3: 6; *Chaim V'shalom* (The Munkatcher) ad loc.

16 *Torah Or, Bereishit* 6a.

17 *Bereishit* 2:18.

על כן יעזב איש את אביו ואת אמו, ודבק באשתו והיו לבשר אחד.

> Therefore a man leaves his father and his mother and clings to his wife, and they become one flesh.[18]

Similarly, eating from the tree ruptured Hashem and humans' relationship. This very rupture allowed humanity to truly *become* "one flesh" with Hashem, only this time of our own volition and through our own efforts. And this was G-d's deepest desire: נתאוה הקב"ה להיות לו יתברך דירה בתחתונים, G-d desired a home, a place where His essence could be revealed, in this lower plane.[19] To fulfill that desire, the home has to be built by humans, Hashem's ambassadors in the lower realm who are, post-schism, characterized by flaws and foibles. Eating from the tree, Chava understood, was the only way to set the stage for the fulfillment of this purpose. Humanity lays each brick of that home following Hashem's instruction against the backdrop of the potential to do otherwise.

In this new reality, there could and would be the capacity to stumble, or to turn away. Adam and Chava recognized their own transformation resulting from having disobeyed G-d's injunction, and they also realized how easy it would now be for them to choose unwisely, again and again. Beset by this shame and the overall possibility of shame they'd ushered into the world, they ran for cover.

Our coupling, now tainted by systemic self centeredness, can easily spiral down into a lust-driven, autonomous activity and might even involve abuse of others. Or it could be elevated to serve the most exalted platform of our lives, our marital bond, and the children we bear (a central facet of creating a dwelling place in the lower realm).

Though rife with challenge, *daat*, is not necessarily problematic. Indeed, when correctly channeled, *daat*, is humanity's ultimate triumph.

Immediately after Adam and Chava's banishment from the Garden, the couple once again is engaged with *daat*. This time the Torah says, והאדם ידע את חוה, Adam "knew" Chava,[20] meaning was sexually intimate with Chava. She then conceived, and gave birth. Here we have *daat*, as it is turned inside out, from self-centered indulgence to other-centered devotion, a true "knowing" of and paying attention to another.

Intimacy is first and foremost about connection on every level, teaches the Torah. It is about listening and sharing; empathy and devotion. Individual identity does

---

18 *Bereishit* 2:24.

19 *Midrash Tanchuma, Parshat Naso*, sec. 16: This can be seen as one of the greatest seeming contradictions in Torah.

20 *Bereishit* 4:1.

not disappear, yet intimacy denotes a constant, comprehensive effort to focus on the needs and desires of the other until the connection is seamless. It is about an other-consciousness so suffusive that it is no longer paramount to separate individual desires from those of your beloved. Instead, your greatest desire is to be one.

Most essentially, this unity is fueled by reverting back to G-d consciousness; by placing the sanctity of the marital bond, a transcendent value, above all else. Sanctified intimacy is about alighting once more to G-d consciousness even as we retain consciousness of the self.

Achieving sanctified intimacy is no simple task. Sexuality presents challenges that the laws of physics help illustrate. Objects of equal weight will fall to the ground with variable velocity and impact force depending on the height from which the object is thrown. If an object falling from great height meets no resistance, it will fall deeply into the ground–far more deeply than if thrown from a lower height. This mirrors a spiritual truism: the more elevated and exalted the potential of the act, the lower it can plummet.[21]

One of the most important tools in achieving holy intimacy is the act of consciously framing our lives, and specifically our intimate experiences, within the rubric of *tzniut*, modesty. Adam and Chava's fig leaves– the first clothing humankind ever wore– along with the couple's sense of sexual intimacy as a private reunion of two soulmates, set a precedent for *tzniut* in navigating intimacy in the post-*chet* world.

The solution to avoiding a great moral plumet in the area of intimacy is not to retreat into asceticism. Hashem does not ask humans to repress our impulses and subvert our sexuality by ignoring or heavily cloaking the body until its natural impulses and contours are unrecognizable. We are called upon, instead, to unlock the potential holiness in each encounter by using it in service of a higher purpose.

---

[21] *Sefer Hamaamorim* 5708. p. 195.

chapter two

Restore and Recalibrate:
OUR LIFE'S MISSION

Siddur Kiddushin:
Marriage contains a hidden compartment;
The kallah and chatan's inexpressible bond

As *kallah* and *chatan* stand under the *chuppah* on their wedding day, an *Or Eloki*, a Divine light, surrounds the couple and fuses their *neshamot*, merging the two souls into an eternal unit. For each person, these holy moments serve as the basis of marriage *and* shape the contours of the couple's lives together. Every aspect thereof is rich with meaning.

At this most important time, the *mesader kiddushin,* the officiant, makes the following *bracha:*

ברוך אתה ה׳ אלקינו מלך העולם, אשר קדשנו במצותיו וצונו על העריות, ואסר לנו את הארוסות, והתיר לנו את הנשואות לנו על ידי חפה וקדושין. ברוך אתה ה׳, מקדש עמו ישראל על ידי חפה וקדושין.

Blessed are You, Hashem our G-d, King of the universe, who has sanctified us with His *mitzvot* and has commanded us [to keep the *mitzvot*] concerning forbidden relations. He has prohibited us [from having relations with] those who are merely betrothed, but He has permitted us [to have relations with] those married to us through the marriage canopy and the wedding ritual. Blessed are You, Hashem, who has sanctified His people Yisrael through chuppah and kiddushin.

Among the many, many *brachot*, this is the only one that concerns a prohibited act.[1]

The *bracha* references *kiddushin*, also known as *erusin*. *Erusin* is defined as betrothal, and is the initial binding stage in the relationship between a man and woman who will eventually marry.[2] Marriage proper is known as a *nissuin*. Nowadays, these two stages in Jewish marriage, betrothal and marriage proper, follow each other with little pause. Just the reading of the *ketubah*, marriage contract, separates the two under the *chuppah*.

The *bracha* on *kiddushin* notes that, at this stage, the betrothed couple are prohibited from engaging in sexual intimacy. Only after the *chuppah*, provided that the *kallah* is *tehorah*, ritually pure, are they permitted to each other. Why, one might ask, have a *halachic* construct that binds a man and woman in an exclusive relationship while at the same time prohibiting them from enjoying intimacy?

The fact that the two stages remain *halachically* separate entities underscores the essential nature of the *kiddushin* commitment.[3] *Kiddushin*, betrothal, establishes the transcendent fact of a couple's soul union. Though less visible than *nissuin*, *kiddushin* shines a light on the exaltedness of the couple's connection, a bond that defies physical expression. Only after this prerequisite, do we proceed to *nissuin*, marriage, which acts as the portal into physical intimacy and life as a married couple.

This *bracha* reveals a profound lesson concerning the Jewish understanding of marriage. *Kiddushin* underscores that marriage is anything but a conventional relationship. In stark contrast to the hook-up culture that gave us the term "friends with benefits," the basis of a Torah marriage is marked by what used to be an extended betrothal phase during which there are no sexual benefits. The couple cannot even be *b'yichud*, alone together, at this point.

Long after the wedding day, *kiddushin* reminds us that even when life is challenging and, in all the mundane ways, our marriage does not seem to be prospering, husband and wife remain one on a more exalted soul level. Marriage is unlike any other relationship that we might end when it does not seem to be serving our purpose. When faced with problems in our marriage we should relate to them as challenges we are facing together.

---

1   Insight based on *Hegyonot el Ami* 2:41.

2   In no way should this *halachic* construct be confused with the modern day engagement which is why we use the rather dated term, betrothal.

3   As illustrated by the fact that both the *kiddushin* and the *nissuin* components of the modern day *chuppah* are preceded by a separate *bracha* of *Hagafen*.

What would I do if my hand was terribly infected or compromised in some way, would I casually have it amputated?

If and when, despite arduous efforts, a marital union has to be terminated, *chas v'shalom*, G-d forbid, the couple cannot simply walk away from one another or merely file a divorce. Even when their marriage appears to have ended, the dissolution of the underpinning oneness, which is the uncoupling of two half *neshamot*, can only happen through a *get*, religious divorce.

As part of *nissuin*, *sheva brachot*, seven uniquely crafted blessings, are recited under the *chuppah*. Indeed, for the first week, whenever a meal in celebration of the *kallah* and *chatan* takes place in the presence of a *minyan*, the *brachot* are recited again. The crucial life messages held in these *brachot* always bear repeating. These *brachot* anchor the couple's newly forged bond within the context of Jewish history, beginning with Adam and Chava's marriage in *Gan Eden* and ending with the ultimate marriage of the Jewish people to *Hakadosh Baruch Hu*, the Holy One Blessed be He, with the coming of *Mashiach*. When these blessings are understood through the lens of chassidut, we glean vital insight and instruction in our quest to build a *binyan adai ad*, an everlasting edifice.[4]

---

[4] *Reshimot* nos. 123 and 149; *Sefer Habayit Hayehudi*. Rabbi Karasik. p. 108-132.

Borei Pri Hagafen: Getting Past a Skin-Deep Connection

ברוך אתה ה' אלקינו מלך העולם, בורא פרי הגפן.

Blessed are You, Hashem our G-d, King of the universe,
who creates the fruit of the vine.

The *chachamim* taught, נכנס יין יצא סוד, when wine enters (is imbibed) it causes secrets to emerge.[5] Marriage is a marvel and a wonder, one of the sweetest secrets of the universe. This *bracha* reminds the *chatan* and *kallah* that just as wine constitutes the most essential aspect of the grape, so too should the couple set their focus on their spiritual and emotional connection. When that essential bond is nourished, physical intimacy flourishes in the most healthy and fulfilling ways. Profound truths emerge only when the proverbial grape is squeezed, through shared life experiences and commitment to shared goals.

During the first years of marriage, a couple could experience a fiery, hormonally charged physical relationship. For some this comes easily, others may have to work through some initial awkwardness. Either way, the initial intensity most often gives way to a deeper, more soulful mellowness. Very much like wine in which the various compounds break down over time and then later reconnect, forming new structure and causing a deeper, finer taste, our marital relationship is constantly evolving. The peaks and valleys of a life traversed together lend our relationship its particular flavor. Through it all, our physical intimacy is a time of unique connection.

Many couples experience their deepest connection through their physical intimacy. It is a shared private escape from the busyness that is life. Intimacy is a safe harbor that offers emotional pleasure and the thrill of being enveloped by someone you love and who loves you. Optimally, it is about soldering our hearts, minds, souls, and bodies. It is a feeling of homecoming and wholeness.

In the words of the *Shelah HaKadosh*, a 17th century commentator and mystic:[6]

ענין הזיווג כשהוא בקדושה ובטהרה הוא קדוש במאוד ומעורר למעלה. מתקדש מלמטה מעט, מקדשין אותו מלמעלה הרבה, ומקיים קדושים תהיו כי קדוש אני ה' אלקיכם. כי כל זיווג הוא מעין זיווג אדם וחוה הנעשה בצלמו ודמותו ית'.

---

5   *Eruvin* 65a.

6   Rabbi Yeshayah Horowitz, *Shnei Luchot Habrit, Sha'ar Ha'Otiyot, ot kuf, kedushat hazivug*, par. 384.

> When a couple is intimate and does so in a holy and pure way, it carries tremendous sanctity and has an effect in the spiritual realms. When you sanctify yourself even just a little, you are granted a far greater level of sanctity from Above, and you fulfill the verse, 'Be holy, because I am holy.' Every union is reminiscent of the union of Adam and Chava, who were formed in G-d's image.

Marital relations are the medium for fulfilling both the great mitzvah of *pru u'rvu*, having children, and the great mitzvah of *onah*, a husband's obligation to provide his wife with sexual pleasure. Chassidut, which emphasizes *hitkadshut*, elevating and consecrating each detail of our lives, highlights that sexual intimacy is a moment when *hitkadshut* is particularly crucial. Especially when sexual intimacy might lead to conception.

The most important sex organ is the brain. The quality of intimacy has to do with feeling valued, cherished, respected, safe, and cared for. What happens in the bedroom is nourished by what happens in every other room of the house. When we are calm, happy, and feel fulfilled, we fuel our intimate relationship. In like manner, the loving expressions we share in our inner sanctum, the kissing, hugging, and cuddling, no less than actual intercourse, lends meaning to every other aspect of our lives. Just as a soul animates a body, a husband and wife's shared emotional bond animates the couple's physical intimacy.

Emotional intimacy, much like physical intimacy, differs for each couple, and even for the same couple, at different points in their life together. Intimacy is always about that feeling of closeness that invites vulnerability and a sense of security. It provides a license to share personal feelings and feel assured that your partner will show understanding, affirmation, and care. Emotional intimacy, like physical intimacy, is about closeness, which includes feelings of trust, respect, tenderness and passion. It contains the powerful elements of exclusivity and safe haven; the assumptions that what you share with this person is unique and that they will always have your back. As the first of the seven blessings underscores, physical intimacy serves as the outer casing or external expression for the profound emotional connection shared by husband and wife.

YOU MIGHT BE WONDERING:

Why an emphasis on being intimate at night and specifically, in the dark?

There is clear preference in both *halachic* and *hashkafic* sources towards intimacy at night rather than during the day.[7] Nocturnal hours are generally quieter; the couple's focus on each other can be sharper, with less chance of interruption or distraction.[8]

Halacha also addresses the importance of intercourse [as opposed to foreplay] taking place in the dark.[9] Darkness makes it easier to achieve single minded, laser sharp focus on the internal landscape; on the feelings for each other that fill our hearts and minds. Light increases the likelihood that our attention will bifurcate and stray to externalities. Even when a woman and her husband might not share this concern, *halacha* guides the couple towards elevating their time together to a higher plane.

Though it's been hundreds of years since *halacha* mandated darkness during intercourse was recorded, its relevance is ever more apparent today. Far too many women suffer inhibition during intimacy because of real or perceived bodily flaws. Today more than ever, women find themselves competing with unrealistic, perfectly airbrushed images. Such worries can cause women to feel self conscious and unable to fully experience pleasure. These fears rob couples of the ability to relax and enjoy this special time together. For this reason and others, *halacha* seeks to nurture a sense of respect as well as mystique. *Mesorah* lovingly advises: if you truly want to see each other, shut the lights on all the externals so you can have your eyes wide open to what is essential. If a couple wants to hear each other, find a special time and a private place to be together.

Rivkah: Years ago, when I was still quite young and new to public speaking, I was addressing a large group about the concept of *mikvah*. A man in the audience who appeared to be completely sane stood and asked: "You spoke so beautifully about the power and holiness of intimacy. Should my wife and I bring our children into our bedroom to watch?" I was so thrown by this question that I remember pretending that the mike was not working, so I could buy a few more minutes to muster a reply.

---

[7] *Shulchan Aruch, Orach Chaim* 240:11.

[8] If the only time you can be intimate is in the morning or some other part of the day, it is best for you, (or your husband, if you prefer) to consult with a Rav or *mashpia* on this issue.

[9] *Shulchan Aruch, Orach Chaim* 240:11.

Restore and Recalibrate: Our Life's Mission

> In retrospect, the reply is so very obvious: If you want your children to see the beauty of intimacy DON'T bring them into the bedroom. Nothing happens in the bedroom that they can witness except for a weird type of callisthenic. It might even scare them. The spectacular beauty and potency of intimacy lies in our hearts, minds, and souls. What happens physically in the bedroom between a couple cannot possibly reflect that truth; it's a miracle that it can even facilitate it! That's why it's true to say: "nothing– no thing– happens in the bedroom.[10]" What happens between a woman and her husband is not a thing; it is an energy that transcends dimension and defies description. It is, in fact, everything.

Are there limitations on touching, caressing, kissing, and cuddling outside of the framework of sexual intimacy?

Sexual intimacy is about much more than foreplay, intercourse, and the afterglow. While not every loving exchange between a couple will culminate in sexual intercourse, every affectionate touch, even a loving glance, nourishes physical as well as emotional intimacy, and is absolutely appropriate and positive. Greetings of hello, goodbye, and good morning/good night are all enhanced by a touch, kiss, or hug. When we are in need of comfort, an embrace and cuddle can mean the world. And there is nothing quite like a hug that accompanies a *mazal tov* or as a show of special appreciation.

Everyone appreciates physical touch within a particular framework that is specific to their individual preferences. For some, extended romantic touch throughout the day may result in less craving for full-blown intimacy at night; for others, this only whets the appetite for more. With time couples learn what their partner enjoys and needs, and this is often different from what the individual prefers. More importantly, couples begin to appreciate that a loving relationship is based on understanding and respecting each other. It most certainly precludes touch that is uncomfortable or unwelcome, due to a particular context. This is an integral part of growing together and finding balance.

With breastfeeding an infant and/or managing children's various needs during the day, some women may feel all touched out and want to limit physical romantic interactions with their husbands. Often, it's not that a woman doesn't want her husband's physical touch, but rather that she craves emotional intimacy as a precursor. If we articulate that want and need, in most cases, the frequency and

---

[10] This quote is attributed to Rabbi Manis Friedman.

quality of the special moments we enjoy together physically will increase as well. Creating quality time during the day for a coffee date, a nice phone conversation, or even planning a little surprise can go a long way towards meeting that need. In that emotional climate, the physical expression will usually fall into place.

When a woman is *tehorah*, any type of physical affection that is pleasing to both herself and her husband is permitted provided that:

1. The exchange does not take place in the presence of others.[11]

2. It doesn't lead the man to be *motzi zera levatalah*, to wastefully emit his seed,[12] which is a serious *issur*, prohibition.[13, 14]

It is important for a couple to be sensitive to each other's needs; balancing the necessary expression of affection with how it impacts the husband's response. His response is specific to his body and will fluctuate based on age, libido, duration of marriage and other factors. While it is not a woman's job to be her husband's monitor or mentor in this area, she is his life partner and best friend. She will be tuned in to his sensitivities and support him in this issue which is to their joint benefit. Although you may enjoy extended hugging or cuddling, if you are not prepared for full intimacy at that time, or it is simply not feasible, make sure your husband knows you are okay with him stopping when he senses it is the right time for him to draw back.

This, arguably, is one reason that in many communities, wife and husband sleep in separate beds even when the wife is *tehorah*.[15] This is not a case of all or nothing; many couples enjoy cuddling and kissing for some time before they each retire to their own beds. On the other hand, there may be times when even couples who routinely sleep apart feel the need to sleep beside each other, requiring physical proximity for additional comfort and security.

Some couples find that sleeping together during the non-*nidah* period actually chisels away at the excitement that surrounds their intimacy. Like the bells on the *Kohen Gadol*'s robe that heralded his entrance to the *Kodesh*, a special

---

11 *Rama, Shulchan Aruch, Even Ha'ezer* 21:5.

12 Defined as ejaculation of sperm outside of the woman's vagina.

13 *Shulchan Aruch, Even Ha'ezer* 23:1.

14 Chassidic men and therefore their wives, guided by the teachings of chassidut and Kaballah, are especially attentive to the issue of *hotzaat zera levatalah*. See *Zohar* I 188b; *Tanya*, end of ch. 7.

15 *Ba'er Heiteiv* on *Shulchan Aruch, Orach Chaim* 238:2. This was the time honored *hanhagah* of chassidim.

aura surrounds the couple's personal *Kodesh* when this holy space is entered, not casually, but consciously. There are also completely pragmatic reasons like different sleeping styles, chronic pain etc. for why a couple might opt to sleep in separate beds when she is a *tehorah*. Sleeping in separate beds is not a commentary on the strength of their marriage, and should not be misconstrued as a breach of *shalom bayit*, in the same way that sleeping in the same bed is not proof positive of a healthier and more vibrant relationship. Each couple will work out what is best for them, keeping in mind that it is the love, devotion, and tenderness they share that is the bedrock of their union.

As noted, this first *bracha* highlights the importance of the inner sphere, the wine, over the external, the grape. This first *bracha* over which we say the *sheva brachot* hints at an essential truth; it teaches that just as the cup of wine serves as a receptacle for Hashem's blessings, so too a couple's physical union serves as a conduit for *Elokut*.

The next *bracha* addresses the symbiotic relationship between the body and soul and helps address the question: where does this leave us in terms of just enjoying physical pleasure?

Shehakol Bara Lichvodo: Everything, Including Marital Intimacy, Was Created for Hashem's Glory

ברוך אתה ה׳ אלקינו מלך העולם, שהכל ברא לכבודו

Blessed are You, Hashem our G-d, King of the universe, who has created all things for His glory.

At this moment, with *chatan* and *kallah* poised at the precipice of building their life together in the presence of a *minyan*, we are reminded that the gathering is for the purpose of bringing glory to Hashem. More profoundly, the *kallah* and *chatan* are told: Your marriage parallels the original six days of creation; the two of you are creating your own new world. This *bracha* reminds us that everything temporal and physical was created to fulfill the desire of our Creator, *Hakadosh Baruch Hu*, and to bring honor and grandeur to His name. This is the task of humanity.

This synergy of body and soul is more than a philosophical platitude; it finds practical expression in *halacha*. For instance, a husband's duty to give his wife sexual pleasure is a *d'orayta*: שארה כסותה ועונתה לא יגרע, he may not diminish her sustenance, her clothing, and her conjugal rights.[16] The three duties of a man as spelled out in the *Ketubah* are to provide his wife with food and medicinal needs, shelter and clothing, and sexual pleasure. This third obligation is most often referred to as the mitzvah of *onah*. Literally, *onah* means a season or time period. In this context, the time that the husband devotes to pleasuring his wife. Alternatively, *onah* may be etymologically linked to the term *la'anot*, to respond or answer. *Onah* is about the husband's responsiveness to his wife's needs and desires. In fact, the *Ramban* explains the above *passuk* as referring in its entirety to this mitzvah: *she'erah* refers to flesh-to-flesh contact during intimacy, *kesutah* refers to the bed and bedding used by the couple during intimacy, and *onatah* refers to the conjugal act itself.[17]

The mitzvah of *onah*, of a man giving his wife sexual pleasure, is a separate mitzvah from *pru u'rvu*. This mitzvah is independently important and holy. As long as a man is married, he is charged with respecting his wife and providing her sexual satisfaction regardless of his wife's ability or inability to conceive, due to infertility, pregnancy, use of contraceptives, or being post-menopausal. Sexual satisfaction is so basic to the human condition that, in our holy texts, it is referred to euphemistically as *derech eretz*, the way of the world.

---

16 *Shemot* 21:10.

17 *Shemot* ad loc. See also *Ketubot* 48a.

Restore and Recalibrate: Our Life's Mission

While a physical child may not be conceived, a holy *neshamah* is conceived, or brought forth, as a result of each and every intimacy enjoyed within the framework of *halacha*. In the words of the *Shelah HaKadosh*:

> דעו בניי יצ"ו, כי מכל ביאה וביאה כשהיא בקדושה, יצא ממנו פעולה טובה. דאף שאין אשתו מתעברת, מכל מקום מעורר למעלה ומשפיע נשמה.

> Know, my children, that each sanctified intimacy brings about a positive result. Even when the woman does not become pregnant, their actions have an effect Above, and a soul issues forth.[18]

The health and vibrancy of the family unit— particularly in its formative stages— is given paramount consideration in Jewish thought and *halacha*. And this is especially so regarding the mitzvah of *onah*.

> כי יקח איש אשה חדשה לא יצא בצבא ולא יעבר עליו לכל דבר, נקי יהיה לביתו שנה אחת ושמח את אשתו אשר לקח.

> When a man marries a new wife, he shall not go out to serve in the army, nor shall he be charged with any military duties. He shall be free for his house for one year, and he shall gladden the wife he has married.[19]

Even when Jews were faced with war, the Torah places great emphasis on addressing the responsibilities closer to home. This finds poignant expression in the Torah's instruction to the newlywed man to spend focused time, without distraction, on nurturing his fledgling relationship with his wife. Even today, this concept and underlying value, referred to as *shana rishonah*, the first year, applies in various ways during the first year of marriage. In a testament to its underlying holiness and emotional potency, the mitzvah of *onah* applies for the entirety of a marriage.

The equation in the Torah of a woman's sexual needs to food and clothing, basic necessities of life, underscores the value the Torah attributes to female pleasure within marriage. At the absolute minimum, a husband is obligated to pleasure his wife upon her return home from the *mikvah*, before he departs from home on a trip, when they are reunited after such a separation, and at any time that he senses his wife's desire.

---

[18] *Shnei Luchot Habrit, Sha'ar Ha'Otiyot, ot kuf, kedushat hazivug*, par. 402.

[19] *Devarim* 24:5.

Outside of the above occasions, *halacha* creates a sliding scale of frequency based on the husband's vocational obligations and abilities.

It is forbidden for a husband to deny his wife her due pleasure.[20] It is considered a heinous form of torment.[21] In fact, in the section of *Gemara* discussing the taking of *shavuot*, vows, we are taught that if a man takes a vow to deny his wife the pleasure of marital intimacy, his vow is automatically null and void; he cannot vow against what the Torah requires of him.[22]

Just as *halacha* details the quantitative dimensions of this mitzvah, so does it address its qualitative nature. It is a mitzvah for a man to gladden his wife, to assure her pleasure and joy to the best of his ability.

It goes without saying that for a man to force himself on his wife is absolutely forbidden.[23] The mitzvah of *onah* obligates the husband to be responsive to his wife's cues as to when and in which ways she desires to be pleasured and encourages a husband to prioritize his wife's pleasure over his own. That being said, the Torah's definition of physical intimacy recalls Adam deeply "knowing" Chava for the first time, and is about focus on the other. If, for instance, a woman feels pressured to climax first— a pressure that detracts from her pleasure instead of amplifying it— that is clearly not a way to fulfill the mitzvah *of onah*. It is in focusing on our spouse's happiness and satisfaction that we access the essence of intimacy.

Much is written about the best way for a woman to convey her desires. אישה תובעת בלב, a woman asks with her heart, teaches the *Gemara*.[24] Aside from pointing to the inherent modesty in this behavior, this teaching underscores a woman's desire to be desired. She does not want to have to solicit attention. At the same time, her husband cannot be expected to read her mind. He is therefore bidden by *halacha* to be ever attentive to her asking him from the heart. This might include her taking extra care with her grooming or using a certain scent. Her hints can also come in the form of more understated cues like body language or even a glance.

---

20 *Halacha* also addresses a woman who denies marital relations to her husband, who is termed a *moredet*, a rebellious woman. A woman is given this title if she denies her husband sexual relations for no reason. In some cases, she would even forfeit her *Ketubah*. This does not include cases of abuse or exhaustion. That said, the burden and primary concern of providing sexual pleasure rests with the husband. (*Shulchan Aruch, Even Ha'ezer* 77)

21 As we say in the Haggadah, וירא את עניינו זו פרישות דרך ארץ, the term "affliction" refers to abstinence from marital intimacy.

22 *Kiddushin* 19b.

23 See essay "I'm So Confused. Am I Being Abused? Guidance for the Orthodox Jewish Spouse and Those Who Are Trying To Help" for more information on marital rape and abuse.

24 *Eruvin* 100b.

Restore and Recalibrate: Our Life's Mission

Sometimes couples, especially newlyweds, agree on some form of subtle but specific code with which she conveys her intention. The *dinei harchakah*, when reversed, can inspire behaviors a woman might engage in precisely when she is interested in intimacy.[25]

Such signaling to initiate intimacy is not only permissible but is seen as virtuous. In *Bereishit*, Leah models this practice in initiating intimacy with Yaakov and is rewarded with the conception of her son Yissachar, the *shevet* blessed with the highest caliber of *talmidei chachamim*.[26]

The mitzvah of *onah*, however, still places the responsibility for his wife's sexual satisfaction on the husband. This concept is as primal as the words of Hashem to Chava following the *chet*: ואל אישך תשוקתך והוא ימשל בך, you will desire your husband, yet he will dominate you.[27] Rashi's commentary on these words reframes the meaning of these words, applying them to one specific area in life. As he explains, the desire mentioned is the will for marital relations. Although you will desire relations with your husband, you will not have the boldness to demand it outright from him. Rather, he will dominate you, namely, you'll need him to tune in to your intimations and take the initiative in this matter.

Here, too, chassidut, deepens and widens our perspective.[28] The Rebbe explains that the symbiotic dynamic of *mashpia*, the initiator, and *makabel*, the receiver, informs all aspects of creation.[29] Take, for example, the sun and moon. The sun is the central light. The moon reflects its light. Thus, it would seem that the moon is nothing more than a conduit in a different form for the essential light of the sun. In truth, the moon offers a specific form of light that can illuminate even the darkness. Moreover, there are certain types of vegetation that are nurtured exclusively by the moon's light.[30]

As the dynamic noted above suggests, the essential nature and focus of the *mashpia* is on bestowal. And yet, the *mashpia* can only receive the gift of acceptance and appreciation from the *mekabel*. When a woman expresses her desire for her husband, when she draws on his innate will to satisfy her sexual desire, she grants him a unique opportunity to access a new dimension. The *mekabel*, thus, influences the *mashpia*, as

---

25 See chapter seven, "*Dinei Harchakah*: Pulling Apart; Staying Together" for more.

26 *Eruvin* 100b.

27 *Bereishit* 3:16.

28 *Maamar Lechah Dodi* 5714, par. 5-7.

29 The word *mashpia* is etymologically related to the term *shefa*, flow.

30 *Rashi* on *Devarim* 33:14.

expressed in the *passuk*:³¹ אשת חיל עטרת בעלה, a woman of valor is the crown [above the head] of her husband.³²

The delicate intertwiment of physical and spiritual is not a simple task, particularly when it comes to sexual intimacy. זכר ונקבה ברא אותם, male and female he created them.³³ To be human is to be a sexual being. Neither tangential nor peripheral, our sexual urge is one of the three key drives, along with an impulse toward self preservation and social interaction that influence our behavior. The word *adam*, man, is etymologically rooted both in the word *adamah*, earth, and *edameh*, as in the term *edameh l'elyon*, likened unto Hashem.³⁴ These dueling parallels suggest that humans are not animals driven by instinct. Nor are we *malachim*, angels, innately disposed towards unceasing service of the Creator. We are pulled constantly downward towards earth and upward towards the heavens. Having been created *b'tzelem Elokim*, in the image of the Divine, we can control our urges and live in a more elevated fashion. As humans, we are Hashem's only creation vested with *bechirah chofshit*, the ability to choose.³⁵

Sexual intimacy calls forth the human need to choose. On one hand, intimacy involves the organs we objectively consider the most base. The actual coupling of those organs does not require particular intellectual acumen, emotional maturity, or spiritual refinement. On the other hand, these organs are the conduit through which our most important relationship is nourished and our families are built.

---

31 *Mishlei* 12:4.

32 An even deeper interaction occurs as well. The moon, unlike the sun, constantly waxes and wanes. One might think, says the Rebbe, that the relationship between the two luminaries would reach the ultimate point of connection exactly at mid month, when the moon is fullest in its reflection of the sun's light. However, the exact opposite is true.

During the first half of the month, the two celestial bodies move away from each other. It is only where there is distance between the two that reflection can occur which results in the waxing of the moon. It is during the second half of the lunar cycle that the two move closer to each other, though the moon appears to us to be "shrinking." At the point when the moon can no longer be seen, the discrete specificity of the two luminaries fades, leaving one unified whole. The push-pull of the *mashpia-mekabel* vanishes; they are both *mashpia* to and *mekabel* from each other simultaneously. In this essential place, there is no need for outward expression. At the center of the sun, we see no rays of light. At this moment there is only essence united with essence. On this level, the proverbial "sun" and "moon" revert to the equality they enjoyed upon their creation. This is a Mashiach'dike plane, a consummate level of union.

While, in practical *halacha*, it remains the husband's obligation to give his wife conjugal pleasure with the wife welcoming his overture, the celestial union described above reveals the possibility of an even higher plane, where there is no longer me and you; there is just a single unit. *Sefer HaSichot* 5752, vol. 1, pp. 157-158.

33 *Bereishit* 1:27.

34 *Yeshayahu* 14:14.

35 Rav Yaakov Emden saw significance in the fact that is specifically, *siman* 240, *resh mem*, where these *halachot* are outlined in the *Shulchan Aruch* in *Orach Chaim*. He noted that when intimacy is framed within *kedushah* it is indeed *ram*, exalted. Conversely, *chas v'shalom*, it becomes *mar*, bitter. *Siddur Yaavetz, Mitot Hakesef*, ch. 7, 3:17.

Restore and Recalibrate: Our Life's Mission

Chassidut teaches that כל הגבוה גבוה יותר יורד למטה מטה יותר, whatever is exceedingly lofty descends to a very low plane.[36] When properly harnessed, sexuality generates great joy and pleasure, and gives rise to an ultimate sense of wholeness. As the above principle indicates however, sexuality can conversely find expression in depraved actions and give rise to profound pain and a deep sense of violation.

Halacha provides a framework for navigating sexual expression in a healthy and holy manner. It is a way *in*; our guide to achieving *kedushah*, happiness, and emotional health. Additionally, chassidic teachings can assist couples in navigating the inherent tension in the juxtaposition of the physical and the spiritual.

In the preface to his *Mishneh Torah*, the *Rambam* describes each of the fourteen books in this work. Concerning *Sefer Kedushah*, which includes the *mitzvot* related to forbidden sexual relations and forbidden foods, he writes:[37]

בשני עניינים האלו קידשנו המקום והבדילנו מן האומות - בעריות ובמאכלות אסורות, ובשניהם נאמר "ואבדיל אתכם מן העמים", "אשר הבדלתי אתכם מן העמים."

Through these two matters G-d sanctified us and separated us from the nations: through forbidden relations and forbidden foods. Regarding both it is written, "I have set you apart from the nations,[38] and "Who has set you apart from the nations."[39]

One might think that a book called *Sefer Kedushah* would have included *halachot* about the *Beit Hamikdash* and the *korbanot*, ritual sacrifices, or a discussion about *Yom Kippur* and other holidays. Instead, the *Rambam* focuses on the most basic, organic aspects of our existence. In so doing, the *Rambam* presents the concept of *kedushah* as the symbiotic relationship between the *guf*, body, and the *neshamah*, soul. He counsels us to seek the middle road in satisfying our physical needs and pleasures, even within the realm of what is permitted.[40]

---

36 Quoted many times in chassidut. See, for example, *Likkutei Torah, Shir Hashirim* 23a.

37 *Siddur Yaavetz, Mitot Hakesef*, ch. 7, 3:17.

38 *Vayikra* 20:26.

39 *Vayikra* 20:24.

40 The Gemara assures us that if we strive to achieve this we will be helped and merit a reciprocal response from above: תנו רבנן: "והתקדשתם והייתם קדושים". אדם מקדש עצמו מעט מקדשין אותו הרבה. מלמטה מקדשין אותו מלמעלה. בעולם הזה מקדשין אותו לעולם הבא. Citing the verse, "Sanctify yourselves and you will be sanctified. (*Vayikra* 11:44)" our Sages taught: If you sanctify yourself even a little, you will become greatly sanctified. If you sanctify yourself below, you will be sanctified from Above. If you sanctify yourself in this world, you will be sanctified in the World to Come. (*Yoma* 39a)

In one of the Rebbe's teachings on the liberation from Egypt, he explains that liberty is about giving expression to one's essence. In so doing, he introduces an understanding of freedom that transcends the conventional constructs. Typical understandings of freedom comprise a binary: Either "freedom from," which is negative liberty, i.e. freedom from slavery, freedom from cravings, or freedom from authoritarianism. In other words, this type of freedom is tantamount to an exemption from certain constrictions. Or the opposite, "freedom to" or positive liberty. Positive liberty means that in addition to being unshackled from constraints, one has the ability to act on one's aspirations. In the Rebbe's specific definition, freedom takes the form of living in sync with the values and aspirations that emerge from, and are defined by, one's deepest core.

For inanimate matter, existence is synonymous with freedom. Vegetation, however, has more complex criteria; to achieve freedom, it must possess the capacity for growth. Lacking firm rooting, most vegetation finds itself restricted and strangled. For animal life, in contrast, firm rooting in one place equals a prison sentence. Animal life requires freedom of movement in order to find food, mate, and protect itself and its young.

Finally, a human's needs include all those required by animals and more. To be fully free, a person must use her/his intellectual and emotive faculties in a creative and purposeful manner. To merely have access to and satisfy our animal needs is not enough.

For Jews, having all of the opportunities available to the rest of humankind still does not equate to freedom and can never prove fulfilling. Our freedom flows from living in alignment with our *neshamah*. In the words of the Rebbe:

It is self-evident that harmonious and total freedom cannot be achieved in a way of life whereby the soul, which is truly a part of G-d (the G-dliness in man), would be subordinated to the body, and both of them (body and soul) to the material world. The superior cannot serve the inferior and be content to do so. The highest aspect of human life, the soul, will never acquiesce in subservience to the body. The obvious conclusion, therefore, is that true freedom can be achieved only when the lower constituents of human life – the body and material environment – will be elevated to the highest degree of affinity with the soul and its aspirations that is possible for them, while the soul, on its own level, will liberate itself from everything that hinders her fulfillment. [41]

This definition of freedom suggests that Hashem's commandments are designed to provide maximal function, success, and happiness. The soul, which is a part of Hashem,

---

41 Letter dated 11 Nissan, 5722, printed in *Igrot Kodesh*, vol. 22, p. 204.

Restore and Recalibrate: Our Life's Mission

longs to fulfill His commandments. Observance of *halacha* is a way to embody our truest selves, for the soul to gain expression and spiritualize the body that houses it. Far from suggesting we acquiesce to the myriad *halachot* that govern daily life out of a sense of *kabbalat ol*, submitting to Hashem's desire, this knowledge fills us with joy. It allows us to appreciate that holiness can suffuse every aspect of our lives and reminds us that everything is created for Hashem's glory.

YOU MIGHT BE WONDERING:

Does a wife have an obligation to give her husband pleasure?

Onah, a husband's responsibility to give his wife sexual pleasure, is a mitzvah *d'orayta*. As already discussed, a husband is responsible to attune himself to his wife's desires and meet her overtures.

A woman, too, has a responsibility *d'Rabanan*, from rabbinic sources, to go to the *mikvah* and not to deny her husband sexual pleasure.[42] Intimacy's place in the *halachic* hierarchy is underscored by the prioritization of woman *toveling* at the first possible opportunity.

In a healthy relationship, a woman will welcome and reciprocate her husband's overtures and not, generally speaking, rebuff them. Certainly, this is not carte blanche for her husband to make unreasonable or unequivocal demands of her and vice versa.[43]

It is completely normal for a man or a woman's libido to fluctuate. Health, medication, hormonal changes, stresses related to work, marriage, children, or other causes can all be contributing factors. A lessening in desire should not be equated with a weakening of their relationship.

A woman might find that her desire for intimacy does not necessarily precede foreplay. Sometimes it's about responding to her husband's overtures. Often, a woman can be surprised by how much she can enjoy a positive sexual interlude even if and when she was not initially awash in desire.

If, however, a woman consistently seeks reason to delay her *tevilah* or is completely uninterested in intimacy with her husband, an underlying physical or emotional

---

[42] Rambam, Hilchot Ishut 14:9. Zohar II 111a.

[43] See Rambam, Hilchot Ishut 14:8: אינה כשבויה שתבעל לשנוא לה, a wife is not a captive that she should be made to have relations with someone she hates.

issue or profound fissures exist that need to be resolved. Most often, this will necessitate the assistance of a licensed therapist.

If you feel intimidated to say no to intimacy out of fear that your husband will respond aggressively, you should seek assistance in how best to deal with that type of behavior without delay. Be wary of codependent behavior patterns which aid and abet this behavior instead of putting an end to it. You will need professional guidance in safely and effectively combating abusive, addictive or otherwise dysfunctional behavior.

What if I am not in the mood and I can tell my husband wants us to be together, or I am in the mood but he seems out of it?

Even when a wife and husband love each other dearly and are profoundly devoted to one another, their desires and preferences will not always align. We can, however, take practical steps to bring our sexual desires more in sync with each other.

Generally, two people who are committed to each other, or who want to deepen their commitment, will seek to meet each other halfway. The first step is to clearly communicate and listen carefully to each other. In the case of a pronounced variance in desire, you want to better understand the disparity; what factors contribute to lack of desire, and what can be done to remove those factors. Sometimes, one will yield to the other's preference. Sometimes, the answer will still be no; but the way that "no" is delivered can make all the difference. When you say: "Tonight doesn't work for me, but I would love to take a raincheck for another night," for instance, it articulates your needs without the sting of rejection. That kind of reply signals the overall value intimacy holds in your life, even if it's not right at that moment. Often enough, when we indulge our spouse's overtures, we are swept along by the tide of that desire. The physical pleasure is deepened by the sweetness of knowing you have done something special and meaningful for and with someone you love.

Ultimately, you are the best arbiter of your strength and stamina; your physical, emotional and psychological bandwidth. You should never be afraid to say no if you feel unable to engage in sexual intimacy. At the same time, be aware that not every intimate interlude needs to be lengthy or outfitted with every bell and whistle. Perfect is the enemy of good. Knowing that sometimes your time together will be short and sweet can give you the license to say yes when you are tired or you know you have to get up early the next morning. It can make your husband happy, and even, sometimes, get you into the mood as well.

> **Sara**: Think about Shabbat. It comes once a week, always after Friday, if you are ready for it or not. Most of us put effort into Shabbat meals, some of us more than others, of course, but a Shabbat meal is by definition special. Sometimes your Shabbat meal will be extra fancy. You will spend days thinking about the menu, you will splurge on wonderful extras, you will take pains with a dessert that necessitates many steps and five different bowls. This usually means you have a cherished guest or are celebrating a special occasion. But sometimes, for whatever reason, you have no strength, time, or interest to cook much at all. It's still going to be Shabbat. You are still going to honor Shabbat by having a *seudah*. You still love your family immensely. And you are still going to enjoy it even if your meal is not "insta-worthy."

There is a lot of talk about the need to compromise in marriage. Chassidut, in contrast, speaks of the importance of *bittul*, self effacement; the ability to yield one's own desire in the face of a higher value. If our highest value and deepest desire is the constant deepening of our marriage, we have gained exactly what we want, even if and when, in a particular instance, we have yielded our desire to that of our spouse (assuming, again, the scenario is a healthy one, as noted above).

This should not be conflated with mercy or pity sex, wherein one person aquieces simply to appease the other; that kind of behavior most often boomerangs. What is being suggested is welcoming sexual intimacy even if that was not initially high on your priority list for that precise moment. You do so because you value your spouse and your relationship.

It has been said, tongue in cheek, that spontaneity is too precious to be left to chance. We all recognize the wisdom in appointed times, especially for the most important things in life. The intimacy you share with your husband IS the most important thing. Plan accordingly so that you can welcome and enjoy your special time together. If that means taking a nap, make the time to do that. If it means scheduling some alone-time on your calendars, do that. If it's something else you need, make sure to put that into place.

There is a Yiddish folktale about a mother who would periodically lock herself into a room much to the chagrin and immense curiosity of her children. One of those times they clamored at the door, insisting that she tell them what she was doing. "*Ich mach far eich a mamme*" she replied in Yiddish. *I am making for you a mother.* She was taking the time to nurture herself.

Especially on *mikvah* night, or those times you know are uniquely special for both of you, see what you need so that you can give and receive optimally and wholeheartedly. Share with your husband what it is you will need from him in terms of hands on support. In doing so, you will be "making" for your husband a wife; a loving, romantic partner. And you will bring out the best in him; the loving, romantic partner you deserve.

For mothers, making time for yourself is immensely challenging. In those times akin to living in survival mode, many women require a build-up to intimacy. Make sure you communicate with your husband what you need for intimacy, whether that means specific help with the kids, lingering glances, or kind words throughout the day. Ensure that you feel loved, supported, and taken care of, so that intimacy feels like a joy as opposed to a chore.

If your hesitance is arising because you experience sexual pain, reach out to a doctor or licensed sex therapist who can help you understand what is happening and guide you on practical solutions.

The second of the seven *sheva brachot* reminds the *chatan* and *kallah*: you have the privilege to build your world together in a way that brings Hashem honor. This lofty goal is accomplished not in some abstract way, but in suffusing every aspect of your lives including intimacy with consciousness of this mandate. This itself begs a question: I understand that we have all been sent into this world with an overarching mandate, but does *halacha* allow any room for individuality? Are we stuck in a circumscribed box? The next *bracha* provides an answer.

Yotzer Haadam: Honoring the Individuality of Each Couple

ברוך אתה ה' אלקינו מלך העולם, יוצר האדם.

Blessed are You, Hashem our G-d, King of the universe, the Creator of man.

This *bracha* draws attention to the fact that, unlike all other species, which were created in pairs, Adam, was created alone.[44] It reminds *kallah* and *chatan* that before they become one unit, each must maintain some level of focus on him or herself as an independent entity. While marriage represents a reunion and a fusion, it is not about one being subsumed in or by the other. Nor is marriage a reform school with the goal of fixing the other.

The Gemara teaches קשוט עצמך ואחר כך קשוט אחרים, first fix or adorn yourself, and only then, when warranted, give advice to others.[45] This is true even– or maybe especially– when that other is your other half. Valuing the way in which our spouse is different from us, celebrating those differences rather than rebuffing them, is an important part of marital success.

Our distinctiveness asserts itself in every aspect of our lives and sexuality is no exception. Just as people possess different degrees of appetite for food, dexterity of motion, and rates of metabolism, our libidos vary as well. Although, generally, the male libido is considered more obvious and consistent than that of a female, sometimes the opposite is true.[46]

Overall, women's sexual arousal and satisfaction is much more responsive, that is to say, it is more dependent on context and environment. Said differently, for women, desire might come as a result of a sexually charged overture or experience, rather than as a precursor. A man's desire for sexual expression can be quite spontaneous. Many women, on the other hand, yearn for the experience of intimacy– the combination of both the emotional and physical sensations, hugging, caressing, and snuggling while sharing their thoughts and emotions deeply– and only then does a desire for sexual intimacy begin to stir in them. That is not to say that women cannot experience

---

[44] *Sanhedrin* 37a.

[45] *Sanhedrin* 18a.

[46] *Rashi* on *Ketubot* 64b; Baumeister RF, Catanese KR, Vohs KD. Is There a Gender Difference in Strength of Sex Drive? Theoretical Views, Conceptual Distinctions, and a Review of Relevant Evidence. *Personality and Social Psychology Review Vol. 5 Issue 3.* August 1, 2001.

spontaneous desire or that men cannot have responsive desire, but this is the general breakdown.

If this is true for you, you are not alone. Responsive sexual arousal is no less powerful or potent. It might be difficult for you or your husband to understand this at first. Be sure to explain what you are feeling to him.

Each woman's libido is unique. It is not static. Its waxing and waning is determined by both physiological and psychological factors. In plain English, this means that overall marital satisfaction, life stresses, fatigue, illness, medication, children, hormonal fluctuation attributable to medication, pregnancy, lactation, menopause, mental health, etc. will all play a role in your sexual experience.

Many women suffer the misconception that their sexual response is supposed to mirror or sync with their husband's. Nothing could be further from the truth. The vast majority of women will not climax simultaneously with their husband. On average women need more time than men do, as well as manual stimulation to achieve climax. Perhaps Hashem created our bodies so differently to remind us that intimacy is about focusing on the other. And to underscore that intimacy is in large measure about our distinctiveness.

Finally, each one of us experiences sexual pleasure in a different way. The important thing is that intimacy represents a special time for the couple. Appreciating that each of us is distinctive and will experience life's stages and phases in variant manner, provides just one of many reasons it is harmful to compare and contrast one's personal life with that of relatives, friends, and social media posts.[47] When we tell others what we are doing in our bedrooms, we rob ourselves of the exploration and discovery, the unfurling journey of our unique togetherness. And above all else, the ability to melt into each other's presence in a way and in a place where no one else exists.

On the other hand, should you find yourselves experiencing difficulties, even after open, honest communication between you and your husband, seek guidance. Find someone steeped in Torah (and chassidut, if that is important to you) as well as the interplay of *halacha* and emotional and physical aspects of sexual health, like a qualified therapist, *kallah* teacher, or *mashpia* with expertise in this area.

Even as our *mesorah* values community, we never lose sight of the infinite worth of the individual and the singular gifts each person brings to bear; contributions

---

[47] In analyzing reports of marriage and divorce from more than 50,000 women in the U.S. Government's National Survey of Family Growth (NFSG) they found that women who married relatively young (between 22-30 years of age), and most notably, did not cohabit with their husbands or any other man before marriage, had the lowest incidence of divorce." In Prof. Galena Rhoades estimation, having a history with other cohabiting partners may also make people compare their spouse critically to previous partners in ways that make them discount their husband or wife." (Too Risky to Wed in your 20's? Not if You Avoid Cohabiting First by Brad Wilcox and Lyman Stone, Wall Street Journal Feb. 5, 2022)

Restore and Recalibrate: Our Life's Mission

unattainable through the agency of any other. This *bracha* highlights and celebrates our individuality as well as the individuality of each couple as a unit.

Chazal taught that כל אדם שאין לו אשה אינו אדם, a person is not quite considered a person until they are united with their other half.[48] The third *bracha* hints at the importance of *shalom bayit*. Cultivating such harmony is crucial not only as a precursor to, *b'ezrat Hashem*, building a family, but as a matter of import unto itself. In all the discussion of marriage as the beginning of a *binyan adei ad*, we shouldn't lose sight of the foundation upon which the entire edifice rests, the couplehood. Just as each individual is unique, every couple possesses a distinctive identity and mission statement. They are each other's best friends and confidantes; standing together, always at each other's side. Especially in the face of challenges.

In this spirit, the Midrash relates the story of a pious couple who deeply loved each other but because of their inability to have children together decided, after ten years of waiting, to seek a divorce.[49], [50] When they came before the great Rashbi, Rabbi Shimon bar Yochai, with their decision, he asked to be the one to preside over the *get* process. He advised them to first host a party for their family and friends: "Just as you sealed your union with celebration, so should your divorce be marked." At the meal, the wise woman poured cup after cup of wine for her husband. As his mood gradually lifted, he said to her: "Is there any precious item here that you would like? Please take what you want most with you to your father's home". When her husband fell into a deep sleep, she asked her servants to help him into his bed and carry him to her father's home. Upon awakening, when her husband recognized his surroundings, he asked his wife what had happened. "You told me to take the thing from our home that I wanted most to my father's home, which is exactly what I did! There is nothing in the world that I want more than you!" she said. With that, they returned to the Rashbi, who, seeing their great love for each other, *davened* for them and they were blessed with children.

Even as *pru u'rvu* is a most important mitzvah, and certainly an overarching reason for marriage, its value does not supplant the couple's union. Children, *b'ezrat Hashem*, are the wondrous result of that union; but children are not the definition of marriage nor its sole reason for being.[51]

---

48 *Yevamot* 63a.

49 *Shir Hashirim Rabbah* 1:31.

50 While there is mention in *halachic* sources of the possibility of divorce when after ten years of marriage a couple cannot conceive, divorce is not *halachically* mandated. *Rama, Even Ha'ezer* 1:3.

   While a woman is not obligated in *pru u'rvu*, she can *halachically* initiate divorce if her husband is sterile and she desires children. *Even Ha'ezer* 154:6.

51 See, for instance, *Ramban's* interpretation of *Bereishit* 2:24 as opposed to *Rashi's*.

As we take in the lesson of the third *brachah,* it is important to remember the challenge of primary and secondary infertility. The desire for children is primal and profound, and there is no substitute that can be offered in the face of this painful challenge. The couple, and those who love and surround them, should remain mindful of the fact that first and foremost they are a unit, a holy alliance. No one and nothing can diminish that.

It is especially important that the couple support each other. We *daven* that Hashem will soon bless them with children and life will be a different kind of hectic and noisy. Then too, priority will have to be given to their relationship upon which all else depends.

When fertility treatment is ineffective or not an option, the torment is further amplified if the couple's community broadcasts the message, consciously or not, that marriage is simply a synonym for family; that their union is valued only for the fruit it might bring forth.

In such instances, it's helpful to recall the narrative of Yaakov and Rachel and, in particular, Yaakov's words to his beloved wife. These words may appear discouraging, but they can also convey a message of empowerment akin to that of the third blessing. The Torah says:[52]

> ותרא רחל כי לא ילדה ליעקב ותקנא רחל באחתה, ותאמר אל יעקב הבה לי בנים ואם אין מתה אנכי. ויחר אף יעקב ברחל, ויאמר התחת אלקים אנכי אשר מנע ממך פרי בטן.

> Rachel saw that she had borne no children to Yaakov. She became envious of her sister and said to Yaakov: "Give me children or else I will die." Yaakov, taken aback by Rachel's words, replied rhetorically: "Can I take the place of G-d who has denied you the fruit of the womb?"

In explaining Yaakov's upset, the *Akeidat Yitzchak* teaches that the Torah's first woman is given two names, *ishah* and *Chava*.[53] The first, *ishah,* connotes woman as she derives from man and possesses equal capabilities in the intellectual and moral fields.[54] *Chava*, which comes from *em kol chai,* mother of all living beings, alludes to

---

52 *Bereishit* 30:1-2.

53 *Akeidat Yitzchak, Parshat Bereishit, sha'ar* 9.

54 *Bereishit* 2:23.

the human capacity to bear children.[55] Yaakov was angry with Rachel for forgetting that, without her second purpose in this world, she can still exist, even thrive.

Each couple and the community that surrounds them must keep the words of Yaakov front and center. There are many ways to live, to contribute, and give forth progeny, all of which should be appreciated and cherished.

YOU MIGHT BE WONDERING:

Is PDA, otherwise known as public displays of affection, okay?

> Some couples struggle with the *halachic* ideal that obviates public displays of affection. It seems restrictive and unnecessary.
>
> Part of the difficulty might be rooted in a misunderstanding. Too many mistakenly believe refraining from public displays of affection is a *chumra*, a stringency. However, the *Shulchan Aruch* clearly states:[56]
>
> אין לנהוג אפילו עם אשתו בדברים של חבה...בפני אחרים
>
> Do not act affectionately (even) with your spouse in front of others.
>
> Intimacy between husband and wife represents the most sacred activity. And in Jewish philosophy, the holier something is, the more hidden away it remains. A *Sefer Torah* is belted, covered with a mantle, and placed into an *aron kodesh* behind doors additionally adorned with a *parochet*. The Torah is taken out of this space for the purpose of *kriat hatorah*, reading the Torah, on very specific occasions alone. As soon as the reading is completed, the Torah is once again belted, covered with the mantle, and returned to its place behind closed doors and an additional curtain. The apex of *kedushah* never finds expression in exposure.[57]
>
> The first time Hashem revealed Himself to Moshe at the *sneh*, the burning bush, Moshe covered his face, for he was afraid to behold Hashem.[58] Moshe was not fearful in the conventional sense, but rather in awe of the holiness which he faced

---

55 *Bereishit* 3:20.

56 *Shulchan Aruch, Even Haʾezer* 21:5.

57 There are couples who keep *dinei harchakah* in public even when the wife is *tehorah*. The *Darkei Teshuva* writes concerning this type of conduct that there is nothing more beautiful than modesty. (*Yoreh Deiʾah* 195:9).

58 *Shemot* 3:6.

head on. The appropriate response when faced with *kedushah* is to avert one's eyes, to cover the face.

As the above incident indicates some actions are simply too holy to be witnessed.

Likewise, when Rivkah saw Yitzchak walking towards her for the first time, she recognized the *kedushah* he exuded. In fact, we are taught that he had just alighted from Gan Eden.[59] In response to that holiness, Rivkah covered her face.[60]

The same holds true concerning the celestial realm: *Yeshayahu Hanavi* describes the *serafim*, the angels that surround Hashem's holy throne, as having six wings. Two for flying, the only two that appear to be functional, and four to cover up; two cover the feet and two cover the face when beholding sacredness.[61]

As the *chatan* and *kallah* go into the *yichud* room following the *chuppah*, so too Moshe Rabbeinu, representative of *Knesset Yisrael*, Hashem's bride, went on high, before the Heavenly throne, after *Matan Torah,* the giving of the Torah. Moshe, alone, in seclusion with Hashem.

Later in history, in the *Mishkan,* Tabernacle, and in the *Batei Mikdash*, the first and second Temples in Jerusalem, this same intimacy took the form of the *Kohen Gadol* entering the *Kodesh Hakodashim,* the holiest space in the Temple, on *Yom Kippur.* It was the holiest person, in the holiest place, on the holiest day, *achat bashana*, only once a year. Indeed, it was in the singularly private space of the *Kodesh Hakodashim* that the *keruvim,* the cherubs on the holy ark – which gave three-dimensional expression to the loving relationship of Hashem and *Bnei Yisrael* – were showcased.[62] Significantly, the *Kodesh Hakodashim* is referred to in *Tanach* as the *chadar hamitot*, the bedroom.[63] A master bedroom, like the *Kodesh Hakodashim*, is a private place no one else enters. And even though the children might enter, they don't really enter the *chadar hamitot*. The notion of a private and holy space is reflected in the well known practice in many communities of the wife and husband's beds remaining separated; no one but the couple themselves is privy to their very own *Kodesh Hakodashim*, holiest space.

---

59   *Yalkut Shimoni, Bereishit, remez* 109.

60   *Bereishit* 24:65.

61   *Yeshayah* 6:2.

62   *Yoma* 54a. The two *keruvim* symbolize Hashem and the Jewish people.

63   *Melachim* II 11:2; *Rashi* ad loc.; *Divrei Hayamim* II 23:11; *Torat Menachem,* vol. 30, p. 205.

Restore and Recalibrate: Our Life's Mission

Commenting on the iconic words of the prophet Bilam, מה טבו אהליך יעקב, how good are your tents, O Yaakov, Rashi teaches that the goodness Bilam exclaimed over was the modesty that defined the Jewish encampment in the desert.[64] He noticed the Jewish tents were positioned so that no two doors directly faced each other. This emphasis on privacy is enshrined in *halacha*, which prohibits construction of homes with doors or windows that directly face the doors or windows of adjacent homes.[65] Indeed, the importance of privacy is so deeply ingrained in our national psyche that, each day, we open our *tefillot,* prayers, with this verse!

According to the *Torah Shebaal Peh*, oral Torah, *tzniut* or lack thereof, is a matter of high-stakes. The *Mishna* discusses the category of women who violate *dat Yehudit,* the laws of normative modesty accepted by Jewish women and codified in Jewish law, and, in so doing, forfeit their *ketubah*.[66] In enumerating various forms of trespass, the *Mishna* mentions a *kolanit.* The Gemara explains that this is a woman whose voice can be heard by others regarding matters involving their sexual expressions.[67] This statement can be understood as describing at least two variant scenarios: either that people living adjacent to her home can hear her soliciting or refusing her husband's attention, or that her neighbors can hear the sounds she makes whilst engaged in sexual intimacy. This lack of discretion and modesty is considered so reprehensible that her husband may divorce her over this issue without giving her the alimony normally due to a divorced woman as per her *ketubah*.

The Torah's emphasis on privacy should not be misunderstood as inhibiting sexual expression or as a reason to hold back from seeking counsel regarding doubts or problems surrounding intimacy from a trusted confidante. Ideally, this should be someone older, with life experience, knowledge of *halachic* and *hashkafic* nuances, and the wisdom to properly balance all of the variables. Remaining silent with a pressing question at hand would be a misappropriation of *tzniut,* which could have devastating results.

Intellectual property law may offer additional clarity on the unique value of privacy. The premise is simple: if someone has a great idea, they should have

---

64 *Bamidbar* 24:5.

65 *Shulchan Aruch, Choshen Mishpat* 154:3.

66 *Ketubot* 72a.

67 Ibid. 72b.

the right to protect this just as they have a right to protect their home, car, or bank account. If something belongs to me, it is distinctively mine. As soon as something is in the public domain for all to access, however, it lessens the overall value.

It might be interesting to ask ourselves: Do we feel as passionately about our marriage as we do about our ideas and other assets? Is our kiss, or caress, or even common touch valuable and sacred or something casually flung into the public domain? Is it a work of art signed by our heart and soul, or a cheap copy of which there are millions? Should we not be as concerned with protecting our marital bond as we are with our intellectual property?

To the point: if we reserve intimate touch for expression exclusively within the confines of our bedroom, how much more special does it make it when we walk over the threshold into our inner sanctum and close the doors?

Rivkah: Having lived on a college campus for thirty six years, I cannot for the life of me figure out why young adults who would never share their credit card info, much less their bank account, or toothbrush, are okay with sleeping together. Trust me, I have asked them to explain it to me and they can't figure it out either. We concur that there is a lot of drama and undiluted misery generated by the hook-up culture. But few are willing to buck the tide.

I am even more perplexed, by the propensity for intelligent, *frum*, and even, *chasidically* identified individuals to share details concerning their intimate lives on social media and in person. None of these individuals would share the particulars of their investment portfolios with these same people - sisters in law, cousins, friends. So why share this? Assuming that intimacy is precious, why squander it? If it's exclusive and holy and pure, let's honor that.

If our children never see us hugging and kissing our spouses, how will they know we love each other, and how will they develop an understanding of healthy touch?

Rivkah: If I had a dime for every student who has asked this question of me, I would be a billionaire: "How will your children know that you love Aaron (my husband) if they don't see you hugging and kissing?" Believe me when I tell you that I am touched by their sincere concern for our children. For this reason, I do my best to share my understanding of this matter with them.

Once in a while, when I am feeling provocative I reply: Are you kidding? My children watch us making love all of the time: in the kitchen, in the living room, in the dining room, in the car, in the office, in the laundry room. Ha, I got your attention, right?

What I mean with my response is rather simple. Children are very smart. They can see right through a kiss, hug or caress that doesn't reflect the truth of a relationship. Conversely, they can see the love you share even if they never see you as much as graze your husband's fingers.

Most people do not spend time imagining how they were conceived. This is not because they are ignorant about the birds and the bees. They are not in denial or on hallucinogens. They are simply in touch with a higher truth (even if they are not conscious of it), and that truth for many is: I am not here because my parents did THAT! No, I was conceived out of love and respect and devotion and tenderness and trust and commitment. THAT is really beside the point.

If you want to make sure your children see parents who love each other, take whatever necessary steps to bolster your relationship and make it a truly loving one. Be respectful, be considerate, be tender, be responsible, and be consistent in meeting each other's needs. Show your children through your speech and actions what it means when two people have each other's backs and go out of their way for each other. When your children catch that tender look or shared smile, and they will, you will have shown them true love. You will also have provided the most important backdrop for explaining in an age appropriate manner that married people, including their parents, do indeed enjoy physical expressions of affection and intimacy. The combination of mutual respect coupled with knowledge of the physical dimension gives our children a framework for healthy touch.

Should you get the sense that your kids see and hear you fighting plenty but never get a glimpse of you playing nicely, it's time to change that. There is an almost unmatched anxiety and angst that comes from recognizing that the structure that is supposed to house and protect you is crumbling. You and your children deserve better. Public displays of affection, however, will do little to allay their fears. They are a less effective response than a band aid offered as a solution to full blown cardiac disease.

In our fast-paced society obsessed with instantaneous results and gratification, the most important things in life still take work and time. Hugs and kisses are absolutely precious parts of marital life, but the tapestry of our relationship is woven from a trillion strands of more subtle and routine interactions. Mindful of this truth, every word we exchange, every act of service for the other, every instance of assistance, is the most efficacious public display of our affection for each other.

The third *bracha* tells the *chatan* and *kallah*: you are unique in your capacities and gifts. Hashem created you because there is something specific and integral that He and the world He created needs from you. Embrace and appreciate your distinctiveness. But, you might be thinking, isn't the whole idea of marriage about us becoming one? The next *bracha* explains how and why it is possible for us to merge with our other half, and build something that is unified and eternal.

Binyan Adei Ad; The Heavenly Reach of Sanctified Intimacy

ברוך אתה ה' אלקינו מלך העולם, אשר יצר את האדם בצלמו, בצלם דמות תבניתו, והתקין לו ממנו בנין עדי עד. ברוך אתה ה', יוצר האדם.

> Blessed are You, Hashem our G-d, King of the universe, who created man in His image, in the image of the likeness of His form, and prepared for him an everlasting edifice from his own self. Blessed are You Hashem, Creator of man.

The previous *bracha* speaks of Adam in the singular, a dimorphous being composed of both a male and female aspects. This *bracha* introduces Chava, fashioned from Adam for the ultimate purpose of reuniting and building an everlasting edifice. The *bracha* recalls how Hashem fashioned Chava as an independent person by separating her from Adam, reminding the *chatan* and *kallah* that they experience the very same soul journey as that of history's first couple. Upon being dispatched to this earth, each soul is split in two, with one half in a woman and the other in a man, triggering a sense of fracture and loss. The *bracha* concludes, however, with once again referencing Adam in the singular. It points to the unity that is born from plurality, the exalted oneness that is achieved through marriage and most distinctively in having children. The offspring and their offspring until the end of time, results in an everlasting edifice.

Hashem created each person with a longing for sexual intimacy; for this distinctive type of coming together. *Halacha* positions intimacy as central to marriage, with an emphasis on a husband pleasuring his wife. If deriving sexual pleasure was not a value, why would Hashem create the clitoris, the only organ in the human body with the sole function of providing pleasure?

And yet, our intimacy is much more than the fitting together of anatomical puzzle pieces for the purpose of stimulation and climax. Our physical intimacy is the natural means for conceiving a child, thus fulfilling the great mitzvah of *pru u'rvu*, being fruitful and multiplying. In our fusing and meshing, we become part of something larger; in our transcendence of self, we touch the Divine. We enter into a partnership with Hashem; we come closest to taking on the G-dly attribute of Creator. What can be more exalted than pulling a *neshamah*, a ממש ממעל, חלק א-לוה ממעל ממש, an actual part of G-d Above, into this world?[68]

---

[68] *Tanya* ch. 2.

Every mitzvah is exponentially amplified by *kavanah*, intention, especially this most important mitzvah. We are taught מצוה בלא כוונה כגוף בלא נשמה, a mitzvah without *kavanah* is like a body without a soul.[69] When engaged in intimacy, especially with the possibility of conception, we simultaneously straddle the physical and the spiritual planes. We are but junior partners in the enterprise composed of both corporeal and ethereal components. Not surprisingly, many sources in both the exoteric and esoteric dimensions of the Torah underscore the importance of the parents' thoughts and emotions prior to and during conception and the profound impact of those thoughts on the future child.[70]

The *neshamah* must be drawn down in a most delicate manner. This חלק א-לוה ממעל ממש, an aspect of the Divine, must descend from on high, through myriad spiritual planes, until it reaches its destination in this physical world. To achieve its mission once here on this physical plane, the *neshamah* must be clothed in very specific *levushim*, garments.

In the exact words of the Alter Rebbe in Tanya:[71]

> No *nefesh*, *ruach*, or *neshamah* is without a garment which stems from the *nefesh* of its father's and mother's essence. All the *mitzvot* that a person fulfills are influenced by that garment [i.e. it is through this garment that the soul achieves its ability to affect the body and to perform *mitzvot* involving physical matters]. Even the benevolence that flows to a person from heaven is given through this garment. [Because the soul is so strongly bound up with this garment, the *Zohar* refers to the garment, in this context, as the person's "soul."] Now, if a person sanctifies himself, he will bring forth a holy garment for the *neshamah* of his child [thereby enabling the child to serve G-d more readily].

Today, we can point to the meticulous measures taken to ensure a pristine environment in IVF laboratories as a physical parallel to the spiritual care and intent we invest in preparing ideal soul garments for our children. Modern IVF laboratories enforce strict protocols that control every feature of the environment including temperature, sound, and light. These labs employ novel air purification technology to intercept airborne contaminants and pathogens as well as seemingly benign factors such

---

[69] *Tanya* ch. 38.

[70] *Nedarim* 20b; *Midrash Tanchuma*, *Naso*, ot 7; *Ramban's Iggeret Hakodesh* ch. 5; *Siddur Yaavetz*, *Mitot Hakesef*, 6:8-11; *Or Hachaim* on *Vayikra* 12:12; *Tanya*, end of ch. 2.

[71] End of ch. 2.

Restore and Recalibrate: Our Life's Mission

as perfumes, deodorants, and even odors wafting in from the outside environment, all of which can affect embryonic development.[72]

Understanding the journey of the soul from above to below eludes our human intellect, and yet Hashem entrusts us to partner with Him in this process. Physical intimacy serves as the conduit through which facets of Hashem, *neshamot*, enter this world.

Halachic and Kabbalistic masters guide us in properly welcoming a lofty *neshamah* and providing that *neshamah* with refined *levushim* so that it can successfully complete its *shlichut*, its mission, in this world. Facilitating the descent of these *neshamot*, *bekedushah u'betaharah*, in sanctity and purity, is a weighty responsibility and privilege.

YOU MIGHT BE WONDERING:

I have learned that the thoughts of the parents during intimacy impact the children who will be conceived. Practically speaking, how can I channel my thoughts correctly?

> When compared with many of the most basic *mitzvot* like Shabbat and Kashrut, for instance, there are surprisingly few *halachot* that define the parameters of our intimacies.[73] The guiding principle is that intimacy is about being present, and completely there for the other. Holy intimacy is about connecting physically, emotionally, psychologically, and spiritually. It is the merging of the heart, soul, and mind.
>
> אמרו ז"ל לעולם יקדש אדם את עצמו בשעת תשמיש, וקדושה זו היא טהרת המחשבה שלא יחשוב באשה אחרת ולא בדברים אחרים רק באשתו.
>
> Chazal taught that one must always sanctify oneself when being intimate with his wife. This means that you should purify your thoughts. Do not think about another woman or anything else, only about your wife.[74]
>
> *Halacha* prohibits intimacy when the wife and/or husband are angry with one another, and certainly if they are entertaining thoughts of divorce. Similarly,

---

72 Agarwal N. Chattopadhyay R. Ghosh S. Bhoumik A. Goswami SK. Chakravarty B. Volatile organic compounds and good laboratory practices in the in vitro fertilization laboratory: the important parameters for successful outcome in extended culture. *Journal of Assisted Reproduction and Genetics.* 2017.

73 Within marriage, and when the woman is *tehorah*.

74 *Rabbeinu Bachya* on *Bereishit* 30:38.

intimacy is prohibited if one or both are drunk, or if their thoughts are focused on other people rather than on each other.[75]

In this spirit, as we enjoy foreplay as a prelude to sexual intimacy, we should take some time to focus mentally on the holiness of our togetherness; on the fulfillment of the mitzvah of *onah* or *pru u'rvu*, or both. But the process begins even earlier. *Halachic* sources mention that the first image a woman sees upon ascending from the *mikvah* should be something holy or pure.[76] Surely, then, the time immediately before our togetherness deserves some focused intentionality.

We might think about how fortunate we feel, and how thankful we are to Hashem, to be in a loving relationship. Additional ways to focus one's attention on a source of holiness are suggested in various sources.[77] This focus on holiness affects the purity of the child, providing more refined *levushim* for the child's *neshamah*.[78] Chassidut explains that the more refined these *levushim* are, the easier it is for the *neshamah* to be drawn towards holiness and, conversely, repulsed by unholiness.[79]

Sustaining a spiritually-focused thought process during intimacy is easier said than done. There is a similar analogy with Torah study. Anyone learning Torah is instructed to focus on the *Noten Hatorah*, the Giver of the Torah, as they are learning. But how can you both study and think about the Source? The Tanya teaches that what this practically means is to preface Torah study by setting an intention and remembering the *Noten Hatorah*.[80]

The same is true with intimacy. A brief moment of introspection before intimacy can help us segue into a more elevated type of togetherness. If at any time during intimacy, we feel our thoughts slipping to an unsavory place, we can always return to that moment of introspection to anchor us.

---

75 *Shulchan Aruch, Orach Chaim* 240:3, 10.

76 *Shulchan Aruch, Yoreh Dei'ah* 198:48. Practically speaking, a woman's first interaction after immersion will always be with the *mikvah* attendant.

77 *Iggeret Hakodesh* (Ramban) ch. 5; *Siddur Yaavetz, Mitot Hakesef*, 6:9 mention focusing on images of holy *tzaddikim*, thus evoking a desire to bring righteous children into this world. In addition, see *Shnei Luchot Habrit, Sha'ar Ha'Otiyot, ot kuf, kedushat hazivug*, par. 427 where it is suggested to focus on the names of the *Avot* and *Imahot*. *Midrash Talpiyot, anaf ishah mazra'at techilah* mentions focusing on holy letters of the *aleph beit*.

78 On many occasions the Rebbe reminded us that each person is a *baal bechirah*, a master of [their own] choice, and can *chas v'shalom* choose not to conduct themselves in accordance with Hashem's wishes. This is true of our children as well. It is integral that parents understand this and not automatically attribute their child's less than positive behavior to something they may or may not have done prior to conception. Similarly, this is an important point to remember in regard to *shidduchim*.

79 *Likkutei Sichot*, vol. 13, p. 259.

80 *Tanya*, end of ch. 41.

I have heard something about waiting until after midnight to have relations. And, is it true that intimacy on Friday night is a mitzvah?

The *Shulchan Aruch* mentions the middle of the night as the best time for intimacy, as it is the time most quiet and calm, a time least conducive to distraction.[81] In previous generations, when families often lived in one room, there was a *halachic* and practical reason to wait until the children (and other members of the household) were fast asleep before a couple could engage in intimacy. According to Kabbalah, during the period before *chatzot,* the midpoint of the night, the harshest of spiritual forces dominate.[82] In contrast, the period after *chatzot* marks the beginning of the shining of the light of the coming day. The hours after midnight are, therefore, considered spiritually "sweet" or "light-filled" hours and as such the most ideal time for intimacy and drawing forth the highest *neshamot*. However, delaying intimacy can mean that one or both will be too tired and unable to focus properly, which is an important reason not to wait until after *chatzot*.[83] Additionally, the Rebbe gently reminded us that, nowadays, lacking the spiritual refinement of yesteryear, delaying intimacy by waiting until after *chatzot* might just lead to unhealthy hyperfocus on sexuality and is therefore not recommended.[84]

Friday night is an especially propitious time to enjoy sexual intimacy.[85],[86],[87] Within the context of *oneg Shabbat*, the pleasure of Shabbat, intimacy joins the other bodily delights like delicious food, more beautiful clothing, special attention to the cleanliness and adornment of the home in honor of Shabbat.[88] Kabbalah teaches that our intimacy enjoyed on Shabbat mirrors the celestial

---

[81] *Shulchan Aruch, Orach Chaim* 240:7.

[82] *Reishit Chochmah, Shaar Hakedushah* 7:29; *Shnei Luchot Habrit, Sha'ar Ha'Otiyot, ot kuf, kedushat hazivug,* par. 428-429.

[83] *Pele Yoetz, erech zivug.*

[84] Letter dated 17 Teves, 5743 (printed in *Likkutei Sichot,* vol. 21, p. 455).

[85] *Reishit Chochmah, Shaar Hakedushah* 7:29-32; *Siddur Yaavetz, Mitot Hakesef,* ch. 1, 1-2; ibid., ch. 4, 1:2-4.

[86] On Shabbat, our world, as well as the "upper worlds" (i.e the spiritual planes of *Atzilut, Briah, Yetzirah* and *Asiyah*) experience *aliyat ha'olamot* עליית העולמות; each sphere is elevated to the one above it. As a result, *neshamot* brought down through intimacy on Shabbat are drawn from a higher spiritual plane.

[87] The acronym of the words ושמרו בני ישראל את השבת) alludes to ביאה, a *halachic* term for intercourse. (*Rosh, Bava Kama* 7:1)

[88] *Alter Rebbe's Shulchan Aruch, Orach Chaim* 280:1.

joining together of קודשא בריך הוא ושכינתיה, the masculine and feminine aspects of the Divine.[89]

If, however, Friday night does not lend itself to intimacy for a particular couple due, for instance, to lack of desire, sheer exhaustion, or the very late hour because of a family *simchah*, forcing the issue does not serve the greater purpose. Indeed, a woman feeling obliged to engage in intimacy is inherently oxymoronic.

We all hope for a life filled with *bonei, chayei, mezonei revichi uve'kulom revichi*, blessings of children, good health and sustenance, and all in abundance. The fifth *bracha*, however, recognizes that life's ups and downs and plateaus are inevitable. At times, we might confront situations that pull us away from where we imagined we might be. And yet, all of this is part of our *avodah* of creating the *dirah betachtonim*.

The fifth *bracha* answers an important question and presents insight into another way of understanding the *avodah* of *dira b'tachtonim* on a very personal level: From where can I draw the strength to recontextualize personal lower realm moments as opportunities to rise above– and achieve unity and holiness in– experiences that, at first, seem disunified and disheartening?

---

[89] *Bach, Orach Chaim* 280. *Ketubot* 62b.

Kibutz Baneha: Navigating Life

שוש תשיש ותגל העקרה, בקבוץ בניה לתוכה בשמחה. ברוך אתה ה', משמח ציון בבניה

> May the barren one rejoice and be happy at the ingathering of her children within her with joy. Blessed are You, Hashem, who gladdens Tzion with her children.

While the reference to the barren one in this *bracha* refers to Jerusalem, there is also a deeper strata of understanding that provides an invaluable perspective. Earlier we referenced the primordial closeness of Adam and Chava to *Hakadosh Baruch Hu* in Gan Eden. The pre-*chet* reality was marked by a singular focus on Hashem and, thus, pristine unity. It was barren, bereft of any children, which, according to chassidut, refers to various distractions from *Elokut*, G-dliness. In the Gan Eden era, Hashem was *yachid*, the only reality. The *chet* ushered in a world of disjunction; Adam and Chava suddenly experienced themselves as independent from their Creator.

The fifth *bracha* journeys deeper into the mystery of Jewish marriage. *Chatan* and *kallah* are herewith charged with recreating the pre-*chet* unity of Adam and Chava with each other and with Hashem. This time, the unity is specifically within the plurality and multiplicity that characterize our lives in this world. This is the *avodah* of *echad*, oneness, as opposed to *yachid*, aloneness.[90] It is the mandate to gather and elevate all of the diverse factors that will play out in our lives: the joys and the challenges, the overtly holy and the less so. Only then can we arrive at an authentic union and a happiness born of wholeness. This is a profound level of unity achieved only through reckoning with, and weaving together, life's disparate strands.

Humans have a tendency to wax nostalgic about days gone by and over-romanticize the past. Ever since Adam knew Chava, life has been anything but perfect. Life is best described as complex, messy, and filled with curveballs. The *avodah* of creating a *dirah betachtonim* is about taking what our life hands us in this space, in this time, in this situation, in our unique life, and working it into the larger scheme of Hashem's desire for a home in this world. Resist the ravages of perfectionism by not being overly critical of yourself or your spouse. Instead, be kind, and don't worry about what it looks like to others. Hashem seeks our sincere efforts— not perfection.

This all important *avodah* begins at home, and especially in your bedroom.

---

90   *Torah Or* 55b.

Often it takes a while for a couple to find their groove. Many newlyweds need some time to become more comfortable with the physical sensations and the emotions that are part and parcel of sexual intimacy. In *Shir Hashirim,* Shlomo Hamelech refers to *gan naul achoti kallah*, my loving bride is like a locked garden.[91] Marriage represents the opening of that door to the garden. Enjoying the garden in its full bloom is a process that takes time. Different buds blossom in distinct seasons; many flowers take time to unfurl before you can appreciate their complete beauty. As a young woman grows more comfortable with this new aspect of her life, what might have presented as perplexing or even problematic a few weeks or months earlier falls into place or simply fades away.[92]

Whether you're a newlywed or a long-married couple, if you sense a discrepancy between your and your spouse's *halachic* and/or *hashkafic* approaches to intimacy, it is vital to navigate this tension with utmost sensitivity. Women who love their husbands want to have a harmonious home. Oftentimes, that comes in the form of pleasing our spouse, but it should never come at the cost of our self respect, or our respect for our spouse.

Keeping this in mind, try to resolve differences through honest communication and without a sense of judgment. If you are unsuccessful, consult with someone who has objectivity, sensitivity, wisdom, and life experience to help guide you. This is just as true for misalignments in any other area of life, such as finances etc.

Sometimes, it is as simple as a difference in instruction. It is wise for *kallah* teachers and *chatan* teachers to collaborate for this reason. It is certainly a good idea for the newlyweds to review the *halacha* as well as the *hashkafic* teachings they were taught to mitigate confusion. If that does not prove to be enough, they should most certainly reach out to their *kallah* and *chatan* teachers, respectively, and have them consult with one another and provide you with answers to your questions and/or clarification where there seems to be disparity.

Sometimes tension in this area can portend an underlying, more complex issue. Before you married your husband, you dated him, and presumably had occasion to gauge his overall level of refinement by observing his speech or how he eats, for instance. If a noticeable disjunction exists between his behavior in these other areas as compared to his appetites in the bedroom, this needs to be addressed. Speaking with someone qualified can, as a start, help you articulate what it is you are feeling and dealing with.

---

[91] 4:2.

[92] In the words of the Rebbe: "All the problematic matters about which you write occur very often in the early days of many marriages...These problems then diminish until they completely cease to exist, as long as both parties make a good faith effort." *Igrot Kodesh,* Vol. XIV, p. 62.

Restore and Recalibrate: Our Life's Mission

Hopefully, this person can help you discern if this is just a speed bump in the journey of your relationship or a serious barricade that necessitates professional intervention.[93]

Chazal teach איזוהי אשה כשרה, כל שעושה רצון בעלה, who is a "kosher," valorous woman? the one who carries out the wishes of her husband.[94] While this teaching can rankle our postmodern sensibilities, it is generally understood as a nod to the man as the head of the household paradigm, and not as license for a man to subserviate his wife to his will. The Rebbe underscores this subtlety by turning the orthodoxy of this teaching on its head. The Rebbe taught that sometimes it is the *ishah kesheirah*, the valorous woman, who is *osah*, who creates and fashions, *retzon baalah*, her husband's will to do the right thing.[95]

As a woman and a wife, you set the tone in your home and your bedroom. At the same time, your overtures will only succeed when you and your husband are partners in the home, and neither he nor you feels overpowered or controlled. One cannot create a new will before offering one's spouse complete acceptance and assuring him through words, actions, and body language that you support and respect him. Only then might he be ready to accept your suggestion from a place of security and openness. There are situations that call for more than just the above described good will and earnest, full hearted acceptance. As noted, those scenarios call for specific interventions and behaviors that cannot be undertaken without specific professional guidance.

Sometimes, couples face misalignment in the spiritual sphere. It is normal, within a lifetime, to experience fluctuation; at times, we feel completely aligned with the loftiest Torah ideals, both in general and as it relates to sexual intimacy. And, at times, we experience less spiritual synchrony. As long as we align our actions with what *halacha* asks of us, and we make an effort to bring our minds and hearts in tow, we are doing okay. The Alter Rebbe taught that the pathway of struggle, that long stretch of highway that is the *beinoni*'s route home, is as beloved, if not more, than the overtures of the *tzaddik*.[96] The very process, the painstaking effort, is our *avodah*.

Expounding on this point, the Rebbe taught that life, like the *Mishkan*, is comprised of three domains: the *Kodesh Hakodashim*, the *Kodesh*, and the *azarah*, the courtyard and largest area.[97] The *Kodesh Hakodashim* housed only the *aron*; it was an

---

[93] See Part IV, essays seven and eight, for more on sexual dysfunction, addiction, and domestic abuse.

[94] *Tana Devei Eliyahu* ch. 9.

[95] *Likkutei Sichot*, vol. 4, p. 1069.

[96] *Tanya* ch. 27.

[97] *Reshimat Hamenorah*, pp. 85-110.

area of pristine spirituality. Only the *Kohen Gadol* could enter the *Kodesh Hakodashim*, and only on Yom Kippur. This space and its attendant protocol represent a rather narrow slice of our human experience; a place of utter transcendence from physical enticements and daily distractions.

A less intense level of *kedushah* filled the *Kodesh*. This space represents Shabbat, a space of ascendency, exalted over the everyday. Only *Kohanim* in a state of *taharah* could enter the *Kodesh*. The *Kodesh* housed the *menorah*, the candelabrum, the *shulchan,* the table where the *Kohanim* put the *lechem hapanim*, show bread, and the *mizbeach hazahav* upon which was offered the daily *ketoret,* incense. This was a precinct manifestly defined by holy work and the sensory experiences therein were subtle, refined and elevated.

And then there is the *azarah*, the third area, which beckons to all Jews. The *azarah* housed more earthly work like slaughtering the *korbanot,* ritual sacrifices, washing the priests' hands and feet before they went into the holier spaces, and disposal of the ashes or leftovers from the *menorah* and the *mizbeach hazahav,* golden altar. This physical location literally holds space for the messiness of life. According to the Rambam, this area was the heart of the Mishkan and subsequent *Batei Mikdash*.[98] It was a space where each Jew could bring a *korban,* a radical act of transforming something physical and offering it on the *mizbeach,* altar, to the One up high.

On a figurative level, most of us are not *Kohanim Gedolim*, most of us may not even be able to sustain the level of *Kohen*, but we each can bring a *korban*. When brought with sincerity, our offering gives Hashem great *nachat,* contentment, and joy. Each one of us is a part of the *mamlechet Kohanim v'goy kadosh,* a kingdom of holy individuals and sacred nation.[99]

By way of practical analogy: A bottle of fine wine can be used in a number of ways. It can be used for *kiddush*. In this context its usage is completely holy. A glass of nice wine can also enhance a delicious Shabbat or Yom Tov meal. In this usage, the wine, while not sacrosanct per se, is elevated by its use for the mitzvah of *oneg Shabbat*. But sometimes we just want to enjoy a glass of wine on a Tuesday evening. As long as it is *kosher*, we say a blessing before and after drinking, and it fuels an elevated mood and positive behaviors, this too is part of our *avodat Hashem*. Is there a difference between a cup of wine on Tuesday and *kiddush*? Of course. But not every day is Shabbat or Yom Tov...

---

98   *Rambam, Hilchot Beit Habechirah* 1:1; *Likkutei Sichot,* vol. 11, pp. 120-122.

99   *Shemot* 19:6.

Restore and Recalibrate: Our Life's Mission

The all or nothing standard as applied to *avodat Hashem* is just another brilliant antic of the *yetzer hara*. "You're not that type, you're just not that holy," it whispers, "so why bother at all?" We would never, however, apply that logic to other areas of life. We can all agree that some money is better than none, and a little bit of exercise is superior to a complete absence thereof. Certainly, any overture that enhances our *avodat Hashem*, no matter how insignificant it might seem, is worthy of our effort.

None of us live the picture perfect lives that can be so easily curated on social media feeds. Everyone has stressors, worries, and challenges: chronic illness, infertility, less than ample *parnassah*, imperfect *shalom bayit*, and the additional demands of a child with special needs are some on a much longer list of possibilities. It's easy for these trials to wear down our resolve and drain our happiness.

Just as the *Shechinah* radiated outward from between the *keruvim* atop the *aron* in the *Kodesh Hakodashim*, so does the intimacy shared by husband and wife serve as the vortex of the couple's lives. It deeply impacts every other area and, conversely, is affected by multiple factors. Illness, or drugs used in treatment thereof, can compromise love making, as can anxiety, trauma, addiction, and disabilities, both physical and emotional.

We need to do what we can to make sure our intimacy does not fall prey to "collateral damages" in the face of difficulties. In most cases, those with physical disabilities have the same desires and needs as others, but their unique physical circumstances may pose added challenges in their intimate lives. Emotional disabilities call for a whole different skillset on the part of a spouse: empathy, validation, patience, and positive reinforcement. But as with physical difficulties, emotional challenges don't have to prove a barrier to physical expressions of love. A low or flat libido, sensory issues, unresolved emotional pain, and trauma from unwanted touch or other sources are additional types of challenges that don't have to spell the end of love making. With specialized treatment, shared trust and devotion, and tenacity, most couples can, *b'ezrat Hashem*, find their way. Speaking to a *rav* about your specific challenges will illuminate how inclusive *halacha* really is and can yield surprising latitude in navigating your particular situation.

If you or your spouse suffers a sex addiction, you must seek the advice of a trained addiction therapist.[100] Like with trauma, the absolute touchstone is the addict's ability to honestly acknowledge his/her problem and exhibit resolve in working towards

---

[100] As with any other disorder, it is crucial to seek evaluation by a reputable psychologist, neuropsychologist, or psychiatrist to determine that it is indeed sex addiction, as other syndromes can masquerade in this guise. A misdiagnosis can lead to untold suffering and harm to both the person who has a disease and to his/her spouse. Only after proper evaluation and diagnosis, can a specific treatment plan and support system be put in place.

recovery. And like with many types of traumas, the struggle with addiction– which often is the result of a trauma– is very much in the present. It is a constant, multi-faceted, and formidable force. By utilizing the varied available resources and with ample emotional support and patience, an addict can achieve sobriety and, together with their spouse, experience the joy of a solid marital union.

Ultimately, Hashem is the author of our circumstances, and He empowers us with the ability to succeed. If we are humble, honest, determined, and courageous, we can rise above the pitfalls, transforming the trenches of our most difficult scenarios into a space where Hashem dwells. There are, however, challenges that prove to be insurmountable; they are inherently incompatible with marriage. In such cases, divorce is the solution offered by our Torah.

The Torah, and chassidic teachings in particular, teaches *hashgachah elyonah*, Divine providence, so we might understand cognitively that Hashem orchestrates each aspect of our life, including our specific *nisyonot*, trials. The emotional turmoil of life's tests can still prove profound. When a couple faces challenges, they need each other more than ever. When the difficulties threaten their relationship, pain and suffering amplify exponentially. In such cases, couples must prioritize making time to nurture their relationship and avail themselves of all existing resources. With the exception of dangerous and insurmountable pathologies, there are few obstacles that can strip the couple of their choice to support each other through challenges, and even grow together through the difficult and laborious process. As noted, surmounting such lows with commitment, love, and humility represents the ingathering of the children' mentioned in this *bracha*; the fulfillment of creation's purpose, building a *dira b'tachtonim*.

YOU MIGHT BE WONDERING:

I hear that sometimes couples watch a range of sexually explicit materials together as a form of arousal or just for fun. Is that okay?

> Living in a digital age means encountering more pictures than words; we are literally awash in a sea of images. Popular media and mediums lacking any immodesty thresholds impact us profoundly. In building our home, we want to take precautions, especially in terms of what we see.

All of our senses, and sight in particular, uniquely impact our core subconscious and shift our values in ways that bypass logic and emotion.[101] As such, we are often unaware of the subtle shifts that take place within our internal landscape.[102]

Clearly, it is necessary to be attentive to what we expose ourselves to, especially in relation to how it impacts our marriage and our homes. We don't want immodest images popping up in our consciousness, and certainly not during the moments of great spiritual potential when we are intimate with our spouses. While we have the power to dismiss those thoughts when necessary, why give ourselves an extra challenge?[103]

All of the above concerns the range of sexually explicit materials. The corrosive effects of the scourge called pornography require specific attention. Currently, Western society seems to be reorienting itself in recognition of the deleterious effect negative images can have on our behavior.[104] One example concerns governmental regulation of pornography. While once considered a first amendment issue related to freedom of speech and freedom of the press with regulation kept to a bare minimum, pornography is now framed both as a human rights issue and a civil rights issue for women.[105] Increased data now suggest that pornographic material dehumanizes women, that it causes each gender to lose respect for the other, and that violent pornography violates women's civil rights. Yet the number of both men and women who are consuming pornography continues to rise.

Dr. Nikolaas Tinbergen, a Nobel Prize winner who studied social organization patterns in animals, did extensive research on supernormal stimulus. After identifying which markings on female butterfly wings were most eye-catching

---

101 *Kuntres Ho'avodah* ch. 2. *Likkutei Sichot*, vol. 25, p. 309, fn. 3.

102 The Torah warns in *Bamidbar* 15:39: לא תתורו אחרי לבבכם ואחרי עיניכם, do not stray after your hearts and eyes. Rashi comments: "The heart and eyes are spies for the body." They are its agents for sinning: the eye sees, the heart covets, and the body commits the transgression. The heart and the eyes serve as the entry points for sin, and therefore Hashem says: "When you give Me your heart and your eyes, then I know that you are Mine." (Yerushalmi Berachot 1:5)

103 The *Shulchan Aruch, Yoreh Dei'ah* 198:48, cites the custom of a woman coming in contact with something holy upon emerging from the *mikvah* so that the first image she gazes upon is one of purity. Special attention is warranted before conception.

104 Mounting evidence culled from laboratory-based experimental studies revealed that violent media exposure causes increased aggressive thoughts, angry feelings, physiologic arousal, hostile appraisals, aggressive behavior, and desensitization to violence. Moreover, it decreases prosocial behavior (e.g., helping others) and empathy. Huesmann L.R. Taylor L.D. Huesmann The Role of Media Violence in Violent Behavior. *Annual Review of Public Health Journal*. April 2006.

105 Today's Porn: Not A Constitutional Right; Not A Human Right by Patrick Trueman. *Dignity: A Journal of Analysis of Exploitation and Violence*, Volume 2. Issue 3; Dworkin. A. Pornography is a Civil Rights Issue for Women. *Journal of Law Reform* Volume: 21 Issue: 1 and 2. Fall 1987. Winter 1988. Pages: 55-67.

to males, his team crafted butterflies out of cardboard and exaggerated the patterns on the wings to make them brighter and flashier than would ever be found in nature. Essentially, they created the world's first butterfly supermodels. They watched and charted the male butterflies as they flocked towards the "supermodels" trying to mate with them ignoring the real life butterflies that were all around them.

The lie of pornography is that you can enjoy the immediate gratification of perfectly photoshopped, exaggerated, flashy images, and also have long term satisfaction from a life-long, real relationship. You can't. While sexual intimacy is natural, pornography is anything but. It is a product, a big business that is taking a heavy toll on our relationships. Most simply put, pornography focuses on the body with no regard for context. It is the very antithesis of intimacy.

Despite porn's promise of improving consumers' sexual intimacy, mounting research indicates that compulsive pornography consumption is directly related to sexual dysfunction for both men and women, problems with arousal and performance, difficulty reaching orgasm, and decreased satisfaction. For women, the stakes are especially high. In the words of Dr. Gail Dines, Ph.D.,[106] "the more porn women watched, the more depressed and anxious they became, the less interested they were in having sex with people, and the more body-loathing they experienced."

Additionally, because watching pornography places the user in complete control of the experience, porn consumption leads to the erroneous expectation that sexual relations will be under one person's control. The concept of an intimate relationship is completely lost.

Addiction to porn causes distress, hurt, and worse for the partner. But even when a spouse has no issue with the porn habit, or when wife and husband indulge together, it is still damaging to the relationship.[107]

Clearly, an increased understanding is emerging: noxious exposure to lewd material damages our own sense of health and the health of our relationships.

When we understand the holiness of our marriages and the preciousness of intimacy, when we appreciate the enormity of our responsibility and *zechut* to

---

[106] Dr. Dines is an anti-porn activist and professor of Sociology and Women's Studies at Wheelock College.

[107] Stewart, D.N., Szymanski, D.M. Young Adult Women's Reports of Their Male Romantic Partner's Pornography Use as a Correlate of Their Self-Esteem, Relationship Quality, and Sexual Satisfaction. Sex Roles 67, 257–271 (2012).

have children, the question answers itself. How can exposing ourselves to images that embody all that opposes our cherished and holy values be anything other than unhelpful at best and downright dangerous, even destructive, at worst?[108]

Can we talk about female masturbation?

Masturbation is defined as the erotic stimulation of one's genitals to achieve sexual pleasure which may or may not lead to orgasm. From a purely clinical perspective, masturbation is perceived as natural and completely harmless, even beneficial for some women. Among other things, it can help a woman learn about her body and what she finds pleasurable. There is, however, growing consensus even among secular practitioners that human intimacy is a composite, composed of a physical, emotional, psychological, and even spiritual aspect.[109] The research indicates a widespread longing for the unique combination of intense emotional contact and erotic satisfaction that includes more than physical stimulation. The studies underscore that desire and satisfaction are embedded in relationships; the basis of true eroticism is a deep bond. This of course dovetails with the Torah's definition of intimacy as a union of mind, heart, soul, and body.

A man who masturbates transgresses the grave prohibition of *hotzaat zera levatalah*, releasing seed in vain. In contrast, female masturbation does not fall into the same *halachic* category. The consensus among rabbinic authorities is that a woman does not transgress any *halacha* if she masturbates by stimulating herself manually or with a device, so long as she does not focus simultaneously on illicit sexual imagery.[110] That said, the Kabbalistic master, the Arizal, cautioned that female masturbation has negative consequences.[111]

As we've discussed, sexual intimacy as perceived through a Torah lens is a unique and central aspect of a marital bond. The Gemara teaches that while a prenuptial agreement by the woman to forego her husband's support in terms of food and clothing can be found within the *halachic* rubric, no such agreement on the part

---

[108] A therapist might recommend viewing romantic material to create arousal when a woman is having difficulty enjoying intimacy. Regarding viewing such material for the purpose of strengthening one's marriage, consult a Rav.

[109] See for instance, The 1990 Landmark Study by Dr. Ginda Ogden: "Integrating Sexuality and Spirituality" (ISIS).

[110] Responsa *Torah Lishmah* ibid. Sexual fantasy is prohibited with and without physical stimulation; *Shulchan Aruch, Even Ha'ezer* 23:3; Responsa *Divrei Yatziv, Even Ha'ezer* paragraph 35.

[111] The Arizal in *Shaar Hakavanot, Inyan Derushei Halaylah, derush 7*, teaches that a woman should not masturbate.

of a woman to forego her claim to sexual rights can be recognized.[112] While other rights are associated with mere material goods, sexual intimacy is seen as inherent to the marital bond itself. The Gemara's statement offers insight into how we might view masturbation which is an act of self-pleasuring that (often enough) separates sexual enjoyment and release from the couple's sexual intimacy, and for single women, from the marital context.

From a secular perspective, masturbation is another aspect of a woman's self care; going out with friends, reading a good book, getting a mani-pedi, and masturbation are all of the same category. There is most certainly a place for "me" time, but the question becomes: is our sexuality just another pleasure Hashem has granted us, or is it in some way unique?

It has been noted that the love between parents and children is very different from spousal love. While parental love is in some ways the purest form in that it is inviolable, it does not necessitate close geographic proximity. As long as parents know that their child is safe, thriving and happy, they will be at peace even if they are separated from their child by thousands of miles. Spousal love, on the other hand, is not meant to be experienced from a distance. It is a relationship tightly woven of tiny but constant acts of love, devotion, and service. Marriage thrives on the minutiae of the everyday overlaid with love and deep caring. Spouses want to eat together as often as possible, sleep together, and go on vacation together. More than anything, we want to share in each other's lives– all of it– because we care so deeply. Loving couples discuss not only the big ticket items but the nitty gritty areas of their lives. At the same time, this does not obviate the pleasure of going out with the girls, taking a trip with one's siblings or parents, or sharing a hobby or sport with others.

Our sexuality is different. It was created to be enjoyed within and for the purposes of deepening our marital bond. It is not a stand alone urge and certainly not just another activity or "outlet." The famed Kabbalistic master Rabbi Moshe Cordovero taught that the *yetzer tov*, the good inclination, was given to us for our benefit, but the *yetzer hara*, the negative impulse, often correlated with sexual desire, was given to benefit another.[113] This is yet another meaning of the verse in Bereishit which states ואל אישך תשוקתך, one's desire should be directed to their husband.

---

[112] *Ketubot* 56a; *Kiddushin* 19b; *Rambam, Hilchot Ishut* 12:7.

[113] *Tomer Devorah* ch. 6, based on *Zohar* I 49a. We are extremely thankful to Rav Yitzchak Breitowitz of Yerushalayim for pointing us in the direction of this teaching.

When you orgasm, your brain works to produce and release a cocktail of hormones and neurochemicals. These include serotonin, which is connected to a sense of well-being, dopamine, sometimes called "the happy hormone," and the bond-creating hormone, oxytocin, (which is also released while breast-feeding). When a couple experiences these sensations while together, and only then, their intimacy – both in its emotional and physical expressions – further feeds their bond.

When your sexual pleasure and release is connected exclusively with your husband, you bring the full scope of your desire into the intimacy you share with him. All of the anticipation and tititalion that accrues (for instance, while you are *nidah*, when masturbation might be especially tempting) is poured into your reunion and further fuels a shared love and passion.

There is another aspect worthy of consideration: A man can only truly be a husband when he is in touch with his soul essence, the *mashpia* energy, which is about bestowing upon the other. It is in your intimate life, in particular, that your husband most wants to make you happy; he craves your longing for him. He has a desire that borders on a need to satisfy your desire. As *halacha*-abiding Jews, both you and your husband are each other's sole (human) source of sexual pleasure. Intimacy is not something either one of you can give or receive from any other person. And by definition, you cannot experience intimacy with yourself. Masturbation is pleasurable and, at times, can meet a woman's immediate needs. But, ultimately, it can also detract from this crucial aspect of your relationship: meeting each other's needs.

In some cases, a sex therapist might suggest self stimulation exercises to help a woman achieve climax and generally enhance her intimacy with her husband. Clearly this is in line with Torah values, as the goal is strengthening marital intimacy.

Sometimes, masturbation serves as a self-soothing technique used to alleviate tension or anxiety and even, in some cases, to bolster self esteem. A woman accustomed to masturbating may want to discuss alternate methods of dealing with anxiety and self soothing. Once habitual, masturbation is not something that can be stopped easily or suddenly without the risk of frustration or relapse. A therapist, ideally someone who understands the unique positioning of being a *frum* woman, can often provide guidance and assistance.

What about masturbating for pleasure as a single woman before marriage? This important question can only be answered by taking a long view. If a woman hopes and intends to marry, then the ability to associate sexual pleasure – an exquisite joy in life – exclusively with her husband is an uparalleled gift to the solidity and vibrancy of her marriage.

For a Jew, marriage is undertaken as a most important aspect of *avodat Hashem*. Our sexuality is meant to be embraced in that context; to strengthen and deepen our relationship. Actions that siphon the passion or neutralize the craving for togetherness with our husband–a togetherness the Sages liken to entering the Holy of Holies, as discussed– can compromise that ideal.

The claim that masturbation allows us familiarity with our bodies and makes us better and more satisfied marital partners begs for a cost-benefit analysis. If a woman is accustomed to bringing herself to climax, she might not have the patience to wait for her husband to learn how he can best please her. More urgently, this "lack" can become the sole focus, easily eclipsing what should be the sheer joy of reveling in their new togetherness.

One of the greatest joys of intimacy is the journey of discovery undertaken together. As such, whenever possible, entering a marriage with a *tabula rasa*, a clean slate, bereft of prior sexual experience, is ideal.

The fifth *bracha* expresses the hope that we can recognize Hashem in every time and in every circumstance. Living our lives in consonance with Hashem's guidance to the best of our ability leads to authentic happiness, peace of mind, calm, and equanimity. This ideal often seems too difficult, even impossible. From where will we get the strength?

The sixth *bracha* teaches us that when we are one with Hashem, we connect to a transcendent plane. While this will not erase our pain and difficulties, it allows us to frame our travails within the plan of the Infinite, and, in some way, rise above them. The next *bracha* articulates the request that the *kallah* and *chatan* gain access to the abundant joy and gladness that Adam and Chava enjoyed in *Gan Eden mikedem*, in the pristine wholeness and wholesomeness that preceded the *chet*.

Samach Tesamach: The Joy and Mystique of Intimacy

שמח תשמח רעים האהובים, כשמחך יצירך בגן עדן מקדם. ברוך אתה ה', משמח חתן וכלה.

> Grant abundant joy to these loving friends, as You bestowed gladness upon Your created being in the Garden of Eden of old. Blessed are You, Hashem, who gladdens the groom and bride.

This *bracha* is a request that the *chatan* and *kallah*, the loving friends, be granted joy. The superlative quality of joy is its power to break all boundaries. We live in a world of delineation and demarcation, where each aspect of our existence is governed by specific parameters and categories. So too, each person experiences their own specific boundaries and limitations both internally and in relation to others. Joy grants buoyancy. It allows us to transcend the normative constraints and soar to a higher place. It can suffuse our persona, activate our essence, and change our reality.

The very particular type of joy referenced in the sixth *bracha* is the gladness experienced by Adam and Chava in Gan Eden of "old," that is before the sin.

Ever since the *chet*, we have lived an existence of fissure and tension; we doubt and second guess our choices, and thus, sometimes, even our overall worthiness. Our *mesorah* teaches that there is no joy like that experienced through the resolution or elimination of doubts.[114] Fortunately, we have the Torah for guidance.

The prefix of the English word "happiness" is related to the prefix of words like "happenstance," "hapless" and "haphazard." The implication is that happiness is tied to chance and luck. Not surprisingly, people often feel if they only had more or if their life's circumstances were different, they would be happier.

In contrast, the Hebrew word for happiness, *simchah*, connotes finding purpose and meaning. It is a state of mind. Various sages have expounded on this idea, each in their own way. It has been pointed out, for example, that the word *simchah* and *tzemichah*, growth, are related; happiness comes from growing towards our spiritual potential.[115] The *Zohar* teaches that the words *besimchah*, in happiness, and *machshavah*, contemplation, are comprised of the same letters; happiness hinges on understanding our unique place within the wider world.[116] The word *simchah* can be understood as a

---

114   Quoted often as "an adage of a *chachom*"– see *Shu"t HaRama*, beginning of §5; beginning of *Hemshech Mayim Rabim*, 5636.

115   *Pirush Rav Shamshon Rafael Hirsch al Hatorah, Bereishit* 2:5 and *Shemot* 25:39.

116   *Tikkunei Zohar, Tikkun* 22.

contraction of the words *sham*, there, and *moach*, head. More colloquially, where your head is.[117]

In the Torah, the term *simchah* most often appears in the context of something we do with or for others; it is about something we share. The Rebbe taught that *simchah*[118] and Mashiach share three of the same letters, alluding to the consummate *simchah* we will experience at that time when all negativity will be transformed into goodness.[119]

Ultimate joy, however, will elude us until that time when we have finally reached our destination; when our "who", "what", "when", "where" and "why" are fully synchronized. We do, however, get a glimmer of this intense joy, a taste of the unparalleled sensation of "homecoming", in marital intimacy.

In the iconic words of Rabbi Manis Friedman, "Sex is what you do; intimacy is who you do it with." Chimpanzees mate. Ants mate. Elephants mate. Only humans can be intimate, but because we are corporeal beings our intimacy must also take on physical expression.

Herein lies a deeper truth: marriage is the entrance into a three way bond between wife, husband and Hashem. Each act of intimacy that flows from this union is holy and thus a source of abundant joy. This joy is the joy of wholeness and peace which was experienced in Gan Eden.

Sometimes, children, noses pressed against the glass, look into a bakery shop, eyeing the sprinkle-covered cookies and imagine they would make a perfect breakfast, lunch, even dinner. The children whose parents own the shop, however, know that cookies are best when enjoyed as part of a larger meal. We are the kids whose parents own the bake shop. In fact, our Father created the world and has taught us that the route to emotional satiation and satisfaction lies in the nutritional value of the "meal."

Nonetheless, at times, we fall prey to thinking that without restrictions, without context – without having to factor *tzniut* and *hitkadshut* into our life – we could have so much more fun and enjoy life much more fully. We, who are privileged with a tradition that underscores how the unparalleled potency and pleasure of intimacy is rooted in emotional connection and sanctity, should understand better than anyone else the folly of such thinking. Physical intimacy is a non-negotiable aspect of marriage, its highest point; it *is* a full course meal. Divesting it of its spiritual and emotional depth, however,

---

117   Cited in *Miyad Melachim* by Rabbi Yosef Dahan.

118   Until then, the closest we come to *simchah* is the joy we derive from knowing we are on the right path; that we are doing exactly what we are meant to do with our eser *kochot hanefesh*, the ten powers of our soul (alluded to by the letter yud in Mashiach).

119   *Sefer HaSichot* 5748, vol. 2, p. 627.

relegates it to the status of a stand alone sprinkle cookie. Or, as noted earlier, "a body without a soul."

The assumption that unbridled indulgence brings greater fulfillment is simply not borne out by studies on the subject of sexual satisfaction.[120] Counterintuitive as it may seem, tethering yourself to something transcendent opens you up to a special sort of pleasure and happiness. In the words of the Gemara:[121]

איש ואשה זכו שכינה ביניהם לא זכו אש אוכלתן

> If a man/husband and woman/wife merit, the *Shechinah* rests between them. But if they do not merit, fire consumes them.

Rashi explains that the words, איש, man, and אשה, woman, are almost identical, save for the middle letter *yud* in איש and the final letter *hei* in אשה. These two letters can be joined to form Hashem's name of *yud kei* and represent Hashem's presence in a marriage. If however, the couple do not give the "*yud* and the *hei*" –the Torah's teachings and values– prominent placement in their lives together, Hashem withdraws His name from among them, leaving only אש, a consuming fire.

Fortunately, we have *halacha* (etymologically rooted in the Hebrew word *halichah*, to walk) our navigating system,[122] to guide us through life in purposeful fashion, especially when it comes to this most delicate area. And as the episode described below bears out, we also have our *binah yetera*, the extra measure of feminine intuition, to tap into.

In *Parshat Ki Tisa*, Rashi contrasts Hashem's reaction to that of Moshe when the Jewish women donated their copper mirrors towards the construction of the *Mishkan's kiyor*, the laver.[123] היה מואס משה בהן, Moshe was revolted by the idea of the mirrors serving as the construction material for a holy vessel in the *Mishkan*; he perceived the mirrors as agents of vanity and was inclined to spurn this gift. Hashem, however, said חביבין עלי מן הכל, these are dearer to me than everything else!

It's useful, here, to remember the backstory behind these controversial mirrors. The Jewish women in Egypt faced formidable challenges from without and from within.

---

120 For example, a University of Chicago survey of 3,432 Americans ages 19 through 59 found that monogamous married couples reported the highest sexual satisfaction. Similarly, after surveying 100,000 women, *Redbook* magazine also found that the most strongly religious women were "more responsive sexually" than all other women.

121 *Sotah* 17a.

122 See *Sefer HaSichot* 5752, pp. 32-33.

123 38:8.

One particular internal challenge was that their own husbands, the Jewish men, felt dejected due to their miserable conditions and Egyptian oppression. The men were, therefore, disinclined to continue growing their families. The women, on the other hand, believed unyieldingly in the promise of redemption. And they acted on their faith.

The Midrash describes our foremothers in Egypt going out to meet their husbands hard at work in the fields, and bringing the men food and drinks that they had lovingly prepared. After their husbands were sated and in uplifted spirits, the women used their mirrors, which they had burnished to a shine, in a flirtatious manner to arouse their husbands.[124] Instead of seeing reflections of Jewish misery and affliction in the mirrors, these *nashim tzidkaniyot,* righteous women, saw a reflection of their ancestors, and that gave them strength.

In effect Hashem told Moshe that what he saw as coquettish behaviors or worse, were intentional, sacred acts through which myriads of Jewish children were born in Egypt. What better material than these mirrors to use in constructing the *kiyor,* the laver, which each *Kohen* would make use of in preparation for entrance into the *Mikdash*?

The Alter Rebbe echoed the above sentiment when he taught that the offerings for the *Mishkan* included gold, silver and copper, but nothing sparkled quite like the mirrors presented by the women.[125] While the *kiyor* was the last of the components of the *Mishkan* to be fashioned, it's usage was given great prominence at the start of every day's *avodah,* when the *Kohanim* washed their hands and feet in the *kiyor* before carrying out their holy service.

The Rebbe points out that it is indeed possible to err and construe the behavior of the Jewish women in *Mitzrayim* as less than virtuous, yet theirs was an unflinching *emunah* and purity of motivation as proven from the holy legions, the *Tzivot Hashem,* that they bore.[126]

In yet another discourse lauding the Jewish women in Egypt and their mirrors, the Rebbe explains the novelty of the *Mishkan* and the *kiyor* in particular:[127]

Remarkably, in building the *Mishkan,* the Jewish people took the physical materials of this world and fashioned from them a dwelling place for Hashem. In this way,

---

124 *Rashi* to *Shemot* ibid.

125 Cited in *Hayom Yom,* entry for 16 Adar I.

126 *Torat Menachem,* vol. 27, p. 474.

127 *Likkutei Sichot,* vol. 6, pp. 197-198.

our ancestors created the microcosmic model of the *dirah betachtonim*, fulfilling, in some small measure, Hashem's most fervent desire. However, the *avodah* of *dirah lo yitbarech* necessitates the reappropriation of even the most base aspects of this physical world, the תחתון שאין תחתון למטה ממנו, the absolute lowest dynamic within the lower realm itself. Thus, the mirrors, conventionally used for purposes dictated by the *yetzer hara* – but in this case co-opted by the *yetzer tov* for the sake of Jewish continuity – represent the "final frontier." Using these mirrors marked the ultimate transformation; the rechanneling of natural drives in service of an exalted purpose.

This may also call to mind the point noted earlier: While, on some level, the human drive for intimacy is charged with self-oriented gratification, we can redirect and reframe these "lowest of the lower realm" impulses. In that way intimacy between wife and husband becomes the physical "housing" for spiritual oneness with our spouses and Hashem; our own personal *Mishkan*. The very act of washing off spiritual impurity as preparation for entrance into holy service in the *Mishkan* reminds us to put aside or "wash away" our baser sexual inclinations so that we might enter the "sanctuary of intimacy" with purity and holiness. Naturally, this is not an easy task, but for that very reason, the mirrors were Hashem's most beloved item in the *Mishkan*.

The sages describe two modalities of *nevuah*, prophetic perception of the Divine: most *neviim*, prophets, experienced their encounter with G-dliness through what is described as an *aspaklaria she'eina meira*, a lens that is unclear and dark. That is to say, their experience of *nevua* was one in which Hashem was still shrouded – a partial rather than full revelation. Notably, Moshe Rabeinu (and a select few others[128]) experienced their vision of Hashem through an *aspaklaria meira*, an illuminated lens which allowed for a clear, pristine, and focused prophetic perception.

The Rebbe teaches that an *aspaklaria ha'meira* may be likened to a clear window, while an *aspaklaria she'eina meira* recalls a mirror. Each possesses an advantage the other one lacks. In the case of a mirror, the material that coats the glass on one side prevents one from seeing through it; it is no longer a clear looking glass. And yet, precisely because of this seeming disadvantage, a mirror, unlike a window, holds the capacity to reflect. On the other hand, while reflection is a novel and powerful tool, it must be remembered that a mirror offers only a likeness of the image rather than the real thing. Moshe experienced prophecy the way one views an object through a clear window. Others were privy only to a "mirrored" view of the Divine.

In the realm of our spiritual work, the model of *aspaklaria ha'meira* relates to our observance of *mitzvot*; each one a holy commandment, a flawless and unsmudged

---

[128] *Sanhedrin* 97b.

window into our soul, into the Divine itself. In contradistinction, the *aspaklaria she'eina meira* model recalls the many opportunities we are afforded to elevate aspects of our life not overtly holy or governed by explicit Divine instruction.

The *aspaklaria she'eina meira avodah* does not entail pristine Divinity itself (the window experience) but the Divine as *mirrored* in or refracted through the prism of decidedly human drives we've attempted to subordinate and spiritualize. That is to say, spiritually, the mirror modality is analogous to what can be accomplished through refining the *nefesh habehamit*, our animal soul, through sublimating its intense power and passion to a G-dly rather than selfish end. Here is the Divine *mirrored* in lust transformed to selflessness. The Divine mirrored in the least likely place. Likewise, this type of *avodah* draws a novel and higher celestial energy (a sublime reflection) into this world. Because this energy results from wrestling with the animal soul, it lacks the clear, pristine, and perfect qualities of spiritual light drawn down through *mitzvot*—it is but a reflection. Nonetheless, the mirror energy's potency surpasses that of the pure light associated with a mitzvah.

In creating our individual homes, both types of *avodah*, mirror and window, are necessary. For Moshe who perceived Hashem on the level of *aspaklaria ha'meira*, the mirror model appeared subpar, even revolting. Hashem, however, exclaimed: these "mirrors," this *avodah* of transforming the mundane—and channeling that energy into holiness, is more precious to me than anything else.[129]

The mirrors of our mothers in Egypt held the power of the *aspaklaria she'eina meira*, the rebounding or mirrored light, and with it they built a Divine community, birthing scores of Jewish children who received the Torah. We too have the same capacity.

Unique among the other *keilim*, vessels, in the *Mishkan*, the *kiyor's* dimensions are not delineated in the Torah. The *Ibn Ezra* explains that this reflected Hashem's desire that each mirror offered by the women be included.[130] The *kiyor* would simply be as large as necessary! This is a remarkable testament to the spiritual import of these mirrors in a general sense, and to the distinctive devotion of each individual woman.

Each one of us, equipped as we are with the trademark feminine traits of *binah yeteirah* and *emunah peshutah*, pure faith, will discern the correct way to use our

---

[129] Kabbalah and chassidut discuss many aspects of the Divine-human relationship in terms of *or yashar* (a direct light) and *or chozer* (the rebounding light). Hashem's creation – and constant vivification – of this world is the ultimate bestowal of light and energy. And yet Hashem awaits our overtures, the *Or Chozer*, the light that ricochets upward to Him as a result of our service. This light, while sourced in our finitude and extreme imperfection is the most precious of all. This is sometimes explained by way of analogy to the act of concentrating sunlight by having it reflect off of a mirror. In so doing, the potency of the sunlight is magnified many times over, even to the extent of igniting a fire. (*Maamar Heichaltzu* 5659, Chapter 15)

[130] *Shemot* 38:8

Restore and Recalibrate: Our Life's Mission

"mirrors" in the unique relationship we and our husbands share. We may face criticism, even disparagement—due to certain behaviors—but our source of strength lies in the Torah. And we know that just as Hashem trusted our mothers in Egypt, Hashem trusts us to find the right way, in the right time, in the proper balance.

Specifically, how wide a berth is there in terms of behaviors in our bedrooms? The *Shulchan Aruch* is comprised of four *sefarim* or sections.[131] Generally speaking, the sexual behaviors permitted by *halacha* are outlined in the first section, *Orach Chaim*. However, in the third section, *Even Ha'ezer*, there is somewhat more latitude. Often, people ask, if there is a section in *halacha* that allows for it, why can't we indulge? The truth is, just as with every other area of life and *halacha*, it's a matter of each person's free choice. The chassidic approach is first and foremost to live in consonance with *halacha* and to appreciate that the pathway of *halacha* is Hashem's gift to us and our *shalom bayit*. The original meaning of the term chassid, is someone who lives their life *lifnim mishurat hadin*, going above and beyond what *halacha* dictates in order to reveal and experience Hashem's presence in each act. Especially in regard to the act of intimacy whose spiritual potential surpasses that of any other mitzvah. In the words of the Ramban: כשיהיה החבור לשם שמים, אין דבר קדוש ונקי למעלה הימנו, when a husband and wife unite with the proper intent, there is nothing holier and more virtuous than it.[132]

It's also worth reiterating that the above mentioned section of *Orach Chaim* is the default setting for every Jew, not necessarily a chassid or one striving to exceed the minimum guidelines. Yes, there is a time and a place to apply the latitude cited in *Even Ha'ezer*,[133] but that is not our original point of departure.

And yes, in moments of strong desire, you might feel *halacha* is a system of restrictions from which you would like to escape. At these times, you might take a deep breath and remind yourself of a more accurate and profound conception of *halacha*: It is Hashem's pathway through which He is personally leading me, not only so that I and my husband can welcome Him into our lives, but just as surely, for our overall benefit.

Chassidim and those striving for deeper spirituality can turn as well to the *Reishit Chochmah*,[134] a Kabbalistic book that the Rebbe instructed *chatanim* to learn in

---

[131] *Orach Chaim*. Way of Life, covers prayer, Shabbat and holidays, and other issues encountered in day-to-day life. *Yoreh Dei'ah*, He Shall Show Understanding, includes the intricate laws of kosher, usury, vows, and other areas in which a rabbi is generally consulted. *Even Ha'ezer*, Stone of Assistance, contains laws of marriage, divorce etc. *Choshen Mishpat*, Breastplate of Justice, is devoted to monetary laws, torts, and other issues relevant to a rabbinic court.

[132] *Iggeret Hakodesh* (Ramban), ch. 2.

[133] With rabbinic consultation.

[134] Authored by Rabbi Eliyahu Vidash, a student of the famed kabbalist R' Moshe Cordevero.

preparation for marriage. The Rebbe advised study of two specific chapters that teach about *kedushat hazivug*, consecration within sexual intimacy.[135]

In studying these teachings, we are reminded of the *keruvim*, one male and one female, which, at certain times, were, miraculously enough, locked in an embrace. The image of the *keruvim* – that of a male and female – placed specifically atop the *aron*– reminds us that intimacy shared with our spouse represents the holiest aspect of our lives. Furthermore, our lovemaking is intrinsically intertwined with – and should always always be guided by – the *aron Hashem*, our holy Torah.

A couple who decide that they wish to uphold many, or most, or all of the Kabbalistic teachings related to intimacy should not fall prey to thinking that they are "missing out" on sexual excitement and sensual pleasures. On the contrary, they are fortunate indeed. As explained earlier, happiness flows not from freedom to do whatever we wish but from the expression of our essence, which is bound up with our souls and the Torah. Though not always easy or popular, no path proves more fulfilling or purposeful.

At the same time, it is most important to remember that intimacy can only be sanctified when you and your husband are able to relate to each other in a loving fashion. If any of the suggested behaviors cited in Kabbalistic sources cause friction or make it difficult for you to enjoy your special time together, clearly that is not the right path for you at this time.[136]

Communicate clearly with your husband regarding your desires; tell him what you need or want, what you like or don't like. You can use your words or guide his hand to show him what feels good. Do not expect him to be a mind reader or even to read your body language. Your husband wants to please and give you pleasure but will likely need your assistance in this process. As women, we are sensitive to and strive to (sometimes subconsciously) decipher unspoken cues. Generally speaking, this is harder for men. It is unfair to expect what he can't deliver. This is especially true during the first years of marriage. But any time a change ensues that impacts your relationship and your intimate desires – no matter how long you have been married – communicate, communicate, communicate.

Sometimes you might need to discuss these issues with a *mashpia* and/or a professional; listening to their combined advice is the best course of action. Doing

---

135   *Shaar Hakedushah*, ch. 16 and 17.

136   Kabalistic sources beyond those *halachically* required.

so should not be understood as a concession or *chas v'shalom,* G-d forbid, serve as a catalyst for guilt. On the contrary, that is exactly what Hashem wants.

The commandment of *Kedoshim tihiyu, you shall be holy for I, G-d, am holy* is Hashem's instruction to tether the earthy to the sublime.[137] Within the rubric of our holy Torah, achieving *Kedushah* and *taharah* while experiencing pleasure and joy in intimacy are interdependent values.

YOU MIGHT BE WONDERING:

Why are there so many hanhagot, suggested behaviors, concerning what a couple does in the bedroom? Isn't sexuality all about uninhibited expression?

> One of the most basic ideas in chassidut is that everything in this world, including human behavior, is a pale reflection of a celestial reality. If this is true for pedestrian aspects of life, how much more so is this true concerning sexual intimacy. The unparalleled holiness of sexual intimacy shared between husband and wife can be gleaned from the following teachings.
>
> Reb Yaakov Emden taught:[138]
>
> One should never be intimate without first embracing and kissing his spouse. There are two types of kisses. The first is before intimacy, through which the husband arouses the love between them. The second is during intimacy itself. At that time, kissing unites the couple as well as the heavenly *sefirot*. The *Sefer Hagilgulim* elaborates on the mystical dimension of this practice.
>
> The *Reishit Chochmah* teaches that before our sexual organs are joined, there is to be a union of the upper part of the body with lips united in kissing, and the arms embracing.[139] The combination of a husband's and wife's four lips complete the *Shem Havayah*, one of G-d's sacred names, which is comprised of four letters. Their four arms intertwined parallel the *aleph, daled, nun* and *yud* completing the *Shem Ad-nai*. When we embrace and kiss at the same time, we have the *shiluv*, the intertwining and synergy, of both, *Shem Havayah* and *Shem Ad-nai*.

---

137 *Vayikra* 19:2.

138 *Siddur Yaavetz, Mitot Hakesef,* ch. 7, 2:6.

139 *Shaar Hakedushah* 16:21, quoting *Tikkunei Zohar, Tikkun* 10.

It is a powerful and holy moment, and as per Kabbalistic teaching, a prelude to their full sexual union.

The *Reishit Chochmah* references the iconic words in the Torah, ודבק באשתו והיו לבשר אחד, he shall cleave to his wife, and they shall become one flesh, and quotes the *Zohar*, which illuminates that these words also serve as instruction for the truest type of intimacy.[140] דכך דרכה לאתיחדא דכר ונקבא בקרוב בשר.. בלא לבושא כלל, for this is the way in which male and female unite, with skin touching skin...with no clothing separating between them.[141] This, again, resembles what is true *lemaalah*, in the celestial heights. When there is unity of *Kudsha Brich Hu,* the male aspect of G-d, with *Shechinta*, the female aspect of G-d, there is no separation between them. As a Jew prays *shemoneh esrei*, standing before the wall with nothing between her and Hashem, so too, during the union of husband and wife, should there be nothing between them.

At the same time, there is emphasis on comporting oneself in *tzniut* before *Hakadosh Baruch Hu*, with the couple being covered during intercourse.[142]

During intercourse, there is the same silence as during *shemoneh esrei*.[143] Preceding *shemoneh esrei*, however, we are told, קול מעורר הכוונה, the sound of the voice arouses concentration.[144] When it comes to the *shemoneh esrei* itself, however, we lower our voices to a bare whisper. At that point in our union with Hashem, any noise becomes a distraction and impediment; it compromises the profundity of the union. In like fashion, words of love and affection are shared during foreplay, but at the crescendo, when the feeling of oneness is absolute, words cannot contain the emotion.[145] Only silence can honor that exquisite moment.[146]

Once we understand the holiness of sexual intimacy as taught in the teachings of Kabbalah cited above, and once we contextualize what it is we are actually discussing, it's easier to understand the individual teachings in *halacha* pertaining

---

[140] *Bereishit* 2:24.

[141] *Shaar Hakedushah* 16:23, quoting *Tikkunei Zohar, Tikkun* 58. See also *Siddur Yaavetz* (*Mitot Hakesef*, ch. 7, 3:3) who quotes the Gemara in *Ketubot* 48a: "There must be close bodily contact during intercourse. This means that a husband must not treat his wife in the manner of the Persians, who perform their marital duties in their clothes."

[142] *Reishit Chochmah, Shaar Hakedushah* 16:22. *Siddur Yaavetz, Mitot Hakesef*, ch. 7, 3:3.

[143] *Reishit Chochmah, Shaar Hakedushah* 16:20, quoting *Tikkunei Zohar, Tikkun* 10.

[144] *Reishit Chochmah, Shaar Hakedushah* 15:111. *Igrot Kodesh Admor Ha'emtzai*, pp. 173-174 (in new ed.).

[145] To the exclusion of topics unrelated to their feelings for each other and intimacy. *Shulchan Aruch, Orach Chaim* 240:9.

[146] *Siddur Yaavetz, Mitot Hakesef*, ch. 7, 2:3. Certainly, however, if they need to practically convey something to each other, they should do so.

Restore and Recalibrate: Our Life's Mission

to intimacy. And to appreciate how these practical guidelines facilitate an unparalleled soul experience. Our tradition is not a cage, but rather a key for unlocking the door to ultimate closeness with your spouse and your Creator. Therefore, if the teachings cited present obstacles to your intimacy or overall relationship with your husband, do not hesitate to speak with a *mashpia* and/or *rav* about this.

It is important for us to continually strive for better and higher in the realm of *halacha* and *minhag*. It is just as critical, however, to recognize that our *shalom bayit* is paramount and that a particular *hanhagah*, ideal behavior, might simply not be something we can incorporate in our lives at this time, or perhaps ever.

Every person knows the truth about their particular life circumstances. Remembering that *v'hinei Hashem nitzav alav,* Hashem knows our hearts and understands our life circumstances, should give us peace of mind and obviate any sense of guilt.[147] As *Pirkei Avot* teaches, *Asei lecha Rav*, make for yourself a *rav*.[148] The Rebbe taught that in addition to a *Rav moreh hora'ah*, this means a *mashpia,* a life coach for spiritual matters and questions.[149] Once you have followed this Torah prescription and consulted with a *mashpia*, there is no room to second guess or feel apprehension or feel any sense of culpability. In fact, you have determined that, for you as a couple, this is the Torah ideal and not *chas v'shalom* anything less than that.

Coming back to practical instruction regarding intimacy itself, the *Shulchan Aruch* teaches that the proper setting for intimacy is within a private space, and intimacy is prohibited when the couple is in an unenclosed space outdoors (i.e. in a tent would be fine).[150] Engaging in intercourse directly on the ground or anywhere a person would not normally sleep is deemed undignified and thus discouraged.[151]

The prefered position for intercourse is the missionary position with the husband on top of his wife.[152] This reflects what transpires *l'maalah*, in the heavenly realm, where the male energy is *mashpia* and female energy is *mekabel*. In this position

---

[147] *Tanya* ch. 41.

[148] *Pirkei Avot* 1:6.

[149] *Torat Menachem* 5747, vol. 1, pp. 206ff.

[150] *Shulchan Aruch, Even Ha'ezer* 25:4.

[151] *Ketubot* 60b. *Ramban* to Shemot 21:9.

[152] *Shulchan Aruch, Orach Chaim* 240:5.

each faces their source: the man faces downward towards the earth and the woman upwards, towards the man from whom she was taken.[153] Other positions, while not *halachically* forbidden, are discouraged during actual entry, especially during an opportune time for conception.[154] Certainly, however, if there is a need (such as during pregnancy, or due to physiological makeup, or if you cannot experience pleasure in this position, and certainly, if it is painful) do not hesitate to consult (or have your husband consult if you are more comfortable with that, and don't forget that you can always calls anonymously) with a *rav* or *mashpia* about shifting to whatever position/s works best for you.[155] No matter in what position, the couple facing each other, *panim keneged panim,* in a deep and innermost manner remains a *halachic* value.[156] This *halacha* mirrors what we are taught about the *keruvim* which faced and embraced each other, depicting the closeness between Hashem and the Jewish people.[157]

In addition, a man is prohibited from gazing at his wife's genitals;[158] oral sex is likewise forbidden.[159] The *Chachamim* saw this type of behavior as antithetical to *bushah*, the finely honed sense of modesty, that is an inherent trait of each Jew.

In the words of the *Shulchan Aruch*:[160]

> ...שכל המסתכל שם אין לו בושת פנים ועובר על והצנע לכת ומעביר הבושה מעל פניו, שכל המתבייש אינו חוטא, דכתיב ובעבור תהי' יראתו על פניכם זו הבושה לבלתי תחטאו.

> Gazing at the genitals demonstrates a lack of inner shame and is deemed immodest. By doing so, you are deliberately removing your inner shame from within you. This shame protects you from sin. We see this from the verse, "…so that His fear will be apparent on your face, preventing you from sinning."[161]

---

153   *Niddah* 31b.

154   *Sefer Chassidim* §509.

155   *Bris Olam* to *Sefer Chassidim* ibid.

156   *Ba'er Heiteiv, Orach Chaim* 240:15. quoting *Zohar* II 259a. *Reishit Chochmah* 16:28. *Siddur Yaavetz, Mitot Hakesef,* ch. 7, 2:2.

157   *Rashbam* to Bava Batra 99a.

158   There are other authorities that understand this to be equally true for women gazing at their husband's genitalia and pleasuring husbands orally. *Sheyikadesh Atzmo,* p. 449 and fn. 11. Ibid., p. 455 and fn. 16.

159   *Shulchan Aruch, Orach Chaim* 240:4.

160   Ibid.

161   *Shemot* 20:17.

It is most important to note that the discussion regarding *bushah* in this context is not, as conventionally understood, shame or embarrassment. Nor is it about promoting prudishness or self consciousness. It is, rather, about retaining a refinement that makes it harder to veer from the course of Torah and *halacha*. The above is generally considered the default *halachic* ruling.[162]

One might suggest the *halacha* noted above seems to reflect an asymmetry: there is more resistance to a man pleasuring his wife orally than the converse. At first blush, this seems unfair. Why the discrepancy? In reply, one might point to other examples of this asymmetry in *halacha*: the prohibitions against a man hearing a woman's singing voice, watching a woman dance and gazing at a woman during *davening*. Within the realm of *harchakot*, we similarly find this dynamic: while a woman may not lie on her husband's bed in his presence, a man must refrain from even sitting on his wife's bed and this remains the case, even when she is not present.[163] These examples, and many more, point to *halacha's* pragmatic approach. When it comes to sexual arousal, men and women are soft and hard wired very differently. For men, visual and tactile stimuli are potent. For women, arousal is more nuanced; more than anything else, the process hinges on how she is made to feel by her partner. While, for a woman, it is difficult to separate the sexual experience from whom she is with, for men it is quite possible. There is, therefore, marked *halachic* reticence towards actions that might chisel away at a woman's dignity– that might veer towards sexualization rather than intimacy.

האוהב את אשתו כגופו והמכבדה יותר מגופו

A man is taught to love his wife as much as he loves himself and to respect his wife even more than he respects himself.[164]

By definition, *kavod*, respect, means seeing the complete humanity of the other; seeing them in the totality of their personhood rather than as objects for the purpose of sexual gratification.[165] Chazal were attentive to these considerations when they discouraged staring at a woman's genitals and orally pleasuring her.

---

162   If pleasuring each other orally emerges as integral to the fulfillment of the mitzvah of *onah* or to a couple's overall *shalom bayit*, and provided that this does not make the spouse uncomfortable, and it does not lead to issues of *hotzaat zera levatalah*, discuss this issue with your Rav. Similarly, the third section of the *Shulchan Aruch, Even Ha'ezer* (25:2), includes allowance for occassional anal penetration provided that the woman agrees to this form of sexual expression. However, the *nosei keilim* discourage this conduct, and they also refer to the Kabbalistic texts that strongly disapprove it. *Shulchan Aruch* ibid. *Beit Yosef, Even Ha'ezer* 25:2. *Elya Rabbah, Orach Chaim* 240:10. *Yeshuot Yaakov, Even Ha'ezer* 25:2.

163   *Shulchan Aruch, Yoreh Dei'ah* 195:5. *Taz, Yoreh Dei'ah* 195:6. *Pitchei Teshuvah, Yoreh Dei'ah* 195:8.

164   *Yevamot* 62b.

165   We thank Rabbi Yitzchok Breitowitz for this explanation.

With time, couples learn more about each other's physical preferences as well as spiritual sensitivities. If your husband expresses interest in behaviors that make you uncomfortable, or, conversely, he is adverse to pleasuring you in certain ways you desire, this will have to be navigated with the *binah yeteirah*, the extra measure of discernment and discretion, that is granted to a woman. You might ask yourself: is this behavior true to who I am or to who my husband is? Is this a sexual expression we have quite spontaneously discovered? Is this something we learned of and believe can enhance our relationship? If it has not emerged from organic exploration, and certainly, if it does not conform to *Shulchan Aruch* or our tradition of *kedoshim tihiyu*, why am I doing this? What purpose does it serve? Self reflection and open communication with your spouse, and if need be consulting a *mashpia*, should help you come to a decision.

Rivkah: During the very first years of our *shlichut*, we hosted students in our home dining room and living room. We had, of course, hung a beautiful picture of the Rebbe on the wall and its prominent placement prompted many questions. Often enough, some student would say something like, 'isn't it idol worship to hang a picture of your rabbi on the wall?'

On one occasion, I ended up in the dorms, where life sized posters of Farrah Fawcett (of Charlie's Angels fame, which was all the rage then) were ubiquitous. Aha, I noted: a picture of the Rebbe is idol worship, a huge likeness of a pop culture icon is not idolization; it is just plain normal.

If I had a penny for every time I have been asked about my fanaticism, almost always politely, as in "why don't you eat everything that is marked with an O-U, if you concede that it is kosher" etc – I would be a trillionaire!

I have noticed something: If you spend upwards of $300 on a wheel of cheese you are respected for being a gourmand, $800 on a bottle of wine will earn you the title of connoisseur, spend a few thousands dollars on the last tickets to a game, everyone will understand that you are an aficionado, and certainly if you drop a few million dollars on a painting, you will be courted like nobility as you are a "patron of the arts."

Only, when one displays what is considered undue attention and enthusiasm to matters of religion is there a less than positive reaction. One is summarily derided as a wild-eyed fanatic!

It is time for us to proudly own our truth: Yes! We are Jews who are (or try our hardest to be) punctilious in observance of halacha. Yes, we are concerned with finer points, we care about the subtleties, and appreciate the nuances. Yes, this is our passion.

Restore and Recalibrate: Our Life's Mission

> Yes, some of what we do is technically unnecessary by *halachic* structure; they are, however, holy *hanhogot*, behaviors, and we will not cut corners. *Avodat Hashem* is the definition of our lives, and it is in this sphere that we will be fully invested. So next time someone asks you: "is it really necessary," think, would this same person turn down a gift of a Lamborghini because they already own a fully functional Toyota?

Remember always, that our *shalom bayit*, the fabric of our overall relationship, must be strengthened by the choices we make in the bedroom. Stringencies within this area of life, while designed to amplify both the spiritual and even the temporal quality of intimacy, might not be in order for each couple.

What about lingerie and sex toys?

While we make love with our bodies, the success thereof is dependent, in largest measure, on the goings on in our minds and hearts. The Gemara speaks to this in stating, "There was this man who walked along saying: When our love was strong, we could lay comfortably on the width of a sword. However, now that our love is not as strong, even a bed that is 60 cubits wide is not big enough!"[166]

To feel satisfaction and pleasure, to be "successful" in the area of intimacy, we need to feel safe enough to be vulnerable. We need to trust ourselves and our husband and our anatomy, so we can let go and journey into our truest, deepest depth, both alone, and together. Ideally, we will not be measuring our intimate experiences against any outside metric such as that of a relative, friend or popular media. If we understand intimacy as exclusivity, we will recognize the inherent oxymoron in comparison.[167] Allow your natural sexuality and yen for exploration coupled with inherent *tzniut* and refinement to guide you in this journey.

The term lingerie refers to a very broad range of options; everything from upscale, elegant night wear to decidedly bawdy "costumes." More than anything else, what you wear in your private moments with your husband should reflect you and your relationship.

Quite aside from wanting to strive for beauty and refinement, there is a more profound message here: externalities are exactly that, a topical facade. What lies beneath is what we want to focus on. This is one of the messages of the *bedeken*. With covering the *kallah*'s face before the *chuppah*, the *chatan* reminds them

---

[166] *Sanhedrin* 7a.

[167] *Pesachim* 112a.

both that their relationship is based first and foremost on what lies beneath and remains unseen.

We are not negating the importance of beauty. Beauty is important, and suggestiveness, if that is your style, certainly has an important place in the bedroom. But that is different from coarseness or vulgarity. We want to hit a balance wherein we acknowledge, even honor, a specific occasion— especially our intimate moments— by dressing in a way that reflects how much we cherish this time. We don't, however, want to overwhelm our husbands with visuals that arouse the senses to a point that obscures our personhood.

We live in a world where we are routinely exposed to images of models who weigh 23% less than the average thin woman. Then, there's the issue of image manipulation. The physically perfect specimens seen in photos do not exist. Even these genetically-blessed individuals are treated to rounds of photoshop treatments. Every blemish and wrinkle is removed; their bodies are tightened and trimmed, and legs and arms are often lengthened! This could all be glossed over as harmless, even laughable, if its effects were not so toxic. These images deteriorate women's sense of body image and self esteem, and there is indisputable evidence of their contribution to the mounting incidence of depression, eating disorders and worse.[168] If men have these images in their heads, how can the average woman ever measure up? For your sake and the sake of your marriage, don't buy into this culture. Set the tone of your marriage from the get go: what you have together is deep; deeply beneath your skins. Don't be afraid to bare only as much as you feel comfortable with. Go ahead and be a bit elusive. Romance thrives on the subtle and mysterious. On the other hand, if baring more makes you happy and enhances your intimacy, enjoy!

Sex toys, an assortment of accouterments designed to stimulate sexual arousal and release, are often presented as necessities without which one will be unable to experience pleasure. This is unsurprising given that the larger society in which we live is sexually saturated, jaded, and weary.

In this sense, innocence and lack of prior sexual experience is a precious gift. Revel in the purity and wholesomeness of your body and its natural responses. Beginning with a clean slate means a hypersensitivity inherent in every touch,

---

[168] See, for instance, The impact of the media on eating disorders on children and adolescents (Pediatrics Child Health) by Anne M Morris, MBBS MPH FRACP and Debra K Katzman, MD FRCPC that cites numerous epidemiological studies and The influence of the media on eating disorders (Journal of Human Nutrition and Dietetics) by S. Almond.

and an excitement in every new sensation. Being careful with the *dinei harchakah* introduces an aspect of this clean slate paradigm into each month and allows you to retain sensitivity to touch throughout decades of married life. That acute sensitivity to touch is precisely what eludes so many. Don't feel the need to shortchange yourself and your husband by running after the items that are meant to restore the very gift you already possess.

On the other hand, these tools can be helpful for couples, especially when a partner is having trouble experiencing an orgasm. They may be useful to a couple who, after years of marriage, are looking for something new. Sometimes, couples are just plain curious to see what it's all about. Every human being and every couple is different; there may or may not be a place for these items in your life. In the final analysis, as long as something does not contravene *halacha* (and most sex toys, also known as marital aids, do not), what the two of you need to enjoy a fulfilling sexual relationship, rather than what's "out there" or what "everyone else" is doing, should be the sole determinant!

A rich and nourishing intimate life is informed by two poles: consent and negotiation. At no time should you or your husband feel forced to engage in an intimate expression with which you are uncomfortable. Conversely, there will be times in your relationship when it is entirely appropriate for the two of you to "negotiate" something new. Humans are *mehalchim*, ambulatory; we are constantly moving forward and evolving. Being dynamic rather than static is a hallmark of our humanity.

Don't let social media bully you into behaviors you feel instinctively are not for you. Don't feel cowed into behaviors that seem off. If alarm bells go off in your head, don't dismiss them. On the other hand, don't automatically rebuff an idea just because it's different. Discuss it with your husband and trust your gut.

Regarding the amassment of material assets and physical pleasures, our *chachamim* have counseled us to be happy with our lot.[169] Otherwise, we can never achieve satisfaction; we will always want more, and more, and then still more. With sexual intimacy, this desire is sometimes even more pronounced.[170] The constant urge for the the exotic and erotic, the kinky and fetishized, can obscure what we want most.[171]

---

169   *Pirkei Avot* 4:1.

170   "There is a small organ in man: If you feed it it is hungry, but if you starve it it is full." *Sanhedrin* 107a.

171   Some of these forms like BDSM, also referred to as bondage, are about being in control and giving up control, even welcoming pain. Intimacy,

The first six *brachot* focus on the *chatan* and *kallah*, who, at this moment, begin their lives together. The seventh *bracha* zooms out, placing their personal joy within the larger context of Jewish history.

---

however, is about bonding. Additionally, any activity which includes inflicting pain – even consensual pain – on oneself or another can present serious *halachic* challenges. For more, see *Alter Rebbe's Shulchan Aruch, Choshen Mishpat, Hilchot Nizkei Guf V'nefesh* §4.

Bracha Acharita: The cosmic reverberations of marriage

The seventh *bracha*, is often referred to as the *bracha acharita,* the final blessing:

ברוך אתה ה' אלקינו מלך העולם, אשר ברא ששון ושמחה, חתן וכלה, גילה רנה דיצה וחדוה, אהבה ואחוה שלום ורעות. מהרה ה' אלקינו ישמע בערי יהודה ובחוצות ירושלים, קול ששון וקול שמחה, קול חתן וקול כלה, קול מצהלות חתנים מחפתם, ונערים ממשתה נגינתם. ברוך אתה ה', משמח חתן עם הכלה.

> Blessed are You, Hashem our G-d, King of the universe, who created joy and happiness, groom and bride, gladness, jubilation, cheer and delight, love, friendship, harmony and fellowship. Hashem our G-d, let there speedily be heard in the cities of Yehudah and in the streets of Yerushalayim the sound of joy and the sound of happiness, the sound of a groom and the sound of a bride, the sound of exultation of grooms from under their chuppah, and youths from their joyous banquets. Blessed are You Hashem, who gladdens the groom with the bride.

In invoking ten expressions of blessing upon the *kallah* and *chatan*, this *bracha* connotes culmination and crescendo. The number ten parallels the ten *sefirot*, the ten aspects of each individual's inner landscape, and thus symbolizes completion and consummate joy. It reminds the couple, and all those assembled, that each marriage between a *kallah* and *chatan* brings closer *Yemot HaMashiach*, which will be the ultimate marriage between Hashem and *Knesset Yisrael*.

Human sexuality is a primary force in the lives of a married couple; it is the unique language and expression of the love they share. It is primal and private and as endemic to the human condition as breathing, eating, sleeping and voiding. At the same time, intimacy not only constitutes the backbone of each particular family unit, but also crucially impacts the world at large.

In their private, personal togetherness, each woman and man are creators of peace, harmony and healing—they nurture the basic need for emotional security of their family members and those beyond their immediate circle. The ripple effect of their love and commitment saturates their lives and overflows into their society. Ultimately, it allows and encourages humanity's mandate to arch upwards towards our Creator.

Chassidut and Jewish mysticism teach that creation began with the *tzimtzum*, contraction, of the *Or Ein Sof,* the endless light of G-d, that preceded the existence of the universe.[172] In this process, before time, space, and all delineation, there emerged a binary: male versus female energy. The inherent binary echoes the story of *chet etz hadaat* when self consciousness supplanted the all-encompassing G-d consciousness.[173] That story ultimately sets the stage for a unity that is deeper than and far surpasses the original oneness of Hashem that preceded creation. For, now, unification must entail a paradoxical joining of two opposites, an achievement far more profound than the oneness that prevailed when Hashem was the only Existence; when there was only *Or Ein Sof*. In fact, the power to balance opposites issues from Hashem's Essence, which transcends all categories and, therefore, can fuse the most unlikely combinations.

Unity with our spouse also represents a reunification of souls.[174] Our efforts to unify with our husbands, our "opposites," especially via intimacy, therefore awakens or elicits this Essence power; it touches the deepest "space" in the Divine. In other words, bringing Hashem's ultimate plan to fruition hinges in great measure on the unity we achieve with our other half in marital intimacy. As the *Sefer Yetzirah* teaches, נעוץ תחילתן בסופן, וסופן בתחילתן, the beginning is wedged in the end and the end is wedged in the beginning. Hashem's initial "stirring" or desire for oneness with creation (the beginning) is realized largely in the sanctified act of physical intimacy, of oneness, between husband and wife (the end). Put differently, unification of husband and wife, a balancing of opposites, marks the presence of Hashem's Essence here in the lowest realm, for only Hashem's Essence can contain opposites.

The last of the *brachot* thus speaks to the culmination of Hashem's creation: the time when the male and female aspects of Hashem, *Kudsha Brich Hu,* and *Shechinta,* will be united. In that time we will experience every conceivable iteration of peace and joy because, at long last, humanity will be fully one with our creator.

---

172 *Likutei Torah, Pinchas* 76d.

173 The world would be comprised of this male-female duality: the *kav*, a kaballasitic term for the vector of concentrated G-dly light, and the *reshimu*, the trace, a kaballistic term for the light of G-d that remains in this world after the *tzimtzum*, *orot* (lights) and *keilim* (vessels). *Kudsha Brich Hu* (the male aspect of the G-dhead) and *Shechinta* (the female aspect of the G-dhead), man and woman.

174 *Sefer Yetzirah* 1:7.

YOU MIGHT BE THINKING:

I have not always followed the rules, but I truly want to do things correctly going forward. How can I build my marriage on a foundation of purity and wholesomeness? Is that possible for me/us?

The good news is that the answer is an emphatic yes. Sincere *teshuvah*, deep introspection, and practical integration of those lessons learned, can put you on your desired path forward.

Nowhere is chassidut more radical than in its treatment of the concept of *teshuvah*. The Rebbe teaches that not only is every *yeridah*, descent, for the purpose of an eventual *aliyah*, ascent, but the *yeridah* itself is part and parcel of the ultimate *aliyah*.[175]

Axiomatic to our *emunah* is the conviction that nothing happens by chance As described in *Tehillim*, מה' מצעדי גבר כוננו ודרכו יחפץ, by Hashem are man's footsteps established, and He shall favor his way.[176] Put differently, beneath the surface, the impulses that govern our mundane comings and goings are merely reverberations or echoes of Hashem's will.

At the same time, every person has *bechirah*, free choice, in their *avodat Hashem*. And yet, even outcomes that derive from missteps in our personal *avodat Hashem*, spiritual service, can occur only in consonance with the *hashgachah elyonah*, Divine Providence, and with Hashem's Will.

This delicate point–that we possess free will in our service of Hashem (or lack thereof) while, simultaneously, all that transpires is a matter of Divine Providence– calls for some background: Chassidic thought describes two levels of Divine Will, of Hashem's *Ratzon*. Hashem's primary or inner will, *Pnimiyut Haratzon*, concerns His desire that we engage in Torah and *mitzvot*, *avodat Hashem*. In contrast, His desire for a stage on which Torah and *mitzvot* can be fulfilled, i.e. His desire for a physical world and everything therein, constitutes a secondary or external desire, *Chitzoniyut Haratzon*. To help clarify, we might think of a human example: A businessperson who desires to complete a lucrative financial venture in a distant country wants to book a plane ticket, arrange transportation to the airport, and travel to that far off land. Her desire to travel and make the

---

[175] *Likkutei Sichot*, vol. 5, pp. 57-67. Ibid., vol. 18, pp. 390-398. *Sefer Hamaamorim Melukat* (new ed.), vol. 3, pp. 251-255.

[176] 37:23.

associated mundane arrangements, a desire associated with means to an end, a desire not reflective of her innermost self, constitutes her secondary or outer will. Her core desire concerns completion of the lucrative venture itself.

Naturally, Hashem's external or secondary desire and its interaction with all creation, be it a planet, an animal, or form of vegetation, is relatively removed from His Essence; Hashem's external will is less lofty, less rooted in His transcendent self, and therefore more easily sensed by creation. As such, creation is left with no choice but to yield to the Divine will.[177]

The same is true of all our mundane inclinations not pertaining to *avodat Hashem*. Hence, the Sages say we do not have free will in matters unrelated to *Yirat Shamayim*, fear of Heaven. In contradistinction, man's spiritual *avodah* is innermost to Hashem's Essence and desire. Being so lofty, this level of Divine Will is therefore transcendent and aloof, to the extent that man cannot sense this great force presiding over his *avodat Hashem*. This leaves humanity feeling unencumbered in our choices, even as each action we take is part of G-d's ultimate plan.

And so it is that man can sin; we all misstep and fall. Just as a young child learning to walk might stumble and skin their knees or get a bump on their head, our sins are painful to ourselves but not less so to our Father in heaven. What pains us pains Him infinitely more.[178] The faltering and falling is decidedly not what any parent wants for her child. But holding the toddler won't help the child learn to walk on their own. And so, ultimately, the falling *is* part of what the parent intends; even as it is not the parent's wish that the child be hurt and feel pain.

In the analogue, a given action might indeed be sinful and contrary to Hashem's will (*hepech Ratzon Ha'Elyon*, opposite Hashem's will). Essentially, however, the sinful action does not represent a true descent because the act's consequences and aftermath form part of an ascent which will ultimately follow. (Thus, the overall scenario is, essentially, *lefi hakavanah,* in consonance with Hashem's intention*).*

To further explain, a Jew must know that even when they have sinned as a result of their own ill-advised free choices, and are appropriately pained over these trespasses of Hashem's will, they should not feel depressed nor despondent.

---

[177] This subservience is especially apparent with the celestial bodies. As the *Navi* says in *Nechemia* 9:6: וצבא השמים לך משתחוים, the heavenly hosts bow down to you. The sun sets in the West because the *Shechinah* resides in the West. The sun's orbit from east to west, until it sets, is its form of paying homage and "bowing" to the *Borei Olam*, the Creator of the universe.

[178] *Sichot Kodesh* 5740, vol. 3, pp. 6-7.

Restore and Recalibrate: Our Life's Mission

They should remember that the circumstances of their life, irrespective of their particular choice, are orchestrated by Hashem and must therefore inevitably lead to a greater ascent. In fact, this descent allows them to be *mevarer nitzotzot*, to extricate fallen sparks of divinity, and unleash spiritual lights that would otherwise remain inaccessible had they followed the straight and narrow path. The notion that we can transcend and rewrite our flawed pasts is true, in general, and applies to indiscretions in the area of intimacy as well.

Our masters employ the evocative metaphor of a person walking eastward while aboard a ship traveling westward.[179] Although his own movements take him towards the East, he is in reality traveling towards the West at that very moment.

The entire world is that ship, and Hashem is our captain. We are inexorably traveling towards personal and universal *geulah* even if at a certain moment we may have turned our backs on this plan. If you have meandered and then reoriented, congratulate yourself that you are now in sync with the ship's direction.

When people refer to intimacy as "the mitzvah," it grates on my nerves; can't we just enjoy ourselves?

Rivkah: I remember with clarity how my grandfather (the one I share with Sara Morozow) called me into his office on the morning of my wedding day. In his inimitable, straightforward fashion, he told me *"der velt meint az men hut chassunah tzu huben "fun," uder huben a shaine dirah mit narishe hantecher. Uber men hut chassunah vayl der Aibershter hut azoy bafelt."* Loosely translated from the Yiddish, he said : "The world thinks you get married to have fun and to enjoy a nice apartment with silly towels (he referred to my then obsession with fancy guest towels for the bathroom–the kind you never really want anyone to use). But we get married, he asserted, because G-d so commanded."

I remember feeling irate, even a little angry. Why was he raining on my parade; puncturing my balloon on the day of the grand carnival? But of course, now I understand and appreciate the truly important lesson he was conveying with such love and devotion. I also understand the counterintuitive truth that it is precisely when we move beyond the natural preoccupation with the self and we connect to something higher, that we can experience ultimate happiness.

---

[179] *Sefer Hachakirah* 9a, quoting *Nechmad Vena'im* 1:13.

Marriage is a mitzvah and a mission. It is the institution that makes possible and moves forward the realization of Hashem's most fervent desire: a *dirah lo yitbarech betachtonim,* construction of a home for the Divine in this lower world. We are Hashem's ambassadors, His "construction team." The "home" He desires is actualized only when we spiritualize our physical encounters in this lower realm, including our intimate encounters. It is not the shul but the Jewish home that serves as the primary sphere of our *avodat Hashem*; Jewish familial life is the laboratory in which holiness is incubated.

That is to say, our marriage is so much larger than us. Our desires, our happiness, our pleasure, are all absolutely important, but they are not the central reason for marriage; they are, with Hashem's help, its by-products. We are looking not to fall in love but to climb upwards in love, day after day for the rest of our lives. The foundation is commitment to the institution that is our marriage as defined by *Hakadosh Baruch Hu* Himself. In this context, commitment to each other is cardinal, and surrender of ego, becomes the key ingredient to success. However, as will be seen, self surrender is not as self effacing as we might assume. Quite the contrary.

When we integrate this idea, a simple truth emerges: when I do something for my spouse, I am doing it for myself, for us, for our union, for Hashem. Going out of my way to be considerate is not a chore, and it's not extra work; rather, it is what one does for oneself! When the matter is seen in this light, another point becomes clear: appropriate discussion with those who might help us strengthen our marriage should carry no taboo; on the contrary, it is highly encouraged.

The Rebbe taught: As the *geulah* comes closer, the forces of *sitra achara* seek to sow discord between spouses, as the *shalom* between them mirrors the ultimate union of the male and female aspects of Hashem above, which will culminate and manifest in *Yemot HaMashiach*. At the same time, the Rebbe assured us that we have been given the necessary strength and resilience to confront this challenge.[180]

We need constantly to return to and keep at the forefront of our consciousness the enormity of what is riding on our personal relationships. When we realize how profoundly the health and vibrancy of our individual marital unions impact the entire cosmos and Hashem's innermost desire, we are motivated to put our best efforts forward in this direction. This is the most vital of all *mitzvot*.

---

[180] *Igrot Kodesh,* vol. 4, p. 433.

The realization that our microcosmic marriage causes macrocosmic ripples can take years to process; complete integration of the shocking truth that it's not about us but about something so much larger and more monumental that we are a part of, takes time. But a journey of a thousand miles begins with one step. And then another, and another.

Happiness comes into our lives not when we pursue it but when we pursue our purpose for being. In giving, we receive. In submission, we are strengthened. In gratitude and humility, we are elevated. When these values suffuse our lives, sexual intimacy becomes deeper, more vibrant, rich, and meaningful.

In this light, we can add yet another layer to a point made earlier: marital relations are often referred to not only as a mitzvah but as the *Kodesh Hakodashim*. While, presently, we lack the physical, communal *Beit Hamikdash* in Jerusalem, we can and must build a *mikdash me'at* in our personal lives. Keeping *taharat hamishpachah* and infusing our marriage with *kedushah* is the gateway to this holy ground. It allows us to ascend onto the *Har Habayit*, where the Temple stood, and into the *Kodesh Hakodashim*. And when, as noted, each individual couple nurtures its *mikdash me'at*, the era marked by the rebuilding of the larger *Mikdash* draws ever closer.

chapter three

Gan Eden 2.0:
OUR RETURN

After gaining a deeper understanding of our post Gan Eden existence, the physical world could be considered dangerous to the soul's mission. At most, we might posit Earth as a footstool to heaven. If used properly, it can be co-opted in service of the Divine. Chassidut teaches that the physical world is just as exalted as the heavens above, and in important ways, even more so.

Hashem's ultimate plan and desire for a *dirah lo yitbarech* can only be fulfilled in the Earthly realm. According to the Alter Rebbe, all worlds exist because of and within the framework of Hashem's initial stirring for a home in this world. According to chassidic thought rooted in the *Midrash*, this is the purpose of creation and the justification for the existence of the physical and spiritual universe.[1]

The lower realm is indicative of the rich, spiritual potential of the corporeal world. The fact that the physical universe recognizes a Creator and the fact that each aspect of creation is subservient to the *Or Eloki* that perpetuates its existence, all reinforces that truth. As noted, the *Navi* states, וצבא השמים לך משתחווים, the heavenly hosts bow down to You.[2] The sun sets in the West because the *Shechinah* resides in the West,

---

1 *Tanya* ch. 36.
2 *Nechemia* 9:6.

reflecting an inherent abnegation of the self to the Source of all.[3] The same holds true for all of nature.

When we ponder that within each facet of the world resides *a nitzutz eloki*, a Divine spark, we appreciate the beauty and inherent loftiness in the physical realm. When we apprehend the way corporeal matter is harnessed to its transcendent source, it emerges not merely in the role of utilitarian agent in our spiritual quest but rather as the arena singled out for our service.

Humanity was given the gift to be able to actualize Hashem's plan for a home in this mundane reality via spiritual service. When humans spurn the opportunity to sanctify a physical item or moment, we effectively debase that aspect of existence. Of course, no one is perfect, and everyone will slip up at times. This is by design.

This monumental power of free choice – to elevate or not to elevate – is the most significant legacy of the sin in the Garden, which led to an all encompassing macrocosmic dichotomy.[4] Before the *chet*, the body existed as an extension of the soul much as the world was an extension of He who spoke and brought it into existence. The *chet* was the first act of disconnection. It separated material, corporeal matter including humans from a constant awareness of their de facto G-dly purpose. It turned things inside out and upside down, causing humanity to focus on the body as opposed to the soul.

Like the microcosmic separation of Chava from Adam, the separation of the body from an all encompassing sense of Divine purpose and presence was by design: That design was to facilitate an eventual reunion.

What is the point of a separation that ultimately results in a subsequent reunion? The fact that the post-*chet* reunion far surpasses the pre-*chet* oneness, which was effortless and automatic. Just as man and woman's initial splitting opened the possibility of choosing a profound reunion, so too our present quest to reunite with Hashem through enacting Torah and *mitzvot* yields a richer reunion, the *dirah betachtonim*, the purpose of creation.

From the moment of our banishment, humans have been on a quest to return and to calibrate our perception of reality with the truth. That calibration entails revealing the *nitzotzot*, sparks, that pulsate beneath the surface of all matter, that fill each space and saturate every increment in time. To do this requires approaching life with G-d consciousness rather than the default self-absorption. Especially in terms of intimacy,

---

3   *Bava Batra* 25a.

4   *Sefer Hamaamorim* 5659, p. 22.

this summons does not equate to disengagement from physical life. Rather it requests aiming to unearth the vivifying spiritual sparks beneath the physical surface by doing our best to show up in our relationships.

Our challenge in life is to focus on this calling and let it guide our every decision. It is a constant push-and-pull to stay present amid so many distractions. When we veer from single-minded concentration and are distracted by what obfuscates it, we separate ourselves from the Divine core that animates all.

Imagine ignoring the world-class medical specialist with whom one has been granted a rare appointment after a long wait, in favor of flirting with a good-looking parking attendant. Less dramatically, imagine relating to food only for its taste, color, and texture with no regard to its nutritional value.

Our goal is an eventual state of being in which tension between spirit and matter is erased; a time when matter clearly showcases the spirit that endows it with life. Each time we consciously and mindfully see through the facade and connect with the essence of all matter with its soul, we bring *Yemot HaMashiach* that much closer.

When Adam and Chava donned *chagorot*, when they clothed their bodies, so as to properly concentrate on their souls, they began the work of *tikkun*, of rectifying the result of this sin.

Just as it was for the first couple in history, *tzniut*, modesty in thought, dress, and behavior remains one of the most important ways we preserve the delicate balance between soul and body, the vivifying force and its external encasement. This unique understanding of *tzniut* calls for embracing the inherent holiness of our body, inclusive of our feminine beauty and ineluctable sensuality. *Tzniut* reminds all of humanity to see the female body for what it is: the most miraculous and definitive stamp of Hashem's authorship of creation, and the chosen temple for the human soul. And at the same time, it reminds us how easily this truth can be eclipsed with undue focus on the external. No aspect of our life more profoundly benefits from this prioritization than our sexual intimacy.

Every one of our sanctified acts of intimacy brings us back to that wholeness; that sweet and peaceful primordial, all-pervasive, consciousness of Hashem. The sense of wholeness and peace experienced in lovemaking provides a glimpse into the possibility of this world transformed into Gan Eden. This second version, Gan Eden 2.0, will be the outcome of our overtures; the seeds painstakingly planted, sowed, and watered throughout the long generations since our banishment. At long last, we will welcome the *Shechinah* back to its original abode in this realm, only with a revelation more pervasive and powerful than the one experienced in the pre-*chet* era. The Midrash teaches: "In this world, Hashem's bond with His people was a betrothal—as it is written,[5] 'I shall betroth you to Me forever'…but in the days of Mashiach there shall be marriage."[6]

In our intimate coming together, we mirror not only the original oneness of Adam and Chava, but experience a foretaste of a much deeper and ultimate intimacy; that of humanity and our Creator. We get a glimpse of what it will mean to be reunited and back home.

---

[5] *Hoshea* 2:21.

[6] *Midrash Rabbah Shemot* 15:30.

Part Two
Marriage:
A Study in Three Parts

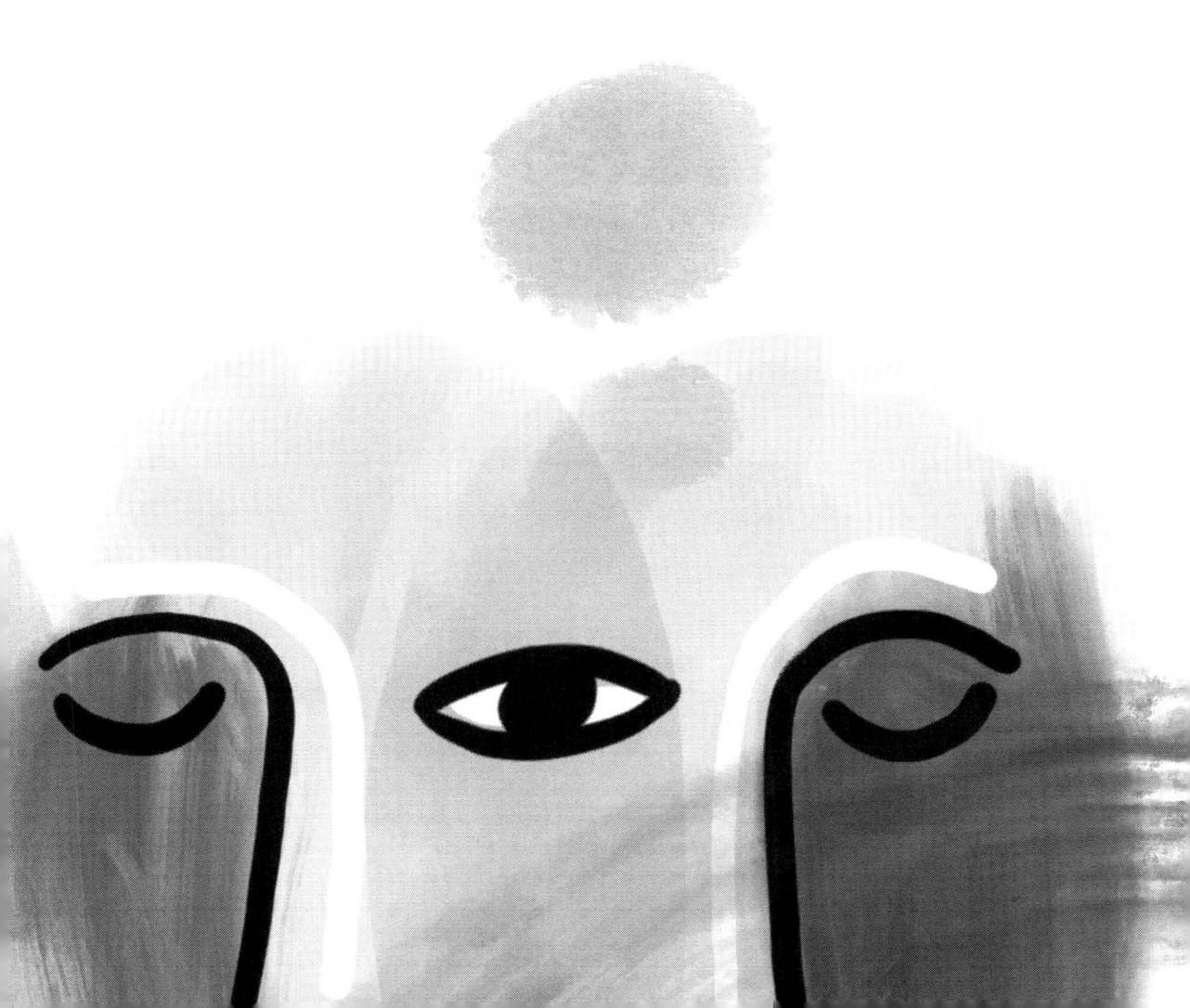

chapter four

When Does Kiddushin Begin?
YOUR CHOICES MATTER

The laws of nature, government, commerce, and society are a few of the systems humans live by. Each of these constructs exists to create order and promote maximum efficacy and benefit to the greatest number of people. As sociological and technological factors evolve and shift, the systems of law adjust to changing realities. Torah Law is different. As cited in *Hayom Yom*:[1]

> There are two kinds of laws: laws that generate life and laws that are generated by life. Man-made laws result from life. That is why they differ in every country, each according to its local circumstances. G-d's Torah is the Divine law that *generates* life. It is the Torah of *truth* – the same in all places and at all times. The Torah is eternal.

Different from every other form of law, Torah law does not react to reality; it creates reality. Said differently, *mitzvot* reveal the essence and truth behind each dynamic of existence.

Globally, marriage is considered one of many possible lifestyle choices. In fact, historically, even the institution of marriage has taken varied forms: a union between one woman and many men, a union between one man and many women, a union

---

[1] *Hayom Yom*, 22 Shevat, citing *Sefer Hamaamorim Kuntreisim*, vol. 1, p. 228.

between two men, etc.[2] At times, marriage was deliberately a temporary union, such as in revolutionary Iran. In China, the definition of marriage once included a union between a living woman and a dead man.

For a Jew, marriage is a central mitzvah that is defined as the union of woman, man, and Hashem in a three-way partnership.[3] Each *kiddushin* is a link in the uninterrupted chain of our history beginning with *matan* Torah; each loving and sanctified union brings all of us closer to the *geulah,* redemption. Indeed, the responsibility and privilege of actualizing the world's purpose rides on the wholesomeness and holiness of the family unit.

Like Adam and Chava in their original dimorphous form, each woman and man is, similarly, one half of a larger whole. We share one soul, which is separated upon birth.[4] Because of this truth, a Jewish wedding is more correctly described as a reunion rather than a union, as the two halves reconnect under the *chuppah*. The merging of these two long lost *ohavei nefesh,* soul lovers, unleashes an unparalleled joy for the entire community that continues for the full week afterwards.[5]

The Arizal taught that a couple is spiritually linked long before they ever meet.[6] When a young woman fulfills a mitzvah, her (future) husband is already included in that act, just as when a young man fulfills a mitzvah, his (future) wife is encompassed in that action. They are one even before marriage.

Because they are a unified soul, their seemingly independent actions impact one another on a basic *halachic* level. The Talmud teaches that אשתו כגופו דמיא, his wife, is considered like his own flesh.[7] The *Zohar* similarly states that a man and woman

---

[2] Aside from the 613 *mitzvot* that Hashem gave the Jews, Hashem issued seven commandments to all mankind. These are called the "*sheva mitzvot bnei Noach,*" the seven laws for the descendants of Noach. Six, or possibly all seven, of these *mitzvot* were originally commanded to Adam; they were re-stated to Noach after the flood, to be passed down to his descendants, the entire population of the world.

Typically rendered as the prohibition against "adultery," this category actually includes far more. Incest, homosexuality, bestiality and other prohibited relationships are all part of this mitzvah. This category also includes the prohibition against castrating any human or animal.

There is another mitzvah that we can easily see was given to Adam before it was restated to Noach. *Bereishit* 2:24 addresses the sanctity of marriage, saying that a man should cling to his wife, and they should be like a single person. It is clear that from the Torah perspective marriage, even for *bnei Noach,* carried particular weight and sanctity.

[3] See *Committed* by Elizabeth Gilbert for a historical survey of marriage throughout the ages. As she writes, "when modern day religious conservatives wax nostalgic about how marriage is a sacred tradition that reaches back into history for thousands of uninterrupted years, they are absolutely correct, but in only one respect — only if they happen to be talking about Judaism." p. 58.

[4] For further discussion about soul mates (including second marriages), see TheRebbe.org, "I Will Write It In Their Hearts," vol. 1, letter dated Thursday, 23 Shvat, 5707. Originally published in *Igrot Kodesh* vol. 2 p. 193.

[5] See *Maamorei Admor Ha'emtzai, Vayikra* vol. 2, pp. 696-698.

[6] *Taamei Hamitzvot, Parshat Bereishit; Likkutei Sichot,* vol. 31, pp. 96-97.

[7] *Talmud Menachot* 93b.

are each *plag gufa*, half of one body [not only one soul].⁸ This is concretized in the *halacha* concerning a woman's recitation of *birkat hamazon*. Although she herself is not circumcised she still includes the words, *v'al britcha shechatamta bivsareinu*, and for the covenant which you have stamped onto our flesh, because it is a reference to the flesh that encases her other half, which is, in the truest sense, also her flesh!

The Rebbe suggests that the female exemption from fulfilling certain *mitzvot* in practice is better understood in light of the Arizal's teaching noted above and the *Zoharic* idea of *basherts*, soulmates, sharing a single soul.⁹

How remarkable that from the beginning, even when housed in two seperate childhood bodies, the female and male halves of the soul already share a bond that allows them to directly impact one another's *avodat* Hashem.¹⁰

When we internalize the delicate and sensitive dynamic of the soul bond, it seems rather logical that we do not approach romantic relationships casually. If, before birth, we are already committed to someone on the most essential level, we must take that bond seriously and live a lifestyle that upholds and safeguards this connection. It is up to us to find that mystery person and to do so in a way that leads, with the best results, to our end goal. As with every other area of life, *halacha* guides our steps in this process.

Being torn away from one's other half forms an innate need and strong desire to reunite.¹¹ With puberty, this magnetic force takes the form of a hormonally induced desire to be together. When a woman kisses, cuddles with, or even thinks about a man in a romantic way, oxytocin floods her system. This hormone is one of a few that constitute the biochemistry of attachment. It becomes hard to think objectively when the brain is drenched in this bonding agent. Recognizing the primal nature of this gravitational pull towards someone does not make it permissible to act upon it, but it does validate the experience and the need for *halachic* boundaries.

Seen from this perspective, there is no benign interaction between a woman and a man. From a spiritual vantage point, since the *chet* marked the beginning of the desire for self-gratification and caused admixtures of good and bad, turbidity and confusion, the powerful drive toward a union with the opposite gender does not always point us toward our soulmate, and even when it does, it may not point at the right time or place

---

8   *Zohar* Vol 3.

9   *Likkutei Sichot*, vol. 31, pp. 93-98.

10 In exploring women's obligations to learn Torah and perform *mitzvot*, the Rebbe delves into the implications of the *basherts'* shared soul bond. Although women are exempt from many *mitzvot*, according to the Rebbe's analysis of a section of the *Mechilta* concerning *Matan Torah*, women did receive and accept all *mitzvot* at *Har Sinai*. As such, they bear a spiritual connection to the whole Torah and all of its commandments.

11 *Maamorei Admor Ha'emtzai, Vayikra* vol. 2, p. 696-698.

for such a reunion. Thus, even a man and woman who speak different languages, have never met nor established any common ground, and are decades apart in terms of age, are prohibited from being in *yichud*, secluded privately together.

The detailed *halachot* that govern intergender relationships reflect a respect for the strength of this attraction and the profound importance of reserving this special connection exclusively within marriage. That said, this area of *halacha* has always been a challenge, and the current cultural climate makes it all the more formidable.

Romantic attraction and entanglement brings a unique thrill and heart-pounding excitement. Even the glance of an eye or a word said with added inflection can be enough to throw us into a happy tizzy. There is also the titillation of curiosity satisfied and forbidden fruit tasted. It feels good to bask in this particular type of attention. And yet, we are much more than bodies hardwired and soft-wired with instinctive and hormonal reactions. In essence, we are a soul, a *nefesh eloki* that has come down into this world with a big job to accomplish and even bigger powers to resist both the pull of our flesh and external pressures.

Halacha aside, physical relationships can get complicated and sometimes, even dangerous. If you sense that your friend or relative has become withdrawn and seems preoccupied and uninterested in the goings on around her, try to see if you can be helpful. Sometimes, a young person might get involved in this kind of relationship, though they know it is prohibited by *halacha*, because she needs validation; she might be seeking assurance that she is desirable and okay. Sometimes it's part of a more general lack of discipline or difficulty with impulse control. Encourage her to speak with a trustworthy adult, and sometimes a therapist, who can offer suggestions for behavior modification that is in line with *halacha*.

If you or your friend/s are challenged with maintaining *halachic* boundaries in this area, know you are not alone. Indeed, even the *beinoni* of the Alter Rebbe's *Sefer HaTanya* shares this struggle. The *beinoni* is the hero of this classic Chabad work who, though he possesses an evil inclination, never actually acts on its predilections.[12] The intensity of the struggle with inappropriate thoughts and desires will vary based on a combination of nature and nurture. As the Alter Rebbe writes in Tanya, Hashem created some with a more overt fiery passion than others. He advises such individuals to shift perspective and ponder a surprising truth: Hashem put some Jews on earth with the mission to overcome struggle! This brings Hashem even more *nachat* than do the pristine actions of the *tzaddik*. Thus, overcoming the struggle draws an even greater

---

12   *Tanya* ch. 12-14.

and holier flow of Divine light into this world than the light generated by one who is naturally pious.[13]

Maintaining proper boundaries also allows both women and men to more easily gravitate toward their soulmate from a less complicated perspective. Unlike the popular Mr. Potato Head, who presents unlimited options for customization, real life is not so simple. No human being is perfect. Unwittingly searching for an unrealistic composite of all the best features you have ever come across can sabotage your best efforts to find your *bashert*. Similarly, having maintained proper boundaries before meeting your *bashert* can help you enjoy a deeper level of exclusivity of focus in that all-important planet known as your own headspace or memory.

YOU MAY BE FACED WITH THIS DILEMMA:

I am having a very hard time with being Shomer Negiah; where does the concept come from and how important is it really?

> Kudos to you for being so self-aware and honest. It's natural and normal to have a difficult time with this. While not every young woman or man will struggle in this area there are at least three factors that make this struggle common enough.
>
> First, let's acknowledge the basic fact of how Hashem created us. At some point in our adolescence, we experience puberty, otherwise known as sexual maturation, which includes both physical and psychological changes all based on a shift in hormonal levels. The adolescent brain triggers the release of adrenal stress hormones, sex hormones, and growth hormones. That alone can make this a challenging, awkward, and confusing time.
>
> Growing research indicates that the brain continues to mature long after puberty into the twenties. Specifically, the prefrontal cortex, where our executive functions, such as planning, and impulse control reside, is among the last areas of the brain to mature. Practically, this translates into it being much more difficult for a teen to hold back from engaging in a new experience that they recognize as dangerous but simultaneously thrilling, such as unsafe driving, experimenting with alcohol or drugs, and sexual experiences.
>
> While there is more emphasis today on age-appropriate sexual development education, not everyone has that advantage. Lacking the benefit of a proper

---

[13] *Tanya* ch. 27.

introduction to this new aspect of life can exacerbate the confusion and lead to unhealthy behaviors that may seem exciting and feel like lots of fun but most often do not lead to happiness or contentment.

All of this inner turmoil is heightened by current societal norms reflected on social media and in every other medium. It is hard, in the throes of maturation, to understand how unrealistic and unhealthy much of this depiction of romantic and married life truly is. Many people get hurt in the process of learning this important lesson.

As we lurch in the direction of straddling the universe and the metaverse, reality becomes harder to identify and hold on to. In a postmodern world where there are no absolute truths and everything is available at the click of a button, upholding *shomer negiah* requires a practice of delayed gratification. It requires diligence.

This practice can be difficult, especially as it requires us to keep our eye on a goal that often seems distant: marriage and holy intimacy.

Fortunately, the Torah provides a clear framework for navigating these desires, through physical and physiological lenses. The Torah recognizes that yes, there is an innate desire and urge to connect with the opposite sex beginning from puberty. This urge is both hormonal, and also is a manifestation of our yearning for reunion with our other half, and thus a reflection of a higher truth.

While recognizing both the physical and spiritual drive for these desires, the Torah asks us to practice discipline that leads to deeper intimacy. To do that, it asks us to channel that desire for sexual connection and expression within a sanctified union.

The Torah lays out healthy markers of development on the path to holy intimacy. First concentrate on growing as a person and developing your inner world: your thoughts and ideas, your passions, your ideals and convictions. Only then is it appropriate to concentrate on joining your inner world with that of someone else. True intimacy is about first connecting with ourselves, and then being able to share that true version of ourselves with someone else. If an individual gets physically intimate with someone before they know themselves, it can stunt or slow one's ability to achieve a greater, more whole intimacy.

As to how important the concept of *shomer negiah* is, and where it comes from: it is hard to overstate just how integral these *halachot* can be in the development of a healthy, wholesome self and the journey towards finding your other half, and just how clearly they are sourced in Torah law. The concept is rooted in three *mitzvot* in the Torah:

לא תקרבו לגלות ערוה

Do not come close [in ways that may lead] to revealing nakedness[14]

We are forbidden[15] from hugging, kissing or engaging in any sensual skin contact with someone of the opposite gender,[16] other than a parent, grandparent, or child/grandchild.[17] Most *poskim* agree that this is a biblical prohibition, an *issur d'orayta*.[18] Because of the gravity of this *issur*, we are careful to avoid any physical contact or touch at all. The detailed laws of *yichud*[19] as well as other interactions to be avoided,[20] provide additional Torah boundaries.[21]

In fact, in the Alter Rebbe's description of a woman's obligation in Torah study, he states that she must be conversant with all of the *halachot* that impact her life, such as *nidah*, *tevilah*, *melicha*, and *yichud*.[22]

Physical contact or touch by physicians, dentists, physical therapists and other practitioners do not present a *halachic* problem.[23] Rabbinic opinions differ regarding the permissibility of a woman using the services of a male beautician, manicurist, hair stylist and make up artist. It is certainly something women aiming for an added measure of spiritual scrupulousness should avoid. In the case of a woman who avails herself of such services, extra attentiveness to the laws of *yichud* and *tzniut* is warranted.

---

14   *Vayikra* 18:6.

15   In this context, *halacha* defines a woman as a girl of 12 or a girl who has started menstruation – whichever comes first. According to some *poskim*, this prohibition applies even as young as age three. Consult with your Rav with any questions. *Halacha* defines a man as a boy of nine and older. Physical touch between siblings is dependent on the situation and type, and should be discussed with one's Rav.

16   *Shulchan Aruch, Even Ha'ezer* 20:1.

17   *Shulchan Aruch, Even Ha'ezer* 21:7; *Beit Shmuel* ad loc.

18   *Beit Shmuel, Even Ha'ezer* 20:1.

19   *Shulchan Aruch, Even Ha'ezer* 22.

20   *Shulchan Aruch, Even Ha'ezer* 21.

21   The Rebbe emphasized conscientiously observing the laws of *yichud* as they impact the home, the workplace, and travel arrangements. The Rebbe recommended that women make use of female drivers when there may be concern with *hilchot yichud*. *Sefer HaSichot* 5751, vol. 1, p. 87, fn. 116.

22   *Hilchot Talmud Torah* 1:14.

23   *Shach, Yoreh Dei'ah* 195:20; *Likkutei Sichot*, vol. 16, p. 589.

לא תתורו אחרי לבבכם ואחרי עיניכם

Do not follow your heart and eyes[24]

This is the prohibition against entertaining focused romantic thoughts of a member of the opposite gender who is not your spouse. The consensus of the *poskim* is that this prohibition, known as *hirhur*, applies to men thinking about women but not the other way around. *Hirhur* is prohibited whether or not it leads to *hotzaat zera levatalah*.

Although this *issur* does not apply to women, the Mitteler Rebbe, the second Chabad Rebbe and the son of the Alter Rebbe, wrote, that women should not make light of this concept.[25, 26] For this reason (and others), chassidim and other groups have always been careful to minimize any relationship with the opposite gender. While these practices could come across as foreign or extreme, if one is honest about the challenges– *halachic* or otherwise– inherent in intergender relationships such precautions may appear less excessive. Emotional entanglement can easily lead to touch, which is prohibited by *halacha*. We want to engage in behavior that honors and helps preserve the unique and exclusive soul bond that binds only the two half souls—a bond that, as noted, exists well before marriage.

לפני עור לא תתן מכשול

Do not place a stumbling block before the blind[27]

The Jewish people are referred to as *komah achat sheleimah,* one single body or organism.[28] In the Torah, there is no concept that each man is an island unto himself, but rather an acute understanding of how profoundly we affect and are affected by each other. Torah makes each Jew responsible for the physical and spiritual welfare of her or his fellow, and prohibits an individual from placing a stumbling block in front of another person. Practically, this means that we are *halachically* mandated to be attentive to how something we do, might adversely affect another.

---

[24] *Bamidbar* 15:39.

[25] *Pokei'ach Ivrim*, ch. 9.

[26] He writes that engaging in these types of thoughts can impact their future children. If you struggle with these thoughts, reach out to a *mashpia* or therapist who can help you navigate.

[27] *Vayikra* 19:14.

[28] *Likutei Torah* 44a.

As such, it is no surprise that the *Shulchan Aruch* discusses the laws of intergender behaviors at great length. Irrespective of age or circumstance, the *halachot* remain relevant to all women and men.[29]

When asked by a young woman, why the laws of gender separation in the Torah are so strict, the Rebbe replied: "The potential power of male-female bonding is like atomic energy. When used in a positive and holy way, there is nothing more powerful and valuable in the world. But when used recklessly and not in a sacred context, it can be the most destructive force in existence. Hence the Torah law."[30]

Halacha aside, maintaining healthy boundaries, being able to say no when necessary, is a crucial life skill and a manifestation of a healthy sense of self. While we have the advantage of Torah giving us unequivocal guidelines, we must also build our own inner resolve and feel empowered from deep within to make healthy, holy choices.

This is not a case of having no recourse but to bow and conform to communal expectations or even Hashem's command. This is Hashem cheering you on and saying, "I know this is hard, I recognize this is challenging, and I also know you got this. I believe in you."

Boundaries are important for healthy relationships, with ourselves, our family, and beyond. A boundary is a personal line that you do not move. A boundary can also be understood as your relationship with yourself. When trying to please someone else by crossing your boundaries, you are actually betraying your relationship with yourself.

In light of the above, it is worth defining your personal boundaries. It is an act of radical self-knowledge and love to do this often difficult activity. Boundaries may also be different for different people. That is normal. What is important is knowing yourself and what you're comfortable with, so that you can build self-awareness, and connect with Torah.

Discipline and self-control are inherent to a Torah lifestyle. In an ever-shifting world where boundaries are constantly changing, *halacha* gives us eternal guidance and guidelines.

Finally, remember that in this struggle like with any other, it should never be all or nothing. Every overture in the right direction is immensely important. Every

---

29 *Shulchan Aruch, Even Ha'ezer* 21.

30 Yehudis Fishman, the young woman in question, relayed this in an interview with Jewish Education Media (JEM) in February 2016.

time you find the strength to say no, to turn down an inappropriate suggestion, you are growing in important ways that have personal and even, cosmic effects.

The Power of Touch

Our sense of touch is designed to gather information about our surroundings as well as to connect and bond us with each other. Studies show that touch signals safety, compassion, and trust. It soothes. This powerful effect on the human being is obvious from the moment of birth, which is why doctors speak to new mothers about the skin to skin benefits to their child. In adults, basic warm touch calms cardiovascular stress. In a study participants laying in an fMRI brain scanner, anticipating an electric shock, showed heightened brain activity in regions associated with threat and stress.[31] Participants whose husbands held their hands while they waited showed a marked reduction in the neural response. In fact, the effect of hand-holding was shown to correlate with the marital quality the couple shared.

Touch activates the body's vagus nerve, which is intimately involved with the emotion of compassion, and can trigger the release of oxytocin, a.k.a the love hormone. The feeling of deep connection is compounded with loving touch. This feeling of connection is not based on a logical choice and is often overpowering.

Chassidut explains that the first six of the seven emotional *sefirot*[32] are correlated with male energy while the seventh is female.[33] The number six depicts the outer layers while the number seven represents the inner core that holds it all together.

The Maharal attributes the symbolism of six and seven to the structure of space: physicality has six sides: top and bottom, right and left, front and back.[34] The seventh dimension is the center, a transcendent dimension that both keeps the external six components united as one and fundamentally reveals the nature of the other six dimensions. The cube, as a geometric shape, readily displays these attributes. Six represents the outer surface and the number seven represents the inner core.

Relationships are about connecting on both the outer layer and at the core; both physically and emotionally. The question is how will this experience begin? Many men

---

[31] Coan JA, Schaefer HS, Davidson RJ. Lending a hand: social regulation of the neural response to threat. Psychol Sci. Dec 2006.

[32] The statement that humanity is created in the image of Hashem is often referenced. According to chassidic thought and Jewish mysticism, this statement teaches us that, just as Hashem projects His pure light through ten Divine *sefirot* in order to interact with and conduct the finite world, so too each individual expresses his or her soul and interacts with the world via ten soul powers. These ten soul powers bear the same names as the ten Divine *sefirot*. Both the ten *sefirot* and ten soul powers include three intellectual faculties and seven emotional attributes.

[33] *Sefer Halikutim*, Tzemach Tzedek, Erech Z"A U'Malchut p 221:6-7.

[34] *Gevurot Hashem*, ch. 46.

tend to engage from the outside in, beginning with the more external, physical aspects; whereas, women tend to engage from the inside out, beginning with a more emotional bond before connecting physically.

A man might test a relationship by initiating touch. In the hook-up model, the woman almost always takes the advances more seriously.[35] Physiologically, the combination of dopamine and oxytocin released in her bloodstream causes a woman to feel attachment and to invest her emotions in the relationship more heavily than her male counterpart might.[36] Oxytocin is the only hormone to have earned such a variety of monikers which include the cuddle hormone, the social hormone, the happy hormone, and the love hormone. Both men and women produce oxytocin. That said, the production of estrogen, the specifically feminine sex hormone, markedly increases the bonding and trusting effects of oxytocin.[37] In these all too frequent scenarios, when the man ends what he understood to be mere flirtation or casual exchange, the woman can be left emotionally distraught, even shattered. Today, sociologists study these incongruous gender dynamics, especially as they unfold on college campuses, where fraternity culture and proverbial players have been associated with actively exploiting young women's emotional sensibilities.[38]

Never forget how much power you have. The first six *sefirot* are correlated with the male energy of initiation and conquest. The seventh, *malchut*, kingship, is aligned with the female energy of *mekabel,* the receiver. It would seem that being the *mashpia,* initiator, puts the power over the relationship squarely in the man's court. But in order for there to be a relationship, there must be both an initiator and a receiver who welcomes the advances of the initiator. If a woman does not welcome a man's overtures, the relationship is effectively over.

If and when a man ignores her cues and oversteps the boundaries, a woman must firmly and clearly state her wishes for him to stop. If he continues, she should turn to a trusted friend or mentor for advice on how to take further action. It goes without saying that should she feel herself to be in a dangerous situation, she should seek help immediately, and call the police.

---

[35] Norval Glenn and Elizabeth Marquardt. Hooking Up, Hanging Out, and Hoping for Mr. Right: College Women on Dating and Mating Today. New York: Institute for American Values. 2001.

[36] Gao S, Becker B, Luo L, Geng Y, Zhao W, Yin Y, Hu J, Gao Z, Gong Q, Hurlemann R, Yao D, Kendrick KM. Oxytocin, the peptide that bonds the sexes also divides them. Proc Natl Acad Sci U S A. 2016

[37] McCarthy MM. Estrogen modulation of oxytocin and its relation to behavior. Adv Exp Med Biol. 1995.

[38] Ram, Alisha K. Masculinity in Fraternities: Impact on Campus Sexual Violence. *PSU McNair Scholars Online Journal*: Vol. 13: Iss. 1, Article 4. 2019.

When dating, it is imperative that we are properly discerning and level-headed. When two people choose to spend the rest of their lives building a home together, they must share the same goals and values. The choice of a marriage partner must be rooted in logic, and enhanced by other factors like chemistry. The introduction of physical contact at this point is *halachically* prohibited and would certainly add complexity to making this important decision from a completely grounded perspective. When touch is introduced, the subconscious desire to connect more strongly is powerful and can easily overrule logic.

Strictly following the *halachot* forbidding physical contact prior to marriage is advantageous in making the most important decision you will make in your lifetime. Practicing self-control at this point and respecting physical, emotional, and *halachic* boundaries lays the foundation for a strong and fruitful relationship. Beyond that, it is the key to success in fulfilling your part in the great enterprise of building and maintaining *kedushat am yisroel*.

Beer Goggles

Halacha prohibits men and women from engaging in lightheaded behavior with someone of the opposite gender.[39] This most certainly includes drinking alcoholic beverages and doing drugs. The Gemara speaks of the disinhibiting effects of alcohol, and more specifically of how it can cause a woman to take risks and acquiesce to prohibited behaviors, often sexual in nature.[40] Contemporary research parallels these ancient ideas in an uncanny fashion. Science has confirmed that attraction is heightened by the consumption of alcohol. A woman will look prettier to a man after he has had a few to drink; she will similarly be more inclined to find a guy interesting after she has had a few shots. This is because drinking affects the *nucleus accumbens,* the area of the brain used to determine facial attractiveness.[41]

Studies suggests that alcohol consumption can increase the likeliness of unwanted sexual contact and assault. Alcohol 'myopia' affects psychological, cognitive, and motor abilities. Without the normal level of alarm that would arise from recognizing risk, a woman does not experience the anxiety or fear that would motivate her to leave a potentially dangerous situation. Because of intoxication, she might experience a variety

---

[39] *Shulchan Aruch, Even Ha'ezer* 21:1.

[40] *Ketubot* 65a. The Gemara discusses the prohibition of a woman becoming intoxicated outside the home and without the advantage of her husband being present.

[41] Monk RL. Qureshi A. Lee S. Darcy N. Gemma D. Heim D. Can beauty be-er ignored? A preregistered implicit examination of the beer goggles effect. *Journal of Psychology of Addictive Bahviors. American Psychological Association.* February 2020.

of psychological barriers that impede assertive resistance. (Even when not drinking in the presence of the opposite gender and even when intoxication is not at a dangerous level, one must take caution with any loss of sobriety.) As adults, we consciously and continuously make choices about letting people in; about with whom, and when, we will allow ourselves vulnerability.

The Gemara teaches נכנס יין יצא סוד, when the wine goes in, secrets comes out.[42] Inebriation causes lack of inhibition, which often causes the lowering of normal guards and disregard for filters in its wake. On a very basic level, drinking impairs our sense of judgment. We may end up sharing or expressing ourselves in a way that is neither dignified nor desirable, or worse.

More profoundly, intoxication allows our core selves to be fully exposed. This can allow for great wisdom, and it can also be extremely harmful. There are stories of great *tzaddikim* who, upon drinking alcohol, revealed great *sodot hatorah,* secrets of the Torah. For them, this was truly a holy experience.

When choosing to drink, a person must honestly examine both their motivation and the most probable outcome.

Once an individual can understand the why, they can work towards making healthy choices, either alone, with their spouse, or with a trusted friend, *mashpia*, or licensed professional.

YOU MAY BE FACED WITH THIS DILEMMA:

I am engaged to be married and my chatan wants us to touch "a bit." This makes me uncomfortable but I don't want to cause problems in our relationship. What should I do?

> First, let's take a moment to recognize that physical attraction is important in a relationship and the desire to touch or go beyond that is entirely normal. Yet, the Torah mandates that we wait.
>
> *Kallot* and *chatanim* have to be especially attentive to these *halachot*. Being emotionally entangled to the point of engagement can make it considerably more difficult to abide by the laws surrounding *negiah* and *hilchot yichud* which are more stringent for an engaged couple precisely because of the natural pull

---

[42] *Sanhedrin* 38a.

between them.[43] For this, and other reasons, the Rebbe counseled that engaged couples limit the time they spend together.[44]

In many cases, the Rebbe directed *chatanim* who lived in close proximity to their *kallot* to leave town and take up residence in another location where they could find a proper framework to support their studies.[45] The Rebbe clearly understood the extent of the *nisayon*, the test, that engagement presents in this regard and wanted to remove the stumbling block with which engaged couples are so often confronted.

We can see this in the Rebbe's written response below:[46]

> **I received a query… concerning your daughter who has become engaged and is now distancing herself [from her chatan], saying that her feelings [about him] have yet to crystallize…**
>
> **I surmise that the reason your daughter's feelings have changed is that they conducted themselves in a manner that is impermissible for Jews to conduct themselves prior to a wedding. This has brought about the opposite result: she is now distancing herself from him.**

In a healthy relationship, the couple respects each other's boundaries and communicates clearly. In unhealthy relationships, one person is often the boundary violator while the other has a difficult time setting and maintaining healthy boundaries. The violator or bully consistently oversteps or ignores the boundaries set by their partner, justifying their actions by asserting that the other person wasn't clear or secure in their boundary and, in any case, seems to be enjoying the overture. The people pleaser has a difficult time saying no and doesn't want to hurt anyone's feelings, so they might tolerate behavior that clearly violates their boundaries. Ask yourself, am I clued into what I really feel about this, and I am communicating what I believe and feel clearly enough to my *chatan*? Many people are non-adversarial and hate confrontation, especially

---

43. It is important for a *kallah* and *chatan* to review these *halachot*. Hilchot Yichud in English is available through the Sichot in English (SIE) publishing house.

44. *Shaarei Halacha U'minhag, Even Ha'ezer*. For more on the engagement period and Chabad customs, see Part IV, essay 10 entitled "*Yakar Mikol Yakar*: The Most Precious Time of Our Lives" by Esther Piekarski.

45. *Torat Menachem*, vol. 39, p. 11, fn. 24; *Me'Otzar Hamelech*, vol. 2, p. 167; *Mikdash Melech*, vol. 1, p. 48.

46. *Igrot Kodesh*, vol. 9, pp. 209-210.

within the context of this most important but still budding relationship, but this conversation is too important to skip.

Even when the couple is mutually comfortable overstepping *halachic* boundaries, this behavior can introduce confusion and insecurity into the relationship.

Additionally, just touching can easily escalate to further and more serious trespass of *halacha* and sometimes lead to deep regrets. Somewhat counterintuitively, some couples who engage in physical touch before marriage and/or are not careful with the *dinei harchakah* within marriage, experience complications in growing their emotional and even physical intimacy.[47]

If your *chatan* cannot respect your feelings on this matter, this could signal overarching issues, and should be discussed with someone you trust and can advise you.

We need to remember that saying NO in response to inappropriate overtures means saying YES to building a *binyan adei ad al yesodei hatorah v'ha mitzvah*, an everlasting edifice predicated on Torah and *mitzvot*. This will necessitate discipline and might make our choices unpopular. Nothing, however, is more important.

> **Sara**: When I was about 18 years old, I visited *Eretz Yisrael*. There I met up with my chassidishe cousins in Bnei Brak. We traveled together by bus to the cemetery in Teveria for the yahrzeit of our holy great grandfather, the Kopitchinitzer Rebbe zt"l. One of my cousins was a *kallah* at the time, and their *minhag* is that from the time that the engagement is announced, until the *chuppah*, the *chatan* and *kallah* do not meet. I was sitting right next to her when one of her friends, while looking out of the window and gesturing to the street below, remarked enthusiastically, "Look! There is your *chatan*!" You would think my cousin would have run to the window to gawk and giggle. Instead, she sat in her seat, her face slowly acquiring the most beautiful blush I have ever seen. All these years later, I still marvel at the untainted purity of her reaction. Can you imagine a young lady in the twentieth century having the sensitivity to naturally blush just at the thought of her *chatan's* proximity?!

In His infinite kindness, Hashem gave us a gift; guidelines for preserving our innate sensitivity to the male/female dynamic and chemistry. Yes, it is healthy to blush just at the thought of your *chatan*.

---

[47] See chapter seven, "*Dinei Harchakah*: Pulling Apart; Staying Together" for a full discussion about *harchakot*.

The Power of Sight

A relationship or touch that contravenes *halacha* never happens in a vacuum. What might bring us to this place? Which experiences are part of the trajectory? Our actions are guided by our conscious thought process, our subconscious, and our conscience.[48]

As individuals trying to live spiritually resonant lives, we want to make sure our conscience remains healthy, strong, and sensitive to *kedushah*. Young children learn by mirroring the behaviors of those around them. No matter how old we get, our mirror neurons, the part of the brain which observes and imitates those around us, continues to significantly impact our choices.

Chassidut teaches that humans gather information via two mechanisms.[49]

The first system works through the agency of our ten *kochot hanefesh*, the ten aspects of our psyche. The human psyche is made up of cognitive abilities, *chochmah, binah* and *daat* and our seven emotive expressions, *chessed, gevurah, tiferet* etc. In terms of absorbing information, one can study a topic intellectually and shift values based on new knowledge gained in the process. Alternatively, one can recalibrate their priorities when emotions, such as love or awe, are stirred. If, for example, you want your children to brush their teeth diligently, you can teach them about tooth decay and hope that logic will compel them to brush regularly. Or you can try the emotive route and extoll the beauty of white teeth, a winning smile, and a pleasant appearance. You can also scare them with the image of an unpleasant visit to the dentist to fill the inevitable cavities.

The second mechanism draws upon our internal ecosystem; namely, that which enters our subconsciousness via our senses.

The expression 'seeing is believing' is conventionally used to underscore that seeing something convinces us of its existence and truth, even if and when that truth is unlikely. But there is more to it. When you see something, that vision becomes your reality in a concrete way, rather than an abstract one. What you see becomes a part of you, and can, for instance, give you immense pleasure, far surpassing the pleasure from intellectual or emotional stimulation.[50]

---

48 Often, people confuse or conflate the concepts of *neshamah* and conscience. A *neshamah* is a *chelek eloka mimaal mamosh*; it is an actual part of Hashem. Nothing can ever compromise or change your pristine core. Your conscience, on the other hand, represents a composite of all the factors that have "capacity to teach." Our conscience will guide our actions throughout our life. In this context it is impossible to overstate the far reaching effects of the media. We are more profoundly impacted by popular and social media than we might ever imagine.

49 See *Kuntres Ha'Avodah*, ch. 2. *Sefer Hamaamorim* 5696, p. 17. *Sefer Hamaamorim* 5699, pp. 97-98. *Torat Menachem*, vol. 27, p. 138.

50 That is why in *halacha* a witness cannot be a judge, as stated in the *Shulchan Aruch, Choshen Mishpat* 7:8. Seeing something causes you to lose all "remove" and objectivity.

The Gemara teaches that the Jewish nation possesses three signs: They are *rachmanim*, merciful; *bayshanim*, bashful, possessed of an innate sense of privacy; and *gomlei chassadim*, perform acts of kindness."[51] *Bayshanut* describes our natural instinct to preserve our privacy and dignity; a healthy sense of restraint and reserve.[52] *Bayshanut* is the quality that makes us discerning and premeditated about how we make ourselves vulnerable; what we will share of ourselves, with whom, and when.

Marriage includes the gift of sharing our most intimate body parts with our one and only husband. When we lose our inner compass and begin to calibrate our intimate choices with external images that have seeped into our minds, everything gets more confusing and complicated. When we are aware of and aligned with our inner core, and preserve that healthy sense of privacy, we can fully trust our instinct as to how much, and in what manner, we feel comfortable sharing.

Consistent exposure to less than modest imagery compromises that innate quality, often without our realizing it.

Consider sunlight. When one looks straight up at the sun, one naturally squints. We instinctively seek to protect ourselves against the powerful rays that can damage our delicate optic nerves. Looking directly at the sun without reflexively squinting, however, does not mean that person's eyes are stronger, rather it indicates optic nerve damage, and thus the unnatural ability to stare right into the glare of sunlight.

Similarly, one sensitive to the concepts of personal and private space naturally feels uncomfortable when exposed to *ervah*, parts of the body that *halacha* says should be covered. With repeated exposure to such imagery, one's sensitivity to private, potent, and intimate visuals is dulled. Outside of marriage, dulled or non-existent sensitivity can lead to regrettable actions that impact an individual's present and future. Within the context of marriage, such overexposure can lead to crude comparisons, objectification of one's soulmate, and loss of mutual respect. Not to mention it can lead to an obvious failure to appreciate and actualize the unparalleled spiritual and emotional connection available to us when intimacy is safeguarded.

There is also the unrealistic expectation of women's (or men's) bodies that can be an unfortunate byproduct of consuming these sorts of images. Studies show that, for far too many, the photoshopped images used in advertisements have resulted in an unhealthy sense of body image and a host of attendant pathologies.[53] There is

---

51 *Yevamot* 79a.

52 *Bereishit* 3:25 *Rashi*; *Nedarim* 20a.

53 Abbadessa, Gina. Airbrushed: Photoshop's harmful effect on girls and the need for legislative controls on advertising. *New England Law Review.*

mounting evidence of the correlation between social media and depression and other mental health issues, especially in young women.[54] The carefully curated pictures everyone is posting to showcase their perfect life yield profoundly negative effects including jealousy, despondency, and low self-esteem. In a number of states, bills have been introduced to incentivize businesses, to use realistic images rather than those digitally altered.

It's more than just our figures that are implicitly being degraded. The alleged perfect life depicted pervasively on TV, in movies, and on social media, prompts fantasies that preclude true happiness. These fantasies often involve a perfect partner or perfect relationship, with no mention of the hard inner work that goes into achieving this goal. This is not reality.

Real life is not an endless string of vacations featuring hand holding and watching the sunset. Long-term relationships rely on the commitment to work together through the drudgery of everyday life and routine. Day after day, week after week, and year after year. When we do not recognize that we might be holding these fantasies as an ideal, it can trigger massive disappointment. The following autobiographical vignette speaks to this point:

> One night in 1953, the then young Chana Zuber (Sharfstein) met with the Rebbe. Initially, the Rebbe asked many questions regarding her college studies. Listening attentively, the Rebbe then asked Chana if she had begun dating. Chana replied that indeed she had met several young men, but none piqued her interest.
>
> "Is there someone you are interested in?" asked the Rebbe. Chana replied that a student who was a popular Hassidic singer had impressed her and that she felt some romantic kindlings toward him.
>
> The Rebbe chuckled lightly, and said, "He is not the right one for you. True love is not that which is portrayed in romantic books. It isn't an overwhelming, blinding emotion. Novels do not portray real life, but rather focus on fantasy, invented worlds, and contrived emotions. Fiction is just that—fiction—but real life is different."
>
> Chana believed the man she would choose to marry would offer her a blissful, exciting, and harmonious life. The Rebbe continued, "Love is an emotion that increases in strength throughout life. It is sharing, caring, and respecting one another. The love that you feel as a young bride is only the beginning of real love. It is building a life together, a family unit and a home. It is through the small daily acts of living together that love flourishes and grows. Therefore, the love you feel after five

---

54 Haidt, Jonathan. The Dangerous Experiment on Teen Girls. *The Atlantic*. 2021.

> or ten years of marriage is a gradual strengthening of the shared bond. When two people unite, with time they ultimately feel completely bonded with the other, so that each partner can no longer visualize life without his or her mate." [55]

Why create confusion of values and expectations only to be disheartened when life doesn't imitate art? The Torah-based values of building a *binyan adei ad*, an everlasting edifice, based on love, commitment and hard work is one that brings authentic wholeness and satisfaction. Nowhere on Netflix can one see the deep happiness that comes with a growing family, the joy and meaning that emanate from *zaide* and *bubbe*, and the exhilaration amidst barely controlled chaos as generations of offspring celebrate together supporting each other through thick and thin.

YOU MIGHT BE WONDERING:

After a day at work, I like to relax on Instagram. Is there a problem with that?

> While there are those who seek to shun social media, even deeming it *assur*, the Rebbe taught that everything Hashem created was created for the purpose of serving Him. This includes aspects of life that can be misused, often with terrible results. From this perspective, social media is not so much a question of right or wrong but an instance of "buyer beware."
>
> Amazing things happen each day on social media: Torah teachings are made easily accessible, consciousness around important issues is raised, and *tzedakah* is collected. It has developed into a communal and powerful space for observant Jewish women around the world to congregate and connect. Additionally, the *parnassah* of many depends on this very platform.
>
> At the same time, it is impossible to overstate the potentially corrosive power of this medium. It behooves us all to critically examine how much time we spend grazing from this smorgasbord designed to keep us coming back. Frequently.
>
> While we might be tempted to describe Insta-culture as simply another form of entertainment and chuckle at its alleged impact, it is no laughing matter. As of 2022, the average social media user worldwide spends 147 minutes per day on

---

[55] Advice for Life: Marriage, a compilation of the Rebbe's guidance on love, dating, the Jewish wedding, marriage and marital harmony, published by Lubavitch Archives.

this pursuit.[56] If you add that up, it's a bit less than two whole days per month! But it's not just the sheer amount of time it takes up; it's the tentacled grip this medium has on us. It has a way of making us blind to the people around us, even to those closest to us, like our spouse and children. It can wreak havoc with our intimacy, and get in the way of our sleep. And that is all before we get into the matter of content.

While the term influencer officially entered the English dictionary only in 2019, the profound influence of association between a prominent person and a product they use was recognized as early as ancient Rome. The history of modern influencer marketing begins with potter Josiah Wedgewood, who in 1760 made a tea set for Queen Charlotte. He billed himself as potter to her Majesty and promoted his pottery as Queensware. Ever since then, the Wedgewood brand is associated with royal luxury.

For a few centuries, only celebrities and other high-profile persons—top level athletes, models, actors, singers and TV stars—were considered influencers. With the advent of social media, however, anyone can become an influencer and share their ideas.

In fact, because most influencers today are regular people without private jets and huge mansions, they earn an even higher level of trust. With their relatable posts about the good, the bad, and the ugly in their lives, their authority has only skyrocketed.

With influencers given the power to sell directly through Instagram, the influencer market, to date, is worth upward of ten billion dollars and climbs every day. But the power of social media as the top conveyor of information dwarfs even its economic sway.

The ubiquitous posts and Instagram stories that nourish voracious appetites for material goods and promise to deliver happiness to your doorstep—including many by *frum* influencers— essentially fly in the face of our cherished values and life goals. As the Frierdiker Rebbe succinctly wrote,[57] "Jewish wealth is not about houses and money. Jewish wealth, which is eternal, is the observance of Torah and *mitzvot*, and bringing children and grandchildren into the world who will observe Torah and *mitzvot*."

---

56   Dixon. S. Daily social media usage worldwide 2012-2022. *Statista*. July 2022.

57   *Hayom Yom*. entry for 9 Nissan.

While many influencers inspire and inform, just as many offer up opinions and information decidedly hostile to Torah ideals. Even innocuous cooking demos that depict unrealistically tranquil domestic scenes, which is a far cry from many of our busy kitchens, muddle our definition of normalcy.

Some of this is, of course, about maturity and discretion; realizing that what we see around us will not always be mirrored in our own reality. And that what someone shares does not have to be embraced as our truth. But even those of strong principles, who have lived many decades, are not impervious to marketing tactics.

That is why being smart and selective in terms of our exposure to social media is important to our emotional health and to building and maintaining a strong marriage. Beyond that, transcending the pitfalls of social media is integral to fulfilling our important mission, as described in the Rebbe's holy words with which he blessed every *chatan* and *kallah*: the building of a *"binyan adei ad al yesodei hatorah v'ha mitzvah kefi sheheim muarim b'maor sh'btorah zuhi torat hachassidut"*, an everlasting edifice on the foundations of Torah and *mitzvot* as they are illuminated by the teachings of chassidut.

The Rebbe stressed the importance of surrounding even young babies with positive and holy imagery and said this was, among other things, in preparation for Mashiach's arrival.[58] At that time, we will live in a utopian reality, and all impurity and negativity will be removed, ואת רוח הטומאה אעביר מן הארץ, I will remove the spirit of impurity from the world.[59] At long last our most potent of all senses, our sight, will be focused with no chance for distraction: ונגלה כבוד ה' וראו כל בשר יחדו כי פי ה' דבר, the glory of Hashem will be revealed, and all flesh together will see that the mouth of Hashem has spoken.[60]

Until that day comes, we must choose what we allow ourselves to see wisely.

---

58 *Likkutei Sichot,* vol. 25, pp. 309-311.

59 *Zechariah* 13:2.

60 *Yeshayahu* 40:5.

chapter five

An Open Letter to the Kallah
(OR ASPIRING *KALLAH*)

Dearest friend sht',

As a *kallah* teacher for over two decades, I write to you from my heart. Oh, how every young woman dreams of her beautiful Jewish home where *shalom bayit* reigns supreme, of being a true *eishet chayil*, woman of valor, an *akeret habayit* that transforms a mere house into a warm, loving, nurturing home. Alas, at the same time, we hear whispers of challenges, difficult transitions, and unexpected hardships that make this journey scary. Besides a heavy dose of *bitachon*, faith, and a strong support system including your personal *mashpia*, I want to share some tips that can help you prepare and transition into married life feeling more reassured and confident.

My first observation is quite simple and logical. If we invest in ourselves properly before marriage, ensuring that we are as healthy as we can be physically, emotionally, and spiritually, we can then use our energy to properly nurture our *shalom bayit* during the *shanah rishonah* period while of course, maintaining our overall health. Everyone has issues; when we come into marriage unaware of our particular tendencies or without the proper tools necessary for change, and without a mind to work on them, it can place unnecessary strain on the fledgling relationship.

Conversely, if we have laid a strong foundation of *shalom bayit* at the beginning of the marriage, once life gets busier with children *b'ezrat Hashem*, and other factors, we can use our more limited time and energy to maintain a balanced home.

No human being is perfect; we are all works in progress. Each of us struggles in at least one area of spiritual, emotional, or physical health. Hashem gave some of us less complex challenges while He gave others challenges in multiple areas. Some of our challenges can be resolved, but others may stay with us until *Mashiach* comes and need to be properly managed. Our goal is to have the necessary tools and support to live a productive, fulfilling life despite these speedbumps.

The first step would be to engage in honest self-assessment. You might want to ask yourself some or all of the following questions. Once you have done so, you can reach out to your *mashpia* to help you strategize and decide where and how to improve, with the goal to make the transition into married life smoother. Once you settle into your married life, you and your husband can jointly use these questions to assess yourselves within the framework of your marriage and decide on how to upgrade specific skills to benefit yourselves as one team.

Physically[1]

How do I feel about my body? Am I content with my body image?

Am I eating, sleeping, and exercising in conformity with my specific body size, weight, and shape (check with your MD)?

Do I practice a healthy routine of hygiene and self-grooming? Do I take care of my physical appearance?

Do I have frequent colds, yeast infections, and other ailments that should be taken care of?

Do I suffer from urinary problems or digestive disorders that I ignore?

Are my periods healthy and regular? Do I bleed or stain between periods, or have periods only rarely? (A healthy period should come every 25-35 days on average, with no bleeding in between, and without extreme pain that is incapacitating.)

Do I have intense hormonal swings? Do I know how to handle them?

How are my basic functioning skills, such as cooking, budgeting, housekeeping, time management, laundry, and organization skills?

Emotionally[2]

Do I, generally speaking, maintain healthy relationships with family members, friends, and co-workers?

Can I communicate my needs clearly and respectfully? Do I do so?

---

[1] See Part IV, essay 1, "Appreciating Our Bodies: Inside and Out" by Rivky Boyarsky.

[2] For a more in depth study of these concepts see A Spiritual Guide to Counting the Omer by Rabbi Simon Jacobson book.

Can I listen attentively to others with whom I have a relationship (even when I disagree)?

Can I make myself vulnerable and trust someone I am close to?

Do I know how to be truly kind and giving, or do I suffer from a sense of entitlement that needs to be addressed? (This connects to the Kabbalistic *sefira* of *chessed*)

Do I have healthy boundaries? Do I overshare? Do I protect my boundaries too tightly? (This connects to the Kabbalistic *sefira* of *gevurah*)

Can I judge favorably? Can I be compassionate? (This connects to the Kabbalistic *sefira* of *tiferet*)

Do I have healthy coping skills? Can I endure discomfort? Do I have a stress management plan? Can I be assertive when necessary to protect my values? Can I wait for delayed gratification, or do I have a need for instant positive results? Am I too rigid or inflexible? (This connects to the Kabbalistic *sefira* of *netzach*)

Do I know how to yield? Do I know how to let go and forgive (including myself)? Can I make room for others? Can I be flexible or am I too impulsive? Am I a doormat? (This connects to the Kabbalistic *sefira* of *hod*)

Can I keep a commitment even when totally inconvenient? Can I bond with others in a healthy way? (This connects to the Kabbalistic *sefira* of *yesod*)

Am I idealistic and realistic at the same time? Balanced? Grounded? Focused? Do I know how to articulate my thoughts and emotions? (This connects to the Kabbalistic *sefira* of *malchut*)

Have I dealt professionally with past traumas or abuse? Can I access that help during the transition into marriage should there be a relapse or flashback?

If I am challenged in any of these areas, do I deal properly with my tendencies towards anxiety, depression, OCD, addictions, and/or eating disorders?

How about my perfectionism and/or anger issues?

Spiritually

Do I know what my values are? Am I happy with and proud of my *Yiddishkeit*?

Do I know how to turn to Hashem for support and *bitachon*?

Do I have awareness of Hashem's presence all of the time, also known as *yirat shomayim*? Am I honest even when nobody knows?

Do I accept the authority of a Rav and/or *mashpia*?

Do I practice Torah-true behavior in my intergender relationships?

Do I treat my parents with the proper respect?

Did I review the *halachot* of Shabbat, *kashrut*, *yichud*, and other realms of *halacha* basics to building a *bayit ne'eman b'yisrael al yesodei hatorah v'ha mitzvah*?

Do I have a healthy way to monitor my self-growth in *ruchniyut*, in spiritual matters?

Do I have the Torah approach and practical skills for healthy dating?

This list of questions is broad in scope and includes issues we continue to work on as long as we are alive! This list, however, is by no means all-inclusive. Please add your own thoughts to ponder, and questions that come to mind, as you tune in to your truest self while making your personal *cheshbon hanefesh*, spiritual inventory taking. The list can be helpful in providing a starting point for a conversation between you and your *mashpia*.

On the other hand, the list of questions is long. Please don't feel overwhelmed by the sheer volume. Take a deep breath and proceed one step at a time. Feel free to use the list as you see fit in your quest to make choices that will benefit your marriage. The pre-marriage period used wisely is an important investment. It is integral to building a strong and healthy foundation with your husband that will last *adei ad*, until eternity, *b'ezrat Hashem*.

You may choose to refer to this list sporadically, after marriage to monitor your growth as well as to set future goals for you as an individual, as a wife and as the *akeret habayit* of your home. It's an unfolding journey.

Sincerely,

Sara Morozow

chapter six

The First Night

BE'ILAT MITZVAH

If you immersed in the *mikvah* before your wedding, there is a *halachic* assumption that you will consummate your marriage through physical intimacy on the wedding night.[1] The thought of intimacy might open up a floodgate of questions and concerns: Can we take it a bit more slowly before consummating our marriage? What if one of us isn't in the mood after the wedding? What if we don't know what we're doing, even though we think we do? Won't it be super awkward?

These important questions deserve consideration and honest replies.

Since touch is forbidden before marriage, there is an immediate shift as soon as you complete the *kiddushin:* you are now permitted to touch and are keenly aware that the wedding crescendos with *be'ilat mitzvah,* the first instance of intimacy.

This is beautiful, and can also be daunting!

Now that your two half-souls have been reunited together through marriage, it is time for you to become one flesh. *Be'ilat mitzvah* is the final *halachic* aspect of the marriage ceremony. This last step of *kiddushin* should ideally be completed without unnecessary delay, just like any other mitzvah. The first instance of physical intimacy

---

1   *Shach, Yoreh Dei'ah* 192:11.

is the doorway into the new home you will build together. It is a mitzvah of towering holiness that finds expression in an act that is natural and instinctive.

At the same time, this is new territory. Anticipation and excitement tinged with trepidation is a very normal mix of emotions to feel at this time. Even as you want to go forward, you might feel something making you draw back a bit. If this is your response, it's normal! This raw and vulnerable experience marks a seismic shift in your life.

Even when we don't feel drawn to engage in intimate relations on that first night, we can and should move forward with pure faith in our Creator who knows what is best and wants only the best for us. While the *halachic* ideal is that consummation takes place on the wedding night, many couples will be unable to do so. That is okay. Give it your best try, and if at any point on this journey you become overwhelmed, take a break and continue trying again soon. You will, *b'ezrat Hashem*, most certainly succeed. Above all, keep an open line of communication between yourself and your *chatan*.

This is the perfect time for you to be there for each other and to set a precedent of support and positivity in your marriage. Moreover, leaning into this new and potentially awkward conversation will begin a pattern of open communication around intimacy.

First and foremost, be attentive to what you need, so you can feel comfortable, safe, and at ease. Only in this way can you welcome your new husband into your life in this unique fashion. When you are relaxed, you can be receptive to his overtures and invite reciprocal calmness from your *chatan*.

Open communication requires clearly expressing your wants and needs, while also actively listening to your *chatan*. In stating your wants and needs, try to broach the topic without judgment or blame, by using personalized statements about your experience and your feelings. When he speaks, listen– do not interrupt. When responding to him, channel a gentle, reassuring, and supportive tone– much like you would want to be responded to, as well. Throughout this exchange, consider each other's wants and needs at the absolute center of the dialogue, so you can step into that higher zone accessible only through abandoning exclusive focus on the self. Indeed, the way you, as a couple, negotiate this new aspect of your life together presents an opportunity to learn best practices for your marriage in all of its dimensions. When "I/you" as individuals becomes "we/us" as a unit, you will have taken a step towards building your very own *bayit ne'eman b'yisrael*.

As important as *be'ilat mitzvah* is, don't take yourself or the hiccups you may encounter too seriously. Don't be afraid to laugh. What better way to undercut possible

The First Night: Be'ilat Mitzvah

nervousness, and be your unmasked, vulnerable self? You only have one wedding night. Whether or not you consummate your marriage that evening, you will want to be able to look back at that night and remember the love and awe that filled you. You want to remember the joy and warmth of your togetherness, and not overwhelming anxiety and physical or emotional discomfort. Even if challenges arise, the experience should be one of gentleness and mutual support. You are in this together.

If you sense that you are not making progress, please do not wait long before reaching out to a *kallah* teacher, *rav*, or other trusted resource for assistance. There is no reason to unnecessarily elongate this uncomfortable state of limbo.

The Gemara teaches:

אשה...אינה כורתת ברית אלא למי שעשאה כלי,

שנאמר כי בועליך עושיך ה' צ-באות שמו.

> A woman only makes a covenant [becomes truly connected] with the one who made her a vessel [through her first act of sexual intercourse], as it is stated: 'For your Husband is your Maker, the G-d of hosts is His name.' [2, 3]

Your first intimacy marks a *brit*; you have fashioned a covenant, a pact, and a spectacularly unique bond.

If you have come to marriage with the sincere intent of building your *binyan adei ad*, everlasting edifice, on the foundations of Torah and *mitzvot*, Hashem surely knows your heart. This is true whether you come into marriage as a virgin or not and whether this is your first marriage or not. The Creator of heaven and earth will undoubtedly affect a covenant of equal or even greater potency to the *brit* referenced above, between you and your husband. Don't allow the *yetzer hara* to drain your resolve to move forward into your marriage with strength and joy.[4]

Either way, your first intimate connection is the beginning of the rest of your lives together. You have entered your own private garden. You have the remainder of your lives to discover and enjoy its beauty.

---

2   *Sanhedrin* 22b.

3   *Yeshayahu* 54:5.

4   For more on the subject of *teshuvah* see the *bracha acharita* section of chapter two.

YOU MIGHT BE WONDERING:

I'm worried about getting my period on or before my wedding day. Is there anything I can do?

According to *halacha*, and as specifically cited in *Piskei Dinim Leha'Tzemach Tzedek*, the *kallah*'s first *tevilah* should take place as close to *be'ilat mitzvah* as possible.[5] The optimum time to go to the *mikvah* is the night before the wedding. If for some reason that does not work, you can go earlier on in the day preceding the wedding. In fact, *halacha* allows for a *kallah* to immerse whether during the day or evening, up to four days prior to her wedding as long as seven complete days have elapsed from a successful *hefsek taharah*.[6]

If your cycle is irregular, or if it is regular, but you expect your period to come at a time that would interfere with your ability to go to the *mikvah* before the wedding, you have the option of regulation through the use of hormonal manipulation. There are various routes that can be taken for regulation purposes, and each person's body is specific in its reaction. It is, therefore, imperative that you do this under the guidance of a physician who has experience with helping *kallot* regulate as well as some familiarity with *halacha*. You should take care of this sooner rather than later during your engagement, leaving time for the physician to tweak the prescription if necessary. This will help you avoid unnecessary long-term problems that can occur by taking a less thought-out approach.[7]

You will want to ask the doctor to regulate you using a method that is most effective and allows you the maximum amount of flexibility. Since a *betulah* becomes a *nidah* through *be'ilat mitzvah*, bringing on your period in the closest possible proximity to when you have completed *be'ilat mitzvah* allows for the two causes of *nidah* (the first due to *be'ilat mitzvah* and the second, your period) to overlap within one time frame. If you are not a *betulah*, your sole concern should be regulating your last period before the wedding so that you have enough days to accommodate the flow followed by seven clean days and *tevilah*.

---

5 *Shulchan Aruch, Yoreh De'ah* 192:2; *Piskei Dinim, Yoreh Dei'ah* 192:5.

6 *Shulchan Aruch* and *Piskei Dinim* ad loc.

7 If you will be using birth control during the initial phase of your marriage, you should share this information with your practitioner as it can have bearing on the method chosen to avoid *chuppat nidah*. Please be cautious both as a *kallah* and as a married woman when making choices surrounding contraceptives. You will want to give paramount consideration to how this method will affect your *nidah* vs *taharah* time. Tahareinu, an organization dedicated to finding medical solutions for women who observe *taharat hamishpachah*, operates a confidential hotline and can be invaluable in this process.

The First Night: Be'ilat Mitzvah

If you are uncomfortable with medicinal regulation, herbal and other homeopathic remedies exist that may be helpful. You may also decide to let nature run its course. No matter how carefully a *kallah* regulates herself or how regular she is naturally, there remains the possibility of a *chuppat nidah*. It is not uncommon for hormonal irregularities to ensue from pre-wedding stress and excitement. If and when that happens, we understand the occurrence to be *hashgachah pratit*, Divine providence. This is not something anyone at the wedding will notice. Only the *chatan* and a few others need this information, and they will maintain discretion. However, since the *chatan* and *kallah* in a state of *nidah* will be unable to be in a state of *yichud* until she goes to the *mikvah*,[8] specific living and sleeping arrangements will have to be made. There are many comfortable and creative options that can afford the *chatan* and *kallah* maximum privacy while not trespassing *hilchot yichud*. This is something the *kallah* will want to discuss with her parents, her *kallah* teacher, and/or a *rav*. The *chatan*, of course, must be informed of her status.

If you should become a *nidah* during the days leading up to the wedding when in many communities, the *chatan* and *kallah* are not in contact, a trusted third party can be used to communicate this sensitive information.

There are instances in which the *chatan* or *kallah* express appreciation for having a *chuppat nidah*, understanding in hindsight how it allowed them some extra time to bond before easing into physical intimacy.

How can I best prepare for "the first night?"

There is one area of life in which lack of experience is not only a virtue but a bonus, and that is our sexual intimacy. What if we are not compatible? People wonder. What if I do the wrong thing and mess us up? They fret. Here is the good news: If you dated intentionally and are committed to building a home together based on all of the values and goals you share, there is every good chance that you will be successful in your intimacy. Sexuality is a natural function. This bears repeating: while sexual dysfunction does occur and can be successfully addressed, most young people find their way quite naturally with some baseline guidance. So don't worry. Hashem created us with a desire, an urge, and a host of physiological responses to stimuli, and we will find our way as innocents can, and have, for millennia.

---

[8] *Shulchan Aruch, Yoreh De'ah* 192:4.

At the same time, this is a good time to say goodbye to the romantic notions you have gleaned from reading or viewing popular materials and say hello to reality. Real-life is not a scripted or choreographed scene spliced and airbrushed to perfection. Real-life is you and your *chatan* finding your way together. It is about commitment. It is goal-oriented towards a long-term commitment. These are but the first moments of, *b'ezrat Hashem*, a beautiful life together.

In this vein, there is NO single NORMAL when it comes to sexual intimacy; it is as individual as each person and each couple.[9] With proper education and self-knowledge, healthy couples will, for the most part, figure it out. It might take longer than you imagined. If that happens, cut yourself and your new husband some slack. Don't compare, don't compare, don't compare! There is only a problem if one or both of you are unhappy.

When you get back from the wedding, take some time to focus on each other and debrief about the wedding, share highlights, and laugh about any surprises or glitches in the plan. If this seems like a good time to convey any specific sensitivities or preferences you have regarding physical touch and intimacy, feel comfortable sharing.

Set expectations together. You're exhausted and in good spirits after the wedding. You're about to engage in *be'ilat mitzvah*. You're both a little nervous and excited. In addition to the huge spiritual aspect of the mitzvah, there is also a physical human aspect as well. You may want to use the following to open the conversation:

Neither of our bodies has done this before. We don't know how our bodies will respond. Let's do it together, we'll figure it out and continue figuring it out. There is no such thing as failure, only step one in this forever process. This is our first experience where we can grow together.

At that point, you may want to ask your *chatan* to help you with the buttons or zipper – or both– so you can take your gown off, or assist you with the latch on your jewelry, or with removing pins from your hair so you can get comfortable. This is a good way to ease into the sensation of each other's touch.

---

[9] There is, however, a range of what can be considered normal. Certain behaviors, or frequency of demand for sexuality can be indicative of a possible addiction or some other disorder and should be discussed with a practitioner. See Part IV, essay seven for more information.

The First Night: Be'ilat Mitzvah

When you change, wear what makes you feel good! Understandably, there is always a lot of thought about what to wear. You should buy and wear what makes you feel beautiful, feminine, and special.[10]

Under no circumstances should you feel pressured into dressing a certain way for your new husband. If you are at ease and comfortable, you will more easily be able to enjoy yourself, and the experience will be that much more pleasurable for both of you. Feeling relaxed and receptive will facilitate arousal and natural lubrication, allowing for easier entry on the part of your new husband.

Trust your (physical) instincts. Allow your intuition to guide your affection and foreplay. This is new and surprising terrain, and will introduce novel sensations and pleasure. With the gradual increase in passionate exchange, you will both become more ready for penetration.

Be mindful of your *chatan's* reaction to you and your body, and encourage him to communicate. He will be attentive to the prohibition of *hotzaat zera levatalah*, and you want to ensure that you're on the same page. It is, therefore best that you take your cue from him in terms of intensity of hugging, kissing, or caressing—certainly before you are in bed together, and reciprocate in kind. Long-term love thrives on making your beloved your priority. You most certainly will want to display sensitivity to your *chatan* on your wedding night. Reassure him that you are in this together.

On the first night, there is a likelihood one of you or both of you will encounter physical speedbumps to your togetherness; you might have issues with vaginal lubrication or pain, or your *chatan* could experience premature ejaculation or could have trouble achieving or maintaining an erection. If either of your bodies does not respond in the way you would like them to, it is not a commentary on your chemistry or the quality of your marriage. Being open with each other about this experience as it's happening will contribute to emotional safety in order to achieve future success. In these moments, convey heartfelt feelings of warmth, affection, and kindness. Mutual reassurance will build safety, trust, and love. (If the issue persists for any length of time, consider reaching out to your *kallah* teacher who can identify resources that will be helpful.)

You might think you are more in love or in sync or evolved or educated than most others. You might project smooth sailing. In truth, until you are in that room together with your *chatan*, it is impossible to know what it actually will

---

[10] To avoid possible *halachic* questions, it is best not to wear white night clothes.

feel like and how the two of you will mesh. Intimacy is natural, the most natural thing in the world. And yet, when it is new it can feel strange and overwhelming. No matter what you read, you cannot be one hundred percent prepared.

Many women experience anxiety around the fact that a woman's first time can be painful. First off, some women experience pain, some experience slight pressure, and some simply experience slight discomfort. Some women may bleed, and some may not. If you do bleed, this is completely normal and is because your hymen has been "broken." Your hymen, which is Greek for membrane, is a thin, flexible, crescent- shape or ring-like tissue located just inside the opening of the vagina and is more correctly stretched than broken. Normal variations of the hymen range from thin and stretchy to thick and somewhat rigid. In many cases, such as if a young woman has used tampons or exercised extensively, the hymen may already be partially or even completely stretched.

There is a truism that the most important sexual organ is your brain. A woman's experience will depend in great measure on her emotional and psychological state of mind. Feeling anxious can cause a tightening of the pelvic muscles, making it difficult to facilitate penetration. Being present in your own body and in the moment will enable you to be aroused and allow your body to work its magic. With arousal, your brain triggers the release of hormones which, among other things, will stimulate additional vaginal lubrication,[11] as well as the expansion and lengthening of your vagina. All of this facilitates penetration. Most important is having a healthy, positive, balanced attitude towards this very new, beautiful, and holy part of your life.

In the event that you feel pain, tell your *chatan*, and stop. Stay attuned to what you're feeling. If you feel up to it, try again. If you do not, do not feel any pressure to try again that evening. Under no circumstances should this become a traumatic event.

With this in mind, when a woman is intimate for the first time, it is normal to experience a minimal level of discomfort, pressure, or slight pain. When you experience this, communicate with your *chatan*.

---

[11] If you experience vaginal dryness, casuing you to experience sexual pain, know that this can be a normal experience. This could be due to stress, hormones, or your body at that moment, and does not reflect your feelings towards your husband. Natural oils and personal lubricants can be very helpful. If the issue persists, consider talking to your doctor or a sex therapist.

Be'ilat mitzvah is a rite of passage that has to be traversed at some time. Your wedding night, or as soon as you are able to after your wedding, is a special time to do so.

Anticipate and embrace the transcendence of this experience. If it does not go as smoothly as you had hoped, stay calm and positive; don't panic or hyper-focus on what went wrong. Communicate openly and directly, and remember, you will figure this out (and even laugh about it in the future)! Sexual intimacy is not something to fear, just something new and out of your comfort zone at this time. If, however, after a number of attempts you are still not successful in consummating your marriage, think of it as an opportunity to set an early precedent of unconditional support and love. Allow yourselves to be distracted by *sheva brachot* and other matters. It is not unusual for successful consummation to take a few tries over the course of a few days, even weeks, and sometimes longer.

Sometimes, your first intimacy feels a bit clumsy and not as wonderfully enjoyable as you had imagined. Remember, like with everything else in life, experience is the best teacher. With time you will learn about your own and each other's bodies. You will feel more comfortable and deeply secure in each other's embrace. The anxiety surrounding the newness will give way to desire, even hunger, for each other. The wonder and pleasure will unfold. Give time, open communication, practice, and other relationship-building skills a chance to work their magic.

Irrespective of the exact details of your personal experience, after complete penetration, or if there has not been complete entry but you are bleeding from the site of the hymen, the virgin bride becomes a *nidah*. You will reunite physically only after your visit to the *mikvah*.

In every other instance, spending time together and basking in the "afterglow" of sexual intimacy is integral. Science is now confirming the importance of the Torah mandate that a man spends time with his wife and not leave her immediately after intercourse.[12] There is growing evidence that cuddling after sexual relations is important to overall sexual satisfaction and the health of a couple's relationship.[13] When a man loses interest immediately after intercourse he may leave his wife feeling used, vulnerable and/or empty.

---

12   *Talmud Eruvin* 100:2; *Rashi* ad loc.

13   Science Proves Cuddling After Sex is Crucial by Kate Moriarty, Women's Health Magazine April 30, 2014.

In this particular instance, after *be'ilat mitzvah*, however, that is not the case. *Halacha* mandates that they separate and the couple must refrain from any touch at all. Not because they want to but because G-d so mandates. When the couple goes into their first intimacy with this understanding, there is not the sting of rejection, but rather a mutual and realistic understanding of what will happen. It still might be helpful for them to talk about how they are feeling and they should certainly go to sleep in a cocoon of emotional togetherness.

This interim stage requires discipline–a new type of maturity and *bittul*. The struggle can feel onerous, even illogical. On the other hand, it is a time to deepen your bond on the emotional level as you process the new terrain of physical intimacy. This slow initiation into sexual pleasure is the converse of the "honeymoon" model. It is not the summit but rather, *b'ezrat Hashem*, the very beginning of a long, happy, pleasure-filled life together. Many couples find that the physical separation after their first intimacy is exactly what they needed.

> **Rivkah**: I still remember the morning after my wedding. In that twilight zone between sleep and wakefulness, I heard our doorbell ringing. It was the couch my mother had ordered for us being delivered at what was, for the rest of the world, a very reasonable hour, but for me, still in the middle of the night. I remember clearly that before I could consciously register that I had just gotten married, I felt a sensation of shock at being in a room with a man—both of us in pajamas—what was this? Years later, I can better identify that feeling as a frisson of excitement or titillation. Even when I did not have the vocabulary, however, I had the feeling that I had just entered a whole new and exciting world. Having some time between the first night and the next time to unpack the newness of it all was helpful.

The world has changed a lot since that night, but human nature has not. The time between the "first night/time" and your next *mikvah* night will give you the opportunity to deepen the special bond you have forged through conversation and shared confidences. Take this time to settle into your apartment, get a head start on thank you notes, and enjoy your *sheva brachot*. Allow the anticipation for a physical reunion to build gradually, and enjoy the process.

Being a *nidah* might make you feel tense and edgy; at least some of the time. This is not necessarily a bad thing—it means you are a human with normal urges. Find ways to channel that pent-up energy.

Depending on your cycle and other variables, it is possible that during the first few weeks of marriage you will find yourself in *nidah* more frequently than you would have liked. This is a passing phase and no reflection of the regular cycles that will mark the rest of your life. Instead of "waiting it out" and allowing tension to predominate, view this as an opportunity to bond in other ways and plan activities for the two of you to enjoy.[14]

How can I/we go from 0 to 100 so suddenly?

Before marriage, *Halacha* limits interface with non-familial members of the opposite sex and prohibits touch. Even sustained thoughts of sexual nature are forbidden. And then after some decades time, all the rules seem to change!

But actually, they don't. All of the *halachot* you abided by until now are designed for just this moment in time. Like layers of tissue paper surround a fragile glass pitcher, protecting it from breakage, so do the pre-marriage *halachot* protect the most precious of all gifts, our marital intimacy. *Halacha* is *not* put in place to guard against sexual expression within marriage. Rather, *halacha* helps get us to and facilitates the most meaningful intimacy possible between husband and wife, ensuring we appreciate and respect that Hashem has gifted this sacred and exquisite form of oneness to soulmates alone.

Once married, you have arrived at a completely new place; a space only you and your husband will inhabit to the exclusion of all others. This is the *Kodesh Hakodashim*, the holy of holies; it stands apart from all other areas, even the others in your personal *mikdash me'at*, your home.

To crystalize this point, it's helpful to consider the notion of *havdalah*, separation, and delineation. *Havdalah,* one of the most important ideas in *Yiddishkeit*, runs like a major artery through every dimension of life: time, space, and person. The realm of time holds sacredness via separation: Shabbat and Yom Tov are distinct and set apart from the weekday. The realm of space entails holiness via separation as well: Israel, Jerusalem, *Har Habayit* represent ascending levels set off from all other spaces and are unique in their sanctity. And the same holds true in the area of personage: even as all Jews are part of the *mamlechet kohanim v'goy kadosh*, the kingdom of priests and holy nation, the *Levi'im, Kohanim,* and the *Kohen Gadol* are set apart, vested with a unique dimension of holiness.

The notion of *havdalah* informs each aspect of our personal lives, as well, including intimacy. Before marriage, there is no sanctioned, holy, physical

---

14   For ideas on how to negotiate your time as *nidah* see chapter seven.

relationship between a man and a woman. Before our *neshamot* are united and become one in the process of marriage, a physically intimate relationship only obscures and compromises what we hope to build together. Therefore, on a *halachic* level, it is *assur*, prohibited. On a more mystical level, chassidut explains that the word *assur*, etymologically rooted in the term for imprisonment and restraint, connotes that, before a *halachic* marriage, the *nitzutzei kedushah*, the sparks of divinity, embedded in the act of physical intimacy are incarcerated and held hostage by the forces of *kelipah*.[15]

Only once *kallah* and *chatan* have joined together through *chupah v'kiddushin* and the *kallah* is *tehorah* can *be'ilat mitzvah*, their first instance of sexual intimacy, complete and finalize the marriage.

על כן יעזב איש את אביו ואת אמו, ודבק באשתו והיו לבשר אחד

Therefore a man should leave his father and mother, and join with his wife and become one flesh.[16]

Not only is the sexual act now permitted, *mutar*, a word etymologically rooted in the term for free and unrestrained; it is, as the *passuk* above mandates, a mitzvah. Furthermore, now that *kallah* and *chatan* have been consecrated to each other, the *nitzutzei kedushah* Hashem has imbued in physical intimacy are accessible to the couple and wait to be unleashed.

This initial intimacy is not only the first of many such expressions in our lives together; it is also the birth of our oneness.

To come back to the initial question: Contrary to some of the ideas peddled in secular culture, the Torah model understands that no incremental physical relationship would or could lead up to marital consummation. With marriage, a new entity is created, and intimacy simply gives physical expression to this newly minted spiritual truth. When consummating our marriage, we are not going from zero to a hundred but, rather, from one hundred spiritually to one hundred physically. We now couple our spiritual unity with a physical union.

---

15   *Tanya* ch. 7.

16   *Bereishit* 2:24.

The First Night: Be'ilat Mitzvah

IMPORTANT NOTE REGARDING TRAUMA

The earlier discussion concerning *teshuvah*[17] is not meant to address the loss of *betulah* status due to rape, *chas v'shalom,* or the wide-ranging types of sexual trauma including, but not limited to molestation and exposure to hypersexual or pornographic images during childhood and young adulthood.[18] These kinds of attacks on your psyche will almost always affect your intimate life. Professional guidance is absolutely critical for someone who has suffered a traumatic experience. Their new spouse will benefit from therapy as well. As you now share one *neshamah* and one life, your experiences are inextricably linked.

Trauma is stored in our bodies until it can be released. This typically leads to pain and can progressively erode one's health. Our bodies store trauma and abuse quite literally.[19] In addition to mental flashbacks, our very bodies respond to new situations that trigger a memory of trauma and the strategies adopted during those trying times.

One can use their energy to hide a traumatic event and its responses, but it won't work in the long term, as the body keeps score, such as the tightening of the vaginal muscles. Alternatively, one can use their energy to communicate about the trauma responses and work through it with a partner and professional.

When this type of information is withheld, it can leave your spouse feeling like a failure, wracked with guilt, hurt, angry, and, at the very best, just plain perplexed by your reaction to his intimate overtures. More profoundly, nondisclosure can lead to betrayal trauma, and enormous efforts will have to be expended to heal the breach of trust.

The good news is that humans are resilient, and it does get better. There is a definite path forward to overcoming past experiences, but you must let your spouse in. You can only meet success in this challenge when you face it together.

Your spouse is your most important support figure and advocate in the journey to complete recovery and lifelong enjoyment of healthy sexual intimacy. Great care should be taken to disclose what must be shared about a situation before engagement. This should be done only with the counsel and advice of a therapist

---

[17] For more about the concept of *teshuvah,* see the *bracha acharita* section of chapter two.

[18] For further discussion about pornography, see the *kibutz baneha* section of chapter two.

[19] For more information on somaticized trauma and moving through it, see *The Body Keeps Score* by Besser Van der Kolk.

who sub-specializes in treating the likes of your particular situation. Only a person with this training is equipped to advise you on what should be disclosed, as well as when and in which manner. When this information is shared properly, it becomes the foundation for healing and recovery. A professional in sexual trauma can guide you as well in pinpointing if and when it is best to include the *chatan* in joint therapy sessions.

If the person who suffered trauma is completely honest about their situation and committed to working towards healing, the chances for success are real and proven. By undertaking the necessary interventions under the care of a licensed and trauma-informed specialist, in collaboration with support services provided within the *frum* community, and, most importantly, the support and encouragement of a loving spouse, the marriage can thrive.

If you or your *chatan* experienced a trauma that stole your virginity and innocence, do not allow that experience to define your present and future. You are, in Hashem's eyes, always His beloved child; pure and whole and precious. A woman who is violated through rape or molestation is *halachically* termed an *ones*, one who was forced; the violation is not attributed to her choices and/or actions. In addition to a professional therapist, a gifted *mashpia* can help you heal from this wound and, very importantly, divest yourself of misplaced guilt and shame you might be carrying. Chassidut teaches us to always look forward and not permit the *yetzer hara* a foothold by dragging us down memory lane.

Move forward with *simchah* and confidence as you build your new home. While we may not always understand Hashem's plan, we know that Hashem directs the footsteps of each person and orchestrates each unique journey.

Part Three
My Home:
Three Guideposts

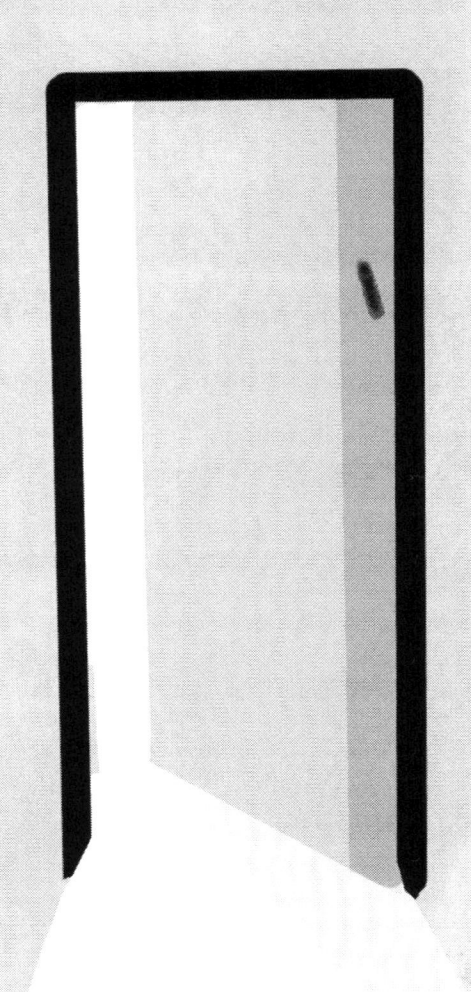

My Home:
HASHEM'S DWELLING PLACE

By all accounts, the *shana rishonah* marks a time of transition and new beginnings. While you remain the same person you always were, you step into a role that is transformative. Newlyweds must acclimate to a set of novel realities which include keeping a home, along with all of the attendant responsibilities, navigating relationships with in-laws, and in some instances, a move to a new geographic location. Whether you adapt easily to change or need to invest concerted effort, this is a time of adjustment for every newlywed.

There is also the shift from a "me" centered existence to a "we" centered life. But that is only the beginning. Marriage marks the founding of a new Jewish home; a holy construct central to the fulfillment of Hashem's goal in creating the universe. Your personal home is essentially Hashem's home.

What distinguishes a house from a home? Conceptually, a house is a form of shelter while a home connotes safety and comfort. The very thought of home is inviting and fills you with happiness and contentment. Marriage presents you with the opportunity to create the future which includes the ideal home for you, your husband, and your children.

As a well-known adage teaches, "you buy a house, but you make a home." Seen through the lens of *Yiddishkeit* and chassidut, we grow a home, incrementally, over time. Our own homes – the home Hashem so deeply desires – take shape and form through reflection and thoughtful choices. A home should be filled with the light of authenticity. It's a home when it feels warm, lived in, and welcoming; not sterile and perfect, like a museum. It's okay if it is marked by the scuff marks of our struggles.

The Rebbe taught[1] that the specifics of each home reflect its owner's choices and preferences. In that respect, it is an outgrowth of its owner. At the same time, a *dirah na'eh*, a beautiful home, enhances the life of its owner in immeasurable ways. *"Na'eh"* does not have to connote extravagance or opulence. It can also describe a simple home that is clean and uncluttered; a living space accented by a bouquet of beautiful flowers, a photo collage of loved ones, nick nacks, or memorabilia. A *dirah na'eh* nourishes the soul in a transcendent way.

That we share a partnership with Hashem is one of the most audacious concepts in Jewish theology. Hashem is not only our Father and King, but as *Shlomo Hamelech* taught in *Shir Hashirim*, He is also our spouse.[2] In part, the spousal metaphor reflects that Hashem desired a relationship with us. Hashem created a dynamic in which He is affected, *kavyochal,* by our actions.[3]

Just as a beautiful home nurtures the human spirit, so too do our efforts to decorate the *dirah betachtonim* elevate Hashem. Consider the analogy of furnishing a home for you and your partner. For your partner to be comfortable in the space, his taste, so to say, must be reflected there. This means everything from the overall aesthetic to the details of the space. Now imagine that Hashem is that partner. Hashem's aesthetic is Torah and *mitzvot*. And Hashem's interior design preferences are our attention to detail of said Torah and *mitzvot*. As the *chachamim* taught, כלים נאים מרחיבין דעתו של אדם, beautiful vessels broaden and expand a mortal human's mind.[4] In like fashion, our attention to details in our observance of *mitzvot* and our quest to beautify them, expands the mind of *Adam Ha'Elyon*, the Supernal Man, Hashem. The Jewish woman, in particular, was gifted with an affinity for interiors; for making Hashem's home truly beautiful. And this work all begins with– and in– our personal homes.[5]

---

1 *Sefer Hasichot* 5752, pp. 354-357.

2 This concept is expounded upon deeply in Kabbalah and chassidut.

3 *Torat Menachem*, vol. 4, pp. 324-327.

4 *Brachot* 57b.

5 In this same vein, the Rebbe highlighted the lessons inherent in the names of Rebbetzin Chaya Mushka: Chaya means life and Mushka is a term associated with perfume, a delightful aroma. Every Jewish woman, taught the Rebbe, has the power to create the atmosphere of her home; to suffuse her household –and the lives of her husband, children and larger community– with her vivifying energy and signature "scent." (*Sefer Hasichot* 5752, p358)

My Home: Hashem's Dwelling Place

In decorating a room or home, the decorating process always begins with what the experts call a statement or anchor piece— something special around which all else will revolve.

The notion of the familial home as Hashem's true dwelling place, and, by extension, a woman's central role in creating that dwelling place, is underscored by the Ramban. The Ramban asserts that the *Mishkan* and *Mikdash* were fashioned after the tents of the *Avot* and *Imahot* rather than the other way around.[6] Those tents were distinguished by the presence of three miracles: *neirot Shabbat Kodesh* that remained lit from *Erev Shabbat* to *Erev Shabbat*, a *bracha* in the dough (which is an allusion to the mitzvah of *kashrut*), and a cloud of glory that hovered above (an allusion to the mitzvah of *taharat hamishpachah*). These miraculous features created the prototype for the *mishkan* and later the *mikdashot*:[7] the *menorah* mirrored candle lighting, the *shulchan* recalled the blessed *challah* and (more widely, *kashrut*), and the *aron ha'eidut* paralleled the cloud, which bore witness to the observance of the holy laws of *nidah*.

A Jewish home is, thus, a *Mikdash* in which the woman, the *akeret habayit*, the anchor of the home, serves as the Kohen Gadol charged with overseeing the execution of all essential details, and then more. Especially the extra dimension of *keilim na'im*.

Indeed, *hadlakat neirot*, *challah*, and *nidah* closely align with womanhood[8] and serve as the undergirding of every Jewish home. Fittingly, this triad of *mitzvot* forms the acrostic *Ha-Ch-N*.[9] Literally, *hachein* means the grace. There are other *mitzvot*, namely *kisui rosh*, the obligation for a married woman to cover her hair, and *pru u'rvu*, the privilege of bringing children, with Hashem's help, into this world, which fit under the larger "*Ha-Ch-N*" umbrella.

You will awaken the morning after your wedding to engage with three new big-ticket items, anchor pieces as it were, around which you will, bit by bit, spiritually decorate your new home. In this section, we focus on the *dinei harchakah* aspect of *hilchot nidah*, *kisui rosh*, and *pru u'rvu*. How you relate to and observe these great *mitzvot* will create the aesthetic of your home, Hashem's home. Conscientious observance of these cornerstone *mitzvot* is important, and it is the passion with which you carry them out that will serve as the *keilim na'im* that turn your house into a warm and inviting home.

---

6   Introduction to *Sefer Shemot*.

7   *Mareh Habazak*, p. 378; *Yalkut Pninim* (Tehillim); p. 417, based on *Nachal Eliyahu*.

8   For more about these *mitzvot*, see the articles on the Three Mitzvot of the Woman on Chabad.org.

9   *Megaleh Amukot Al Hatorah*, Parshat Shelach, sec. *Gimmel Mitzvot*.

In 1959, the Rebbe commented on the story of *bnot Tzelafchad* and highlighted each Jewish woman's power to create an ambiance of *kedushah* in her home. In speaking of their unique *chibat ha'aretz,* the love for *Eretz Yisrael*, the Rebbe identified a unique strain of passion.[10] He saw the love and devotion of *bnot Tzelafchad* as characteristic of all Jewish women who passionately infuse their surroundings with the singular holiness of *Eretz Yisrael*.

Wherever they are, whenever it might be, Jewish women strive to make their homes the land upon which Hashem rests His eyes. As the Torah teaches in *Devarim,* תמיד עיני ה' אלוקיך בה מר[א]שית השנה ועד אחרית שנה, the eyes of Hashem your G-d are always upon it, from the beginning of the year to the end of the year.[11] And from the beginning of the day until the end of the day, in the entire home, including the bedroom!

In the words of the sixth Lubavitcher Rebbe, the Rebbe Rayatz:[12]

> **Hashem entrusted all that is sacred and fundamental to the Jewish nation to the hands of Jewish women to safeguard and develop. This includes giving birth to children and raising them, ensuring the kashrut of food, and preserving the sublime, pure holiness of Shabbat.**
>
> **When a woman fulfills her obligation and destiny in family life, in conducting the home, and in educating her children in the Torah spirit– it is such a woman described by the verse:** חכמת נשים בנתה ביתה, **The wisdom of women constructed her home.**[13]

In the forthcoming chapter on *dinei harchakah*, we focus on the conceptual and practical components of this aspect of *taharat hamishpachah*. In the two chapters that follow, we focus on *kisui rosh* and the mitzvah of *pru u'rvu*. We hope these ideas help ease your transition into the wonders and challenges of married life, and serve as inspiration "photos" for your new home. Through the choices we make in our personal homes, we get to decorate the *dirah betachtonim* and bring expansiveness of mind, *kavyochal,* to the Owner of the universe.

---

10   *Torat Menachem.* vol. 26, pp. 125-126.

11   *Devarim* 11:12.

12   *Hayom Yom.* entry for 26 Adar II.

13   *Mishlei* 14:1.

chapter seven

Dinei Harchakah:
PULLING APART; STAYING TOGETHER

It is forbidden for a woman and her husband to engage in sexual intercourse when she is a *nidah* according to Torah law. This *aveirah* is an *issur karet*.[1] In addition there is another prohibition[2] embedded in the *passuk* that reads ואל אשה בנדת טמאתה לא תקרב לגלות ערותה, and to a woman in her time of *nidah*, you shall not approach to reveal her nakedness.[3] The seemingly extra words "do not approach" teach that the *issur d'orayta* includes physical manifestation of love, such as kissing, hugging, caressing etc.[4] Additionally, *halacha* addresses the twin tensions of a married couple's singular relationship. On the one hand, we can be in a state of *yichud*, alone and secluded with one another, which is unique to a married couple.[5] On the other hand, precisely because of our deep bond and physical proximity, the Torah's prohibition against physical expressions of love during the *nidah* period necessitates extra precaution.

---

1 *Vayikra* 20:18. Sexual relations with an unmarried woman who is a *nidah* is likewise prohibited and an *issur karet*.

2 *Shulchan Aruch, Yoreh Dei'ah* 195:1.

3 *Vayikra* 18:19.

4 *Avot D'Rabbi Natan* 2:1.

5 *Shulchan Aruch, Yoreh Dei'ah* 195:1. This is permissible if the couple has already shared one instance of physical intimacy and will resume their physical relationship after the wife attends the *mikvah*.

At first glance, the *halachically* mandated *harchakot*, laws of distancing, appear to comprise a system of laws designed to put distance between a couple. In truth, the purpose of this system is to put distance between the couple and their trespass, *chas v'shalom*, of this *issur d'orayta*; to create safeguards to ensure we do not transgress the prohibition against sexual relations while *nidah*. Throughout the *nidah* period, this system reminds us that even as we enjoy shared spaces, including our bedroom, there are boundaries that delineate the physical expressions of our inherent closeness.

This is hard. It *should* be hard to abstain from physical expressions of love for your spouse. It takes getting used to. At times in life, observing these *halachot* proves especially difficult, such as postpartum or during a time of loss or other tragedy. Like with so much else, the way we frame these *halachot* will largely determine our experience in keeping them.

We can chafe under the weight of the *harchakot*; we can see them as an annoyance or, worse, a heavy yoke we resent. Or we can embrace and appreciate their necessity in safeguarding what is most important to us.

Most would concede that while not every touch serves as a precursor to intimacy, every instance of intimacy should begin with subtle, loving overtures that build and crescendo into full-blown expression. The system of *harchakot* honors the way that each of our senses can arouse desire. Alternatively, you can frame it as addressing each area of the house which can prompt a desire for intimacy.

Hashem created the human being and He alone is the expert arbiter of when and how we are to express our drives and when and how we must pull back.

Keenly aware of the magnetic power of sensuality, the Gemara offers a startling declaration: אין אפוטרופוס לעריות, no one, not even the greatest and most pious, is in full control over his/her sexual urges.[6] Once triggered, who can say which lines we might cross, with whom, and at what time?

If you are more mystically inclined, it's illuminating to note that, in addition to addressing practical concerns, *halacha* reveals the *Ratzon Ha'Elyon*, Celestial Will,[7] and allows us to touch a spiritual dimension more profound than the human mind can comprehend.[8]

---

6 *Ketubot* 13b.

7 A realm loftier than even the intellectual sefiros – *chochmah, binah and daat* – of the highest spiritual world, *Atzilut*.

8 *Iggeret Hakodesh, siman* 29. According to chassidut and Kabbalah, Hashem's *Ratzon Ha'Elyon* is His innermost core, known in Kaballah as *Keter*, the Divine Crown. Just as a crown sits on top of the head, so too *Keter* represents a Divine space that transcends the reason and logic. *Ratzon Ha'Elyon* is beyond creation entirely. One hint to *mitzvot's* rootedness in *Keter* is evident in *Keter's gematria*, 620, recalling the 613 *mitzvot* plus the seven rabbinic commands.

Dinei Harchakah: Pulling Apart; Staying Together

Ratzon Ha'Elyon refers to a deeply internal and transcendent aspect of the Divine. By way of analogy, think of an inexplicable desire you've felt, not due to a lack, but simply because. A desire that expresses something intuitive, something so beyond the typical parameters of cost and benefit you couldn't explain it to others. Indeed, this kind of desire says more about you than it says about the object of desire. So too, in a sense, Hashem's Celestial Will originates in an internal space within Him that transcends the constraints of reason.[9]

Thus, when resolve to uphold *halacha* wears thin, you might remember that abiding by the *Shulchan Aruch* means reaching all the way up, embracing Hashem as He is in His private core, beyond the created universe. Whether you view *halacha* practically or mystically, the *harchakot* certainly make avoiding serious transgression more tenable.

In every area of our lives, we assume there will be restrictions. We accept these limitations, even if and when inconvenient, because we understand they ensure our safety and the smooth functioning of society. Similarly, the system of *halacha*, includes *harchakot*, safeguards against the practical concern that we might, in a weaker moment, transgress a prohibition.

> **Sara**: When I was a teen living in Canada, our large family of small children used to travel in a station wagon with no seat belts or car seats. In fact, I didn't know that they even existed. But then, one day, our new car came equipped with these strange belts and buckles, and my parents lugged home these new fangled seats for the baby and the toddler. Soon after, seat belts and car seats graduated from modern amenity to law. My first reaction was that these regulations are insane, stifling, and outlandish. Slowly, however, we understood that the inconvenience was a small price to pay for safety. Today, even thinking of driving without buckling up is beyond the pale.

Simply put, *dinei harchakah* are for our own safety. They stop us at the yellow light before we harm ourselves by running a red.

These laws demonstrate a vital lesson about boundaries; the same mechanisms we initially see as constraining give rise to true freedom. Only an instrument with tightened strings can make beautiful music; a loose string on the table is not free but simply useless.

---

[9] See *Sefer Hamaamorim Melukat* (new ed.) vol. 4, p. 24. Sometimes Hashem's pure will, His *mitzvot/halachot*, are logical, but here too, the logic merely serves as external packaging, a garment, in which He enclothes His loftier faculty of Divine will, just as we might later ascribe a reason as to why we desire something we want out of pure will. This is why chassidut tells us all *mitzvot* (including those that appear merely logical) can be categorized as *chukim*.

> **Sara**: I once took my children hiking up a tall mountain. When we reached the top there was a breathtaking view, a stunning natural vista of waterfalls cascading below into a valley. I was petrified for my children to go close to the edge of the cliff to get a better view, for fear that, G-d forbid, they might fall over. And then I saw that on another side of the summit, stood a very sturdy guardrail. I took my children to that spot and allowed them to run freely and enjoy the panoramic view while safe and secure. Rather than functioning as a barrier to free play, the guard rail actually facilitated unrestricted enjoyment of the beautiful falls without worry.

Consistently we find correlation between the importance of a project and the stringency of the protocols surrounding it; the higher the stakes, the more elaborate the safety features employed. Doctors and nurses merely sanitize their hands; surgeons, on the other hand, scrub up before entering the operating room. When we remember that, ultimately, we are *neshamot* in bodies rather that bodies that happen to have souls, we become more aware of how thankful we should be for the *halachot*, for the protocols, for the seatbelts and the guardrails, that safeguard the health of our *neshamot*.

Chassidut illuminates a deeper strata of understanding.

The Rebbe teaches that a Jew can draw an *or pnimi*, an immanent or "internal" celestial light into this world through her observance of *mitzvot asei*, positive actions.[10] There is, however, an aspect of Hashem that transcends what we as limited human beings can access through our actions. That is why Hashem gives us *mitzvot lo taaseh*, the prohibitions. When we desist or abstain, we make room for a higher type of energy; we allow the *or makif*, the transcendent light, to manifest. Put differently, nothingness–absence of action or expression–provides the contourless vessel that holds infinity.

By way of analogy a person can light a candle, even many candles, but they cannot cause the sun to shine; that is beyond our ken.[11] We can, however, remove the impediment to the sunlight by opening the window curtains so that the warmth and illumination (the *or makif*) can flood the room and our lives. When we think in these terms it is easier for us to embrace the prohibitions that are for many of us a challenging aspect of *taharat hamishpachah*.

In a teaching that is thematically related, the Tzemach Tzedek explains that the first letters of the verse from *Tehillim*, נאלמתי דומיה החשיתי, I made myself speechless in

---

[10] *Likkutei Sichot*, vol. 5. p. 224. *Sefer Hasichot* 5751. vol. 1. pp. 305-308. That this particular light can be absorbed in a vessel reflects its limitedness. Similarly, that a *mitzvat asei* - a prescribed action with particular motions, time, and protocol – elicits this light bespeaks a limitation in the light itself.

[11] *Torat Menachem*, vol. 40. p. 208.

silence,[12] form an acrostic for the word נדה *nidah*.[13] In so doing, he takes us far beyond the conventional definition of the term *nidah*, as physically removed or set apart, to an understanding of a higher reality.

The word *nidah* is made up of the three Hebrew letters: *nun, daled, hei* and can be read as a contraction of two words: *nad* and *hei*. *Nidah*, the Tzemach Tzedek explains, describes a spiritual plane in which the *hei* is distanced or set apart. Of which *hei* do we speak? And set apart from what? The *hei* here refers to the final *hei* in the *Shem Havaya*, the name of G-d often referred to as the Tetragrammaton, which is distanced from the three letters that precede it.

The first three letters of *Shem Havayah, the yud, hei and vov*, represent only the potential for outward expression, while the final *hei*, represents impact upon others through speech and actualized expression.[14] The profound mystery and mystique of *nidah* reflects a spiritual state which manifests in the form of metaphoric silence, a lack of external expression.

There are two types of silence: a cold and hostile one, and one born of a depth of emotion that words cannot contain. There are times when every type of conceivable expression will fall short and sully the truth.

In this way, a woman's state of *nidah,* a time during which the couple cannot give full outward expression to the love they share, honors the depth of a couple's oneness; the unity that defies expression. It is a time to focus on the inner secret of this oneness; to step back and focus on a startling truth: Their *neshamah* is interlocked of two components – hers and his – in a way that transcends manifestation.

These teachings introduce a new way of understanding prohibitions. Sometimes, a no is more positive than a yes. Silence can say more than words. When we step back and out of the way, we create room for something larger.

When we choose not to be in the arms of our spouse because we want to fulfill the *Ratzon Ha'Elyon,* we find ourselves nestled in Hashem's embrace.

---

12   *Tehillim* 39:3.

13   *Yahel Or* on *Tehillim* 39:3.

14   In Kabalistic terminology this would be referred to as *malchut* which connotes engagement with an audience outside the self. In a similar vein, *malchut* is associated with Divine speech, and one speaks only when there is another, outside the self, to address.

YOU MIGHT BE THINKING:

Being in nidah is extremely difficult for me; I am moody, lonely, and resentful. Do you have any practical suggestions?

Being in *nidah* can be very tough. While we can bond with our husbands via a number of means, and it is healthy to experience variability in this dynamic of the relationship, taking physical touch out of the equation entails a significant shift.

It is important to own that being in *nidah* can be difficult, while at the same time acknowledging that missing your husband's touch is a positive thing. There is nothing wrong with you if you hate the fact that you cannot touch each other, and you are downright cranky. That's normal and good and healthy. It speaks well of your relationship.

At the same time, it's integral to remember that *nidah* time is not when we put our emotional intimacy on hold. Indeed the Gemara[15] makes exactly this point when it talks about disrupting a couple's privacy and closeness, even during times when they cannot be physically intimate:

אמר רב ברונא אמר רב, כל הישן בקילעא שאיש ואשתו שרויין בה, עליו הכתוב אומר (מיכה ב, ט) "נשי עמי תגרשון מבית תענוגיה". ואמר רב יוסף, אפילו באשתו נדה (עירובין סג ע"ב).

Rav Beruna said in the name of Rav: Whoever sleeps in a chamber in which a husband and wife are resting [thus thwarting their intimacy], the verse says about him: "You cast the women of my people out from their pleasant houses." Rav Yosef said: This applies [not only to a woman who is ritually pure and permitted to her husband, but] even in the case of a man whose wife is menstruating [for even then, although she is prohibited to him, they are more comfortable being alone together].

Irrespective of which end of the cycle they find themselves in, there is so much a couple can do together, and, as noted, there are other forms of closeness to be nurtured at this time. Indeed, the *harchakah* period lends itself to honing communication and relationship-building skills. Having to express the full gamut of emotions without touching skins forces the couple to dig deeper within

---

15 *Eruvin* 63b.

themselves to bridge the gap left by the temporary cessation of physical intimacy. In so doing, they infuse a whole new level of emotional intimacy in their eventual physical reunion. In turn, that heightened and emotionally resonant lovemaking tides them over the next time they need to withdraw physically. In this way, the two poles of the monthly cycle, *taharah* and *nidah*, nourish each other, and, together, strengthen the relationship.

Resist the urge to attribute your *kvetchy* mood to *dinei harchakah* alone.

If you suffer from pain and/or hormonal swings, consider that there are herbs, exercises, and dietary changes that can help alleviate your discomfort. You want to be a happy person, a happy wife, and a happy mother.

At the same time, if necessary, process your emotions and address them. Studies show that recording your feelings in writing, as opposed to typing or even verbally expressing them, can help you understand the underlying cause of your irritation, be it fear of disconnection, loneliness, and/or the need for comfort.[16] You may even be experiencing two opposite feelings at once: that of enjoying healthy space and, at the same time, that of pining for physical affirmation. Sometimes, feelings are intense, such as in the face of tragedy and/or loss, *chas v'shalom*. In these moments, you may feel anger at the "unfairness" of the *halacha* that prohibits you from finding comfort in your husband's touch. Especially when your feelings are strong and multi-faceted, journaling in small increments, so you can identify each feeling and find a way to address each one as needed, can be very helpful.

Communicate with your husband; tell him what he can do to make this time easier for you, and, thus for you both. While sweeping changes usually prove untenable, some simple, specific, easy to incorporate action items may go a long way. At the same time, it's inherently unfair to put the onus of resolving your feelings squarely on your husband.

There are many ways you can boost your mood and change your mindset. Be attentive to your patterns; understanding what can stimulate the secretion of hormones normally triggered by physical touch can be enormously helpful.

Your brain releases dopamine when it expects a reward. This happens when you come to associate a certain activity with pleasure. For this reason, it is often

---

[16] Many of these ideas are based on a workshop by Dr. Miriam Gross LMFT, Brooklyn, NY available on Mikvah.org/audio.

referred to as the reward chemical and is linked to motivation. Identify what forms of self-care will bring you pleasure, and make sure it happens. It can be a mani-pedi, a massage, some shopping, celebrating a special event with a friend, completing a task you have had on your to-do list for some time, reading that great novel everyone is talking about, or even just calling someone you love with whom you have not spoken in a while.

Serotonin is a mood stabilizer released through various forms of exercise as well as meditation and mindfulness. You might want to include some form thereof in your everyday routine, especially during your time of *nidah*.

Endorphins are hormonal painkillers or blockers. You can stimulate their release through laughter and dark chocolate, among other things, to help ease the time.

Finally, oxytocin, the love and bonding hormone, can be stimulated by playing with a baby or any aged child, holding hands with someone, giving a compliment, and even giving yourself a hug!

The important thing is to find effective, prophylactic means that prevent you from falling into a rut of self-pity and irritability. Get practical instead of resentful. Plan purposeful projects you can enjoy with your husband during this time. You can learn together, visit relatives, go bulk shopping, take a walk, do a bit of extra house maintenance, play games, enjoy a paint night, watch a skills-based *shalom bayit* lecture together, and once you start a family, spend extra time with your children. For some couples, especially newlyweds or empty nesters, this is a perfect opportunity to spend more time with friends.

Generally, our disappointments and lack of satisfaction are rooted in unmet expectations. When we understand and remind ourselves that Hashem wants this temporary cessation of physical intimacy, we reorient our emotions to a healthier balance. We understand that our spouse is not withholding something from us, but rather, together, as a team, we are building something larger than ourselves.

Some women are bothered only minimally by the *harchakot* and find it easy to adapt. If you fit into this category, it does not mean your relationship or intimate life is stale or lacking. Everyone is different. You may simply enjoy your own space at times and like the interval of alone time.

If, however, you unduly enjoy this time, if you find yourself anticipating becoming *nidah*, you might want to think about why you would rather run from physical expression. Conversely, if you find the *dinei harchakah* inordinately difficult, even after trying the various techniques mentioned here, a deeper dynamic than simple chafing under the onus of a new discipline may be at work. If, in general, emotional intimacy and proper communication prove difficult for you, you may find the period of physical abstinence especially challenging. A *frum* marriage counselor or sex therapist can be helpful in addressing these issues.

It is entirely normal for the system of *harchakot* to feel awkward and occupy a lot of head space at the very beginning. Like with everything else new, it will take some time before this on-again, off-again rhythm becomes second nature.

If you are feeling self-conscious about the *dinei harchakah* when you are a *nidah*, remember who you are, and take pride in your *yirat shamayim*. Let others think what they may. In truth, the only people who will notice such subtleties are those who are, themselves, aware of the *halachot*. Either they do the same thing, or your example will remind them of the appropriate course of action. It is a win-win proposition.

In keeping *dinei harchakah* you are making the statement that Hashem is the senior partner in your marriage and you welcome that partnership *b'simchah u'b'tuv leivav*, with happiness and gladness of heart. With time and experience, it becomes easier and less onerous to keep the *halachot* discreetly. Every couple finds their groove with *dinei harchakah*; you will too. As you age, as your life circumstances continue to evolve, you will likely continue to assess your behaviors during this time and tweak accordingly.

For a woman coming off of her period, the *shivah nekiyim* might not feel unduly long; most of us do not pine for sexual intimacy while menstruating. And many women appropriate the *shivah nekiyim* as their sacred cocoon of "me" time. You can use this time to pamper yourself, body, mind, and soul. Enjoy more sleep, indulge in some self-care, and tune into your inner landscape.

For a man, the time of separation will invariably feel longer, and the wait may be more challenging. For both men and women, each for their own reasons, navigating the tightrope of emotional intimacy while not giving physical expression an outlet can be hard. Each person must recognize their tipping point, and each couple must find the proper balance for this time. It can be a time of tension, but tension also builds titillation. It is certainly a time for that type of *daat* mentioned earlier: other-centered consciousness. It is a time to show appreciation and compassion; to be attentive and accepting of our spouse's faults. It is the perfect time to model devotion, dedication, and flexibility; to be especially generous and forgiving, and to express gratitude. It's harder to broadcast sympathy, empathy, and validation without physical touch, but it is eminently doable. A sincere compliment, a gentle reminder, and a heartfelt statement of trust are just some of the ways we can offer a loving embrace. For some couples, resolving to go to sleep at the same time can be a form of emotional intimacy and help them feel less estranged, while for other couples, this may not be a possibility due to divergent schedules and other reasons. The important thing is to find what works for you.

Here is a good question to ask yourself: Is it physical intimacy and togetherness that *creates* our sense of closeness, or are our physical expressions of affection an important and distinct *manifestation* of our essential closeness and love for each other? If it is the first, how can I use our *nidah* time to bring us closer in the ways that matter most so that when we return to our physical expression of love, it is a deeper, more soulful, and even more enjoyable experience?

Rivkah: Although decades have passed, and so much has happened since that time, I am still as blown away by this vignette as I was at the moment of its occurrence; the exchange is as fresh in my mind as if it happened today.

The scene is the Women's Center at Our Lady of Lourdes hospital in Binghamton, NY. It was minutes after I had delivered a baby boy, and the nurses were cleaning me up. One nurse casually said: "Can I ask you a question? " To which I replied, "sure!"

"I am just curious," she tentatively began, "and it's really none of my business, but I am just so perplexed. You and the doctor embraced after your birth; you are clearly close with her. And you did the same with your doula. Why...what about your husband?"

Before I could open my mouth to launch into a mini-lecture on the laws of *taharat hamishpachah*, the other nurse in the room injected herself and said to her coworker, "Did you not see the look that passed between them when her husband came back into the room after the baby was born? Boy, did they ever hug!" I was taken aback by how deeply she understood this truth: there is more than one way to express love, devotion, and support. There are physical hugs and kisses, and then there are exchanges that nourish us just as well, or even more deeply.

Authors' note: The Rebbe's *ahavat Yisrael* was legendary; his love for every person simply defies description. Two particularly interesting and poignant expressions thereof include the Rebbe's passionate focus on the scrupulous observance of the *mitzvot* of *kisui rosh* and *pru u'rvu*. A survey of the Rebbe's words and his activism in this sphere reveals, in an almost shocking fashion, just how fervently the Rebbe desired to pour *brachot* into our lives. The Rebbe's words also illustrate his profound understanding of human nature, and how, in a painstakingly sensitive fashion, he sought to resolve and allay varied concerns associated with these *mitzvot*.

Because the Rebbe spoke and wrote about these subjects at such great length and with such passion, we would be cheating you, our respected reader, if we simply synopsized the general ideas. Despite the increasing prevalence of "clips" or "sound grabs", some subjects defy treatment in such a manner. In addition to providing historic context, in the following two chapters, we present to you below – just a drop in the proverbial bucket of – the Rebbe's words on these subjects, with minimal editorializing on our part. We do, however, preface the survey of the Rebbe's words with practical questions and answers.

---

* In the following two essays we reference many of the Rebbe's letters and *sichos*. Since some of these writings have not yet been published in *Toras Menachem*, we have opted to reference them by date.

chapter eight

Hide and Seek:
THE MITZVAH OF KISUI ROSH

A woman's hair is the most striking aspect of her beauty, setting the tone of her overall appearance. The Torah relates how Hashem fashioned Chava after separating her from the back-to-back, dimorphous existence she originally shared with Adam: ויבן ה' אלקים את הצלע אשר לקח מן האדם לאשה, Hashem *Elokim* built the side that He took from Adam into a woman.[1] In commenting on the word *vayiven* in this verse that describes the moment prior to Adam and Chava's first face-to-face encounter, Rabbi Shimon ben Menasya teaches that the Holy One, Blessed be He, braided Chava's hair before presenting her to Adam.[2] From the beginning of time, beauty and the pains it takes to achieve it has been intrinsic to the female experience.

Thus, it should come as no surprise that many young women fully committed to *halacha*, and even to *minhagei chassidut* and Chabad, find it difficult to embrace the mitzvah of *kisui rosh*. Making the transition to a reality in which your hair will never or rarely be exposed to the sun or be blown by the wind is hard. While there are conveniences that come with wearing a *sheitel*, like perfect hair ready to be popped on at a moment's notice, there is simultaneously an unquantifiable constraint that comes with it.

---

[1] *Bereishit* 2:22.

[2] *Shabbat* 95a.

An additional challenge is that even in this day and age of increased Torah study for women as well as men, there are still many observant individuals who do not realize the immense importance of this mitzvah. *Kisui rosh* is often abandoned out of a lack of knowledge and understanding. While this book does not present *halachic* sources and analysis, we present below the five most often asked questions on this subject and make reference to *halachic* sources that we strongly urge our readers to pursue in depth.

Additionally, understanding *kisui rosh* through the prism of the Rebbe's teachings on the subject can help us appreciate the centrality of this mitzvah and its monumental impact on our families. Here, as ever, the Rebbe's approach blends a keen understanding of contemporary concerns with steadfast anchoring in age-old *halacha*. Against this backdrop, the Rebbe emerged as a unique and tireless champion of the modern *sheitel*.

The Top Five Questions People Ask About Kisui Rosh

Authors' note: Different communities have embraced varied *minhagim* in regard to *kisui rosh*, and many opinions exist regarding the specifics of this mitzvah. What we present below is the Rebbe's view which is the accepted *hanhagah* among Chabad Chassidim. The Rebbe's wisdom and blessings are relevant to all, even to those who observe differently. We recommend that each woman consult with her rabbinic authorities as to practical application of the *halacha*.

1. I heard that a married woman covers her hair to "reserve it" specifically for her husband. Is that the reason for the mitzvah of kisui rosh?

There is no reason given in the Torah for why a married woman must cover her hair other than it is Hashem's will. Torah law forbids exposure of the hair of the head by women who are married or were once married (i.e. widows and divorcees) in the public thoroughfare.[3] The *Shulchan Aruch* states[4] לא תלכנה בנות ישראל פרועות ראש בשוק אחד פנויה ואחד אשת איש, Jewish women should not go with uncovered head in the marketplace. The *Aruch Hashulchan* explains ואחת אחת פנויה כגון אלמנה וגרושה, אשת איש, ולילך פרועת ראש ברה"ר אסור מן התורה, the term unmarried women refers to women once married i.e. widows and divorcees[5]… and to married women. To go with uncovered hair in a public thoroughfare is forbidden from the Torah.[6]

---

3   *Tur* and *Shulchan Aruch, Even Ha'ezer* 21:2 and 115:4; *Ketubot* 72a; *Sifri Naso* 11; *Bamidbar Rabbah* 9:16; *Rambam, Ishut* 24:11-12; *Isurei Biah* 21:17. *Smag* Positive Commandment 48.

4   *Shulchan Aruch, Even Ha'ezer* 21:2

5   If the need arises, each woman should consult with her Rav on this matter.

6   *Shulchan Aruch, Even Ha'ezer* 21:4

Hide and Seek: The Mitzvah of Kisui Rosh

A survey of primary sources reveals no reason for this prohibition. There does, however, seem to be a connection between hair covering and loss of virginity.[7] The hair of a *betulah*, a virgin woman, irrespective of her age, is not considered *ervah*, which is the *halachic* term for nakedness, or an aspect of the body considered to be erotic. With marriage, however, a woman is initiated into sexual experience. When she taps into the power inherent in intimacy, the need for an additional aspect of *tzniut* emerges, which is *kisui rosh*.

While there might be poignance and beauty in framing hair covering within the exclusive marital bond, that is not the reason for hair covering, or covering other parts of our bodies referred to in *halachic* terms as *ervah*.[8] Simply put, the exposure of *ervah* contravenes the axiom of *tzniut*.

This mitzvah is inferred from words in *Parshat Naso*,[9] והעמיד הכהן את האשה לפני ה' ופרע את ראש האשה, and the *Kohen* will place the woman before Hashem and he shall uncover the woman's hair. The context of this *passuk* is the description of the protocols surrounding an *Isha Sota*, the suspected adulteress. Rashi explains that in an effort to tire out the woman, lower her defenses, and get her to admit to her sin, she is led from place to place and humiliated. This act of public humiliation sheds a light on the Torah perspective that for a married Jewish woman to expose her hair is shameful. While the *Mishna* fills in additional details such as tearing away the clothing from upon her upper body, the Torah mentions only the exposure of her hair. Apparently, a married woman's bare head is considered the quintessential act of exposure, the single most effective technique for persuading the woman to confess.[10]

In his essential distillation of all of Torah, the *Navi* Michah taught הגיד לך אדם מה טוב ומה ה' דורש ממך כי אם עשות משפט ואהבת חסד והצנע לכת עם אלקיך, [Hashem] has told you, O man, what is good and what Hashem requires of you: Only to do justice, to love goodness, and to walk modestly with your G-d.[11]

Tzniut is not an outfit; it is a worldview. It begins with a constant consciousness of Hashem's presence that fills all time and space. This is why *tzniut* is necessary even

---

7 Tamar put a scarf upon her head after Amnon violated her. *Shmuel II* 13:19; *Bamidbar Rabbah* 9:33.

8 *Shulchan Aruch, Orach Chaim* 75:2. *Even Ha'ezer* 21:1-2.

9 *Bamidbar* 5:18.

10 For a comprehensive overview, tracing the *halachot* of *kisui rosh* from the Torah, through *Mishna*, and Gemara all the way to *Shulchan Aruch* and contemporary *poskim*, see thebatshevalearningcenter.com/textbooks *Kisui Rosh*.

11 *Michah* 6:8.

when we are alone and even in the dark.[12] And it is certainly about carrying ourselves with dignity befitting the daughter of the King of all Kings, when we are with others.

We do not cover our hair to keep it special for our husband, just as we do not cover other private aspects of our body for that reason. A married woman covers her hair to walk with her Creator.

2. *If a sheitel looks just as good or better than your hair, especially with the newest sheitlach looking like they are 'growing out of your scalp', what is the point of a sheitel?*

The Torah mandates that a married woman must cover her hair, and a sheitel allows a woman to do exactly that. Questioning the efficacy of an extremely natural looking *sheitel* is based on the mistaken premise that a *sheitel* is meant to detract from a woman's beauty. This idea is likely connected to the erroneous notion that a woman's hair is covered for the purpose of reserving it for her husband. In fact, if a woman's hair and beauty are solely to be enjoyed by her husband, it might be the case that a *sheitel* or other hair covering should diminish her attractiveness in the eyes of others. This is, however, most definitely not the case.

Beyond questions about the beauty of a *sheitel*, there seems to be concern with just how closely some *sheitlach* resemble a woman's natural hair. In this vein, some argue that wigs might be just as erotically stimulating as one's natural hair, assuming that dynamic poses a *halachic* problem. Centuries ago this very issue was addressed quite pointedly by *Poskim*: The *Shiltei Giborim* wrote that the principle that the sight of a woman's hair constitutes *ervah*, שער באשה ערוה, an erotic stimulus[13], applies only to the hair visibly connected to her scalp but not to natural wigs.[14] Neither does use of such wigs constitute leaving the hair uncovered. It seems to make no difference whether the wig is made of her own hair or from that of another woman, as long as it is made as a hair covering, and is unconnected to her scalp.[15]

Halacha mandates that a married woman's hair must be covered. As to exactly how it should be covered, various *shitot,* opinions, give rise to differing *minhagim*. As long as a woman's hair is completely covered, how she achieves that goal is a matter

---

12 *Kitzur Shulchan Aruch* 3:1.

13 *Brachot* 24a.

14 *Shiltei Giborim* on *Rif, Shabbat* 375.

15 Some Rabbonim prefer that a certain percentage of hair that is not her own be interwoven in such a wig.

of her choice, provided her method does not contravene the *minhag* of her family or community.

The Rebbe's opinion on this matter is abundantly clear. During a *farbrengen* the Rebbe noted:

> **The wearing of wigs became a widespread custom—especially today, when one can buy wigs in many colors, which may look even nicer than one's own hair.**[16]

The Rebbe encouraged women to buy the most beautiful *sheitlach* they could acquire, even paying for some of these *sheitlach* himself (see the stories below). Still, a wig should reflect her overall *tzniut*; modesty and beauty are not mutually exclusive. For example, lacetop wigs look extremely natural and beautiful; that in and of itself is not problematic. From a modesty standpoint, the *sheitel* should however, have a lining sewn underneath the netting section where a woman's hair might be exposed through the small openings so that her natural hair is covered.

No matter how natural a wig might look, *halachically*, it is still not analogous to natural hair attached to the scalp. Rabbi Ovadya Hadaya wrote that man is tempted only by things attached directly to the body of a woman herself, for those things have life. Once the hair is separated from her, it ceases to be forbidden.[17]

The Kabbalistic explanation for the mitzvah of *kisui rosh* adds additional depth to these *halachic* conclusions.

3. What about marit ayin,[18] people mistakenly thinking that my hair is uncovered? Wouldn't a hat or tichel be a better option for obviating this concern?

While some *halachic* authorities express concerns about a hair covering appearing too much like one's hair, *halacha l'maaseh,* practically, most *poskim* concur with the words of the *Shiltei Giborim* who said "Although the wig is an adornment creating the impression of uncovered hair, this poses no problem."[19]

---

16   *Rosh Chodesh* Elul, 1954.

17   *Yaskil Avdi,* vol. 7, *Even Ha'ezer* 16.

18   The concept in *halacha* which states that certain actions which might seem to observers to be in violation of *halacha,* but in reality are fully permissible, are themselves not allowed due to *gezeirot* that were put in place to prevent onlookers from arriving at a false conclusion.

19   For *halachic* sources which discuss natural-looking and specifically, human-hair wigs, and find them unobjectionable, see *Shiltei Giborim* on *Rif,* Shabbat 29a. *Yaskil Avdi,* vol. 7, *Even Ha'ezer* 16. *Igrot Moshe,* vol. 4, *Even Ha'ezer* II, 12.

The Rebbe's focus was squarely on ensuring complete coverage of a woman's hair in a way that was practical and reflected her aesthetic preferences. While the Rebbe's position was seen as stringent, some considered his stance a lenient one. In some communities, wigs are not deemed *halachically* acceptable at all based on their similarity to a woman's hair. In others, women do wear wigs but cover them partially with a scarf or hat so as to signal that they *are* covering their hair. The Rebbe believed that there was no *halachic* obligation to cover the wig.[20] In one of many letters on this subject the Rebbe wrote:

> **As to her wearing an exposed wig (a wig with no hat or other covering over it)—for the past several generations, this practice has become widely accepted. Understandably, however, it is necessary to ascertain the custom of your place so as to ensure that this does not constitute breaking a precedent, G-d forbid.**[21, 22]

On the other hand, the Rebbe was concerned with an aesthetic look that could lead some to think that hair was covered only partially. For instance, Mrs. Esther Sternberg, director of the Lubavitch Women's Candle Lighting campaign, related[23] that when the candle lighting guide was prepared for the year 1984, some felt that the model on the cover should wear a covering over her wig so that it was clear that she was covering her hair; additionally, a covering on a woman's head (very often made of lace) stirred memories for many of a grandmother or mother who lit candles. Once the brochure was printed, however, some commented on the fact that the covering on the model's wig left some of the hair uncovered. Mrs. Sternberg turned to the Rebbe to ask him what should be done. The Rebbe instructed that going forward, the cover photo should feature a woman wearing a wig only and not a kerchief atop her wig. For that year, since 500,000 brochures had already been printed, the brochures were sent back to the press and a sentence: "The woman in the photograph above is wearing a *sheitel.*" was imprinted directly under the photo.

---

[20] Yet, the Rebbe encouraged women who hailed from various chassidic communities to maintain the custom of their mothers vis a vis *kisui rosh*, even after they had adopted a Chabad lifestyle.

[21] *Igrot Kodesh*, vol. 16, pp. 330–331, dated 10 Adar, 1958.

[22] The Rebbe was not castigating previous generations of women who had covered their heads with scarves, as there is no *essential* advantage to the wig over the scarf. As far back as Talmudic times, women wore a *redid*, a larger scarf over a smaller hat, that covered their heads. As such, even if hair protruded from the first hair covering, the strands were covered by the *redid*, as delineated in *Ketubot* 72a.

[23] Related to the authors by Mrs. Sternberg in a 2022 interview.

Finally, Rabbi Moshe Feinstein, a leading American *posek* during the 20th century, negated the concern of *marit ayin* in his responsum on this exact issue, listing three reasons in support of his stance.[24] First, since there is no prohibition against this in the Gemara, there is no grounds for prohibiting it. Second, people can (especially women), in most cases, discern the difference between natural hair and a wig. Finally, it is common knowledge that wigs exist and might be worn as a hair covering.[25]

4. *I have heard that it is not, strictly speaking, necessary to cover one's hair while at home, and that when out and about, some hair can be exposed. Can you help me understand the differing opinions on these two matters?*

For Lubavitcher women, carefully covering the hair at all times is a matter of *halacha* and not only a *minhag*, as per the *psak* of the Tzemach Tzedek:

> **Privately in the presence of her husband, a woman is permitted to expose 'side hairs' which extend beyond her tichel (i.e. her payot - the hair growing in front of her upper ear). While other men are present, however, there is no heter at all to do so.**
>
> **For hair protruding beyond the tichel is halachically identical with ervah, nakedness, just as (or even more severe than) the exposure of the leg....**
>
> **Exposure of the hair outside the tichel is pritzut, licentiousness. Regarding the custom to do so, it is written: [the word] Minhag is comprised of the same letters as gehinom...**
>
> **To expose even the least bit of hair is absolutely prohibited... May this practice be eradicated forever.**[26]

For women who are not Lubavitch, we encourage you to speak with your *posek* regarding this issue. For all of our readers, we present the *halachic* background so you can understand the source of the varied opinions.

---

24 *Igrot Moshe*, vol. 4, *Even Ha'ezer* II, 12.

25 This same logic is at work in a *kashrut* related context. For the first few decades after the manufacture of non dairy creamers, kosher caterers routinely put a sign on the tables at *smachot* informing the guests that the coffee creamer and desserts were not dairy. This is no longer necessary as there is a proliferation of non dairy milk substitutes on the market and everyone is aware of this.

26 Quoted from *Tzemach Tzedek*, Responsa *Even Ha'ezer* 139 and 363; Responsa *Yoreh Dei'ah* 93:10, *Chiddushim Al Hashas* to *Brachot*, ch. 3.

For a married woman to be *b'shuk,* in the public thoroughfare, with her hair completely uncovered is an *issur d'orayta,* otherwise referred to as a trespass of *dat Moshe;* if her hair is partially uncovered, she trespasses *dat Yehudit.* The Mishna rules that a woman who trespasses *dat Moshe* or *dat Yehudit* is divorced with forfeiture of her *ketubah,* alimony.[27] The Rambam writes that a woman who exits her home with exposed hair and enters a public space violates *dat Moshe.*[28]

Regarding a woman whilst in her home, the Gemara relates the story of Kimchit, a famous righteous woman from the Second Temple period.[29] She had seven sons all of whom served as *Kohanim Gedolim.*[30] When asked what she did to deserve this remarkable *zechut,* she replied: "the walls of my house have never seen the braids of my head." This Gemara coupled with the *Zohar* form the basis of the *halachic* discussion regarding hair covering while at home.[31]

Although some *Poskim* maintain that a woman need not cover her hair at home, many conclude that a woman's hair should remain covered at all times.

The *Rama* wrote that it is considered modest for a woman never to reveal her hair even at home, as we find regarding Kimchit, who was rewarded for this.[32] The *Magen Avraham* references the *Zohar* when he urges women to cover their hair even while at home.[33] The *Mishnah Berurah* quotes the *Zohar* as well.[34] The *Bach,* going further, wrote: Leaving the hair entirely uncovered is forbidden, even if she remains in her courtyard…Among Jews the world over, even before the men of her household, a woman will not appear without a kerchief and head covering.[35] And the *Chatam Sofer,* going further still, wrote that a wife requires a kerchief even in her own room.[36]

---

[27] *Ketubot* 7:6.

[28] *Rambam, Ishut* 24:11.

[29] *Yoma* 47a.

[30] Kimchit's son, Rabbi Yishmael, the regular *Kohen Gadol,* was ineligible to serve due to temporary impurity. Over time, each of his brothers had the opportunity to substitute for him as *kohen Gadol.* (*Tosafot Yeshanim, ad loc*)

[31] Rabbi Yehuda said that the exposed hairs on the head of a woman cause another kind of hair [of the *sefirah* of *malchut*] to be exposed [to external impure forces] and impair her. Therefore, a woman should be careful that none of her hair is visible even to the beams of her house, and all the more so outside.

[32] *Darkei Moshe, Even Ha'ezer* 115:4.

[33] The exact words of the Magen Avraham are: But the *Zohar* (*Nasso* p. 239) is very stringent that not a single hair of a woman should be seen and thus it is fitting to practice. (*Magen Avraham, Orach Chaim* 75:4)

[34] 75:14.

[35] *Bach, Even Ha'ezer* 115.

[36] Responsa *Chatam Sofer, Orach Chaim* 36.

From a practical standpoint, the Rebbe reminded us:

> **Repeatedly acting in a certain manner causes it to become second nature. It is possible to forget oneself and act in this manner even when someone else is in the house, then one does this as well in the yard, then on the street! Because it has become a habit, one is not aware.**[37]

He also taught:

> **Since this tale [regarding Kimchit] is related to us by the Oral Torah, it follows that this is not just a story of something that transpired in the past, for "that which has passed is past." Rather, it comes to teach every Jewish daughter how much she is to scrupulously observe tzniut, even when there is no one else in the house, etc. For the Aibershter is in the house with the Aibershter's Torah and the Aibershter's tzniut.**[38],[39]

The Rebbe tirelessly reiterated that this *hanhagah*, behavior, is a wondrous conduit for blessings in our life. May we see these *brachot* come to fruition *b'tov hanireh v'hanigleh*, in a most open and revealed manner.

5. I have heard that the Zohar emphasizes the importance of a married woman's hair being completely covered, and teaches that abundant blessings flow to the woman, her husband, and her children in this merit. Which Kabbalistic teachings can help me understand the importance of this mitzvah?

The mystical implications of a married woman keeping her hair scrupulously covered go beyond ordinary considerations of modesty. The *Zohar's* position connects to broader Kabbalistic ideas according to which hair – most generally – and a married woman's hair, in particular, is associated with *dinim*, harsh judgment, and is thus uniquely vulnerable to *kelipah*, negative energies. A married woman's scrupulousness

---

[37] *Chai Elul*, 5742.

[38] *Chai Elul*, 5742.

[39] Even if it were solely about fulfilling the Rebbe's *horaah*, we have been taught (20 Av, 5710) that a *minhag* that a Rebbe establishes is a *d'orayta* for his chassidim. The Rebbe made it crystal clear that this is what he wanted of us, and for us. In a letter that the Rebbe wrote on Gimmel Tammuz, 1950, he defined the term *nassi* as one who "radiates both inward and encompassing influence – in Torah, in *avodah*, and in the practice of good deeds; and conveys blessings both spiritual and material."

in covering her hair acts not only as a protective device in warding off these unwelcome energies, but as a conduit for the most important *brachot* in life.

Before we can understand the spiritual implications of hair in Kabbalistic teachings, it is helpful to remind ourselves how Kabbalah works, more generally speaking. An apt metaphor might be the microscope, an instrument that provides an enlarged image of a small object, thus revealing details too small to be seen by the naked eye. As with every other aspect of existence, Kabbalistic teachings approach the topic of hair seeking to understand its ability to attract or conversely repel spiritual energies. Perhaps surprisingly, hair occupies a rather prominent place in Kabbalistic teachings and practice.

The forces of *kelipah* – translated literally as husks or shells, forces that cover and conceal the Divine oneness that underpins all of creation – are always seeking access to *kedushah*, especially through the Jewish body. To persist and flourish, the *sitra achra*, the other side, of which *kelipah* is a part, must siphon vivifying energy from the side of holiness. *Kelipot* can be compared, for example, to weeds which will never be watered by the owner of the garden, and must therefore derive their succor from the water poured lovingly over the rose bush.

The inherent *kedushah* of a Jew, however, repels these unholy seekers or parasites, overwhelming them with holy light, thus keeping them at bay. The hair, however, different from all other aspects of the anatomy, is not connected to the brain; it has neither nerve endings nor blood vessels.[40] Not quite alive but not completely dead, hair holds the minutest amount of living energy. In Kabbalistic terms, we would associate this minimized energy with the process of *tzimtzum*, contraction. As such, hair provides the only port of entry for the *kelipot* who seek desperately to siphon energy from the holy. Hair also provides the *kelipot* with the energy in a proportion they can comfortably ingest. *Tzimtzum*, which derives from Hashem's power to limit or withhold, gives rise to *dinim* or *gevurot*, severity, and often deleterious energies. *Tzimtzum* needs to be handled with great care.

To understand how this relates to the mitzvah of *kisui rosh*, it is helpful to review the Kabbalistic teachings concerning a man's hair.[41] These writings emphasize the need for a man to keep his hair short, in this way guarding against providing the *kelipot*

---

[40] Tiny blood vessels at the base of every follicle feed the hair root to keep it growing. Once the hair is at the skin's surface, the cells within the strand of hair aren't alive anymore. This is why we feel no pain when our hair is cut.

[41] The following is based on the book *HaShabbat* by Rabbi Y. Karasik. Vol 1 p. 165-179.

For an in depth study, refer to the extensive sources referenced in this book on page 166 footnotes 8, 10 and more.

with a place to take root and from which to siphon energy *(Yenikat Hachitzonim)*.[42] A male's long hair attracts and beckons to the *kelipot*; their presence on one's person can precipitate all types of spiritual ill effects. This scenario, Kabbalistic writings warn, must be avoided.[43]

There is, however, no mention in Kabbalistic literature of the spiritual qualities of a female's hair separate and apart from the hair of a married woman. What accounts for this difference, and what changes vis a vis a woman's hair when she marries?

To answer those questions, we need to reference one of the most basic of all Kabbalistic axioms. We are taught that the entire world was created in binary fashion, with the *mashpia* and *mekabel* as perhaps the most prominent binary in the system. Generally, the masculine is associated with the modality of *mashpia*, bestowal, or filling, while the feminine modality is associated with receiving, providing vessels that welcome the bounty. We can now understand why, when the *kelipot* seek to parasitically feed, they will approach the male; they are drawn to the source of bestowal. The female's hair, on the other hand, holds no such attraction for the *kelipot*.

All of this changes, however, when a woman enters marriage. At that time, husband and wife become, in the *Zohar's* holy words, *chad gufa*, two halves of one body, in addition to two halves of a soul.[44] Given this "new body" from which to draw succor – comprised of both a male and female aspect – the *kelipot* prefer to feed off of the woman's hair. This is because, Kabbalistically, the feminine is associated with the *sefira* of *malchut*, the final *sefirah* of the ten *sefirot* and the one associated with the most intense contraction of Hashem's light.[45] As noted, hair connotes *tzimtzum*. Women's rootedness in the *sefirah* of *malchut*, also associated with *tzimtzum*, creates *tzimtzum* within *tzimtzum or tzimtzum* to the second degree. Thus, a married woman's hair proves especially appealing to *kelipah* in that, through marriage, she absorbs the more abundant energy of the *mashpia* but, at the same time, makes this energy available in bite-sized or doubly contracted dosages. The holy energies, delivered in tiny increments make a woman's hair perfectly conducive for *kelipot* seeking nurture. By means of analogy, consider a sippy cup for a toddler or, even before that, how small the hole in the nipple must be to accomodate the newborn. We note that while Kabbalistically a

---

[42] *Pelle Yoetz, Likutei shoshana Parshat Naso* by the *Noam Elimelech, Tzava'at Reb Yehuda Hachassid*.

[43] In sharp contradistinction, a man's beard attracts and facilitates the downward flow of spiritual bounty.

[44] *Zohar* III 7b.

[45] Hashem's light passes through the hierarchy of the *sefirot* and various spiritual worlds in diminishing measure via a process of *tzimtzumim*, or contractions.

man is bidden to keep his hair short[46] a woman, even after marriage, need not do the same; it is enough that she covers it.[47]

When a woman covers her hair punctiliously, she blocks the entrance and impedes the arrival of these *kelipot*. In fact, by carefully covering every strand of her hair she not only blockades the *kelipot* but weakens them.[48] This action becomes a conduit for the most magnificent blessings, as delineated in the *Zohar*.

Below, we cite the exact words of the *Zohar*[49] [50]:

> Rabbi Yehuda said that the exposed hairs on the head of a woman cause another kind of hair [of the *sefirah* of *malchut*] to be exposed [to external impure forces] and impair her. Therefore, a woman should be careful that none of her hair is visible even to the beams of her house, and all the more so outside.
>
> Come and see! Just like for the masculine aspect [*ze'eir anpin*] hair represents the harshest of severe judgments. So it is by a woman [whose hair has a stronger attraction to external forces, and thus is necessary to not be revealed since that empowers them].[51]
>
> ...Therefore, a woman's hair should be covered even in the innermost parts of her home. If she adheres to this, it is written: בניך כשתילי זיתים, your children are like olive plants.[52] What does "like olive plants" mean? Just as an olive tree does not lose its leaf cover in winter or summer and always has more value than the rest of the trees, so will her sons be elevated in respect to other people. Her husband will also be blessed in everything, with blessings above and with blessings below,

---

46   But a man is encouraged to let his beard grow unhindered. According to Kabbalah a man's beard represents channels for divine abundance and acts as a conduit for the thirteen attributes of Divine mercy.

47   *Halachic* authorities have recommended and encouraged that a woman wear her natural hair cut short, although it is covered anyway. See *Sdei Chemed, Klallim* Lamed, 116; *Darkei Teshuvah* 198:91 and others. Among the explanations offered: Longer hair cannot be constantly contained and covered (especially while wearing a hat or a *tichel*), as is mandatory. Also, proper immersion in the *mikvah* is more difficult with long hair. [½-1 *tefach* has been quoted as the preferred length] *Kovetz Yagdil Torah* (N.Y.), 2:10 (22), in the name of the Rebbe Rashab of Lubavitch; Op. cit. 13 (25) in the name of our Rebbe, *Kvudah Bat Melech* 1:19.

48   *HaShabbat* by Rabbi Y. Karasik, Vol. 1, p. 169-180.

49   *Nasso* p. 239

50   Translated and annotated by Rahmiel-Hayyim Drizin from the *Zohar* selection in *Chok L'Yisrael*. Copyright 2003 by KabbalaOnline.org, a project of Ascent of Safed.

51   In keeping with the Rebbe's emphasis on the positive, we do not here cite the words of the *Zohar* on the deleterious effects of a married woman's hair remaining uncovered.

52   *Tehillim* 128:3.

with wealth, children and grandchildren. This is what is meant by [the continuation of this psalm]: הנה כי כן יבורך גבר ירא ה'. יברכך ה' מציון וראה בטוב ירושלים כל ימי חייך. וראה בנים לבניך שלום על ישראל, behold, thus shall the man who fears Hashem be blessed. Hashem shall bless you out of Zion, and you shall see the good of Yerushalayim all the days of your life. You shall see your children's children, and peace upon Yisrael.[53]

---

53 Ibid. 128:4-6.

Blessings from Above and Blessings from Below:
The Rebbe's Teachings regarding Kisui Rosh

A Brief History of the Rebbe's Focus on This Mitzvah

Living in the twenty-first century, it is sometimes difficult to conceptualize the vastly different religious landscape that dominated America and the greater Jewish world less than one hundred years ago.

In her definitive study of Orthodoxy in America between the years of 1880 and 1945, Jenna Weissman Joselit notes:[54]

What animated and sustained that experience was not a lasting preoccupation with Jewish law or a collective nostalgia for the piety of an earlier, parental generation but rather an ongoing romance with modernity. Instead of shunning modernity, the interwar Orthodox embraced it, deferred to its strictures, and fashioned their institutions in accord with its dictates… Keeping outwardly distinctive practices to a minimum, Orthodox Jews of this era did not publicly demonstrate or proclaim their Orthodoxy. "It was certainly not a time when you showed your Judaism outside," related one rabbi. "It was a time when you kept your Judaism to yourself. There was no such thing as wearing a *kippah* on the street."[55] The absence of distinctive dress was a hallmark of that era.

In the same book, in a chapter on women titled "The Jewish Priestess and Ritual: The Sacred Life of American Orthodox Women," the practice of married women covering their hair goes entirely unmentioned.

When the Rebbe assumed leadership in 1950, the Lubavitch presence in America was relatively small, depleted, like many European Jewish groups, by the events of the previous decade. With relatively few young women among the ranks of Lubavitch in those days, many of the young chassidim married into "American" Orthodox homes where the mitzvah of *kisui rosh* was honored more in its breach than in its fulfillment. Even many of the young women who came to America from Russia along with their chassidic families were not committed to this mitzvah whose observance had declined

---

[54] New York's Jewish Jews: The Orthodox Community in the Interwar Years. p. 20-21.

[55] Rabbi Haskel Lookstein. Ramaz School Oral History Project. 1986. p. 2.

Hide and Seek: The Mitzvah of Kisui Rosh

under the Communist regime. In an era when standing out as Jew incurred dreadful consequences including death, it was difficult for most to perform the mitzvah.

Through the Rebbe's correspondences and public addresses, it becomes clear that he carried out a systematic campaign to promote and restore the mitzvah of hair covering as *de rigueur* for all married women. In this regard, it is important to remember that the Rebbe was not a spiritual leader only for the select group of individuals who considered themselves Lubavitcher Chassidim. From his published volumes of correspondence,[56] it is apparent that the Rebbe's influence extended over the widest cross-section of world Jewry.[57]

During the early period of his leadership, the Rebbe sought to establish that hair covering for a married woman was a matter of *halacha* and not an obscure *minhag*, a relic that belonged to another age. Furthermore, the Rebbe asserted that *halacha* requires all of a married woman's hair be covered.[58] And he unabashedly championed the *sheitel* as the optimal way for a woman to fulfill this crucial mitzvah.

The Rebbe's approach to promoting *kisui rosh* entailed a balancing act: He wanted to supplant the widespread aversion to appearing different and too Jewish with a strong sense of Jewish identity and pride. At the same time, he was acutely sensitive to many women's concerns about maintaining a fashionable and contemporary appearance. The Rebbe worried that most women, even those more *frum*, would not wear a scarf consistently and in a manner that covered all of their hair. It appears that, even then, the Rebbe foresaw the eventual swell of observant women whose professional and social involvements would preclude covering hair with scarves or hats. Certainly, without the option of a *sheitel*, many professional women might not consider observing the mitzvah of *kisui rosh*.

An early example of the Rebbe's thinking in support of *sheitels* is articulated in the following excerpts taken from his public address, or *farbrengen*, on Rosh Chodesh Elul 1954:

The difference between a wig and a kerchief is the following: It is easy to take off a kerchief, which is not the case with a wig. For

---

56 To date, thirty three volumes of the Rebbe's correspondence have been published under the title *Igrot Kodesh*, Kehot Publishing. They include selections from his correspondence through 1977-78.

57 According to Susan Handelman, a professor at Bar Ilan University, as cited by Mendel Kalmenson in the Chabad.org article "Local is Global," "The Rebbe would receive—and personally read and answer—around four hundred letters a day. And probably equally as many telephone calls, with questions for him and requests for blessings, would come in each day from around the world." Kalmenson adds, "Purportedly, research done by the New York Postal Service in the '80s found that the Rebbe received second to the most (non-commercial) mail in all of New York State!"

58 *Magen Avraham, Orach Chaim* 75:4. *Tzemach Tzedek*. Responsa *Even Ha'ezer* 139.

instance, when one is at a gathering and wears a wig, then even if President Eisenhower were to enter, she would not take off her wig... Let the woman ponder this matter... Why doesn't she really want to wear a wig but only a kerchief? Because she knows that a wig cannot be taken off when she is walking in the street or at a gathering, while a kerchief can be moved all the way up and sometimes taken off entirely.

It is possible that she will say that she will wear a kerchief properly. If she does so, then surely it is well. But...why place oneself in the path of temptation? We beseech G-d prior to our prayers, "Do not bring us to temptation."[59]

Not surprisingly, at first, the Rebbe's stance proved unpopular. Many women simply did not want to cover their hair while others found the notion of a wig utterly foreign, associating it with an outdated homeliness. Displaying patience and uncanny sensitivity to the psychological and sociological issues at play, the Rebbe persisted in his efforts. Eventually, it paid off. By the late 1960s, the Rebbe's ardent promotion of wigs led to adoption of the *sheitel* as a norm in most Orthodox circles.

Clearly, the Rebbe wished to inspire women to wear wigs and to stand firm in this observance in the face of the unique social pressures of the hour. A more careful reading, however, uncovers additional nuances worthy of mention. For instance, the Rebbe's attentiveness to how, for many women, identity is linked to physical appearance. He understood this dynamic as a critical factor when women considered whether to cover their hair. The Rebbe's *farbrengens* were serious affairs often lasting many hours; occasions when he discussed multi-layered Torah insights, sometimes deep into the night. Attending the aforementioned gathering were hundreds of men and relatively few women.[60] Yet given *kisui rosh's* universal importance, the Rebbe did not seek to obfuscate what is often construed as a solely feminine issue in *halacha* while addressing every audience.

The Rebbe went so far as to state that wigs might even be more attractive than one's own hair. At the time, the statement was meant to encourage and educate women who assumed all wigs were aesthetically unflattering. In comparison to what women might have worn in earlier generations, the new wigs, the Rebbe said, were attractive. (Here, it's worth recalling that the Jewish conception of modesty does not equate to

---

[59] *Likkutei Sichot*, vol. 13, p. 189.

[60] In stark contrast to the later years when thousands of women attended regularly.

unattractiveness but largely entails covering areas of the body deemed *ervah*, nakedness, which, for a married woman, would include her hair.)

Today, when the highly sophisticated, proliferating wig industry offers truly beautiful options in synthetic and human hair alike,[61] it is instructive that the Rebbe had no objection at all to wigs that enhanced a woman's appearance so long as they completely cover the hair. On the contrary, he encouraged women to take advantage of their availability.

The Rebbe did not miss an opportunity to promulgate the mitzvah of *kisui rosh* and to promote the particular way he felt it was best observed. During the first decade of his *nesiut*, leadership, from 1950–60, the Rebbe served as the *mesader kiddushin* at numerous weddings.[62] Among the conditions he set for doing so was the *kallah's* commitment, once married, to wearing a *sheitel*. It was a great *zechut*, merit, to have the Rebbe be *mesader kiddushin*, and this opportunity inspired many young women to commit to wearing a *sheitel*. The Rebbe relentlessly championed this cause in conversations with *kallahs* and *chatanim*, their parents, and others who would come to him for *yechidut*. According to numerous accounts, the Rebbe urged young couples to make buying a *sheitel* a high priority in pre-wedding planning. The Rebbe made a point of reminding the *kallah* to buy the most beautiful *sheitel* she could find, and to some, he specifically stressed the need for two, so that if one was serviced, the other would be available.[63] In some cases, the Rebbe made the *chatan* responsible for this purchase. The Rebbe even went so far as to pay for the *sheitlach* of some young women during this period.

One such woman was Chana Sharfstein. In her own words:

> Just a few days after my affirmative response [concerning wearing a *sheitel*] had been given to the Rebbe, we received a phone call from Rabbi Yehudah Krinsky, a member of the Rebbe's secretariat, that there was something important waiting for us at the Rebbe's office. Of course, my husband immediately went to his office, and I impatiently awaited his return. In a small white envelope was a personal check from the Rebbe, and with it came a special message that I should buy the most beautiful *sheitel* I could find; he said I should wear it in great happiness and joy. In a large flowered wig box on the top shelf of my closet is that first *sheitel*. It was custom-

---

61   For *halachic* sources which discuss natural-looking and specifically, human-hair wigs, and find them unobjectionable, see *Shiltei Giborim* on *Rif, Shabboat* 29a; *Yaskil Avdi*, vol. 7; *Shulchan Aruch, Even Ha'ezer* 16; *Igrot Moshe*, vol. 4; *Shulchan Aruch, Even Ha'ezer* II. 12.

62   The Rebbe was *mesader kiddushin* at weddings before this point, but not in his capacity as Rebbe, and he did make an exception for a few couples between 1960–63. After this time, because of the exponential growth of the Lubavitch community and the Rebbe's myriad involvements, the Rebbe no longer officiated at weddings. See *Mekadesh Yisrael* for more.

63   *Mekadesh Yisrael*, Kehot Publications, p. 291.

> made by an outstanding wig stylist in Williamsburg. I wore it and wore it and wore it until the netting on the inside began to shred. Then I carefully mended it with loving care and patience. I always felt very special wearing that *sheitel*. And no matter how many *sheitlach* I have had since then, none were more wonderful than the first one. I always wore it with great happiness and pride and whenever someone would remark that I had lovely hair or a beautiful hairstyle, I would smile and respond with confidence that I was wearing a wig because I was an Orthodox Jewish woman.[64]

The Rebbe contributed to the purchase of Crown Heights resident, Mrs. Zelda Nemes' *sheitel* as well. In the summer of 1958, when Rabbi and Mrs. Zelda Nemes were expecting their eldest son Mendel, they merited to go into the Rebbe for *yechidut*. Mrs. Nemes was wearing a half wig, known as a fall, with a hat which completely covered the front part of her head. The Rebbe looked at her and said: "a half *sheitel* is half a *bracha* and a whole *sheitel* is a whole *bracha*." The Rebbe showered the couple with tremendous *brachot*, and he said he could even give more...

The Rebbe then asked to speak to Rabbi Nemes alone, at which time he took a large amount of money out of his drawer and told Rabbi Nemes to go to Manhattan and buy the most beautiful *sheitel* he could find from a wig maker that serviced the Hollywood actors and actresses.[65]

Rabbi Shmuel Lew, a *Shliach* in London, England since 1965, recounts that shortly after the Rebbe let it be known that he would be *mesader kiddushin* at his wedding to Hindy Jaffe in 1963, the Rebbe's secretary Rabbi Chaim Mordechai Aizik Hodakov asked him a number of questions.[66] "One of the questions was: Does your *kallah* have a *sheitel*? I answered yes. The next question was: How many? I said two. Rabbi Hodakov said, 'That is what I wanted to hear. She should have another *sheitel*, so that even when one is being washed, set, etc., she does not go without a *sheitel*.'"

While the Rebbe communicated with individuals about the mitzvah, he simultaneously promoted its observance on a more communal level, "opening the door" for the modern day *sheitel* industry. Mrs. Freeda Kugel, whose name is synonymous with wigs, related the following:[67]

---

[64] Excerpted from *The Letter* by Chana Sharfstein, printed in the N'shei Chabad Newsletter, December, 1993.

[65] Related in private conversation to the author by Rabbi Mendel Nemes.

[66] In an interview with the N'shei Chabad Newsletter.

[67] In a phone interview with the author conducted in Summer 2000.

I came from Israel as a young woman with small children, and at the time, my husband was unable to find work, so I became the breadwinner. In 1970, I had a small business as a wig stylist, and on one occasion, in *yechidut* with the Rebbe, I complained about how difficult things were. I worked long hours and did not bring in enough money. The Rebbe told me not to worry, that my line of work would become very lucrative because every woman would need at least one *sheitel* for every day and one for Shabbat. The Rebbe then said that there will come a time when wig salons the world over will order wigs from me. I was stunned by the Rebbe's words. First, because women were not buying multiple *sheitlach* at that time. The human-hair wigs of the 1960s were truly ugly, and synthetic wigs had just come onto the scene. [At the time, Fashion Tress produced a line called Look of Love; this preceded the wig business of Georgie, Yaffa, and others.] Even more astounding was the Rebbe's reference to an international business, which was beyond my wildest dreams.

Shortly after this exchange, women started traveling from the affluent Upper West Side to have their *sheitlach* done at my salon in Crown Heights. I considered this a direct result of the Rebbe's blessing.

In 1980, with the Rebbe's words echoing in my mind, I went to Korea in an attempt to start my own line of synthetic wigs. I was not particularly successful with this line; in fact, I was tired and discouraged, and with my husband now established in his own line of work, I took a hiatus from the *sheitel* business.

But with the advent of glasnost, my husband urged me to travel to the Soviet Union in search of European human hair for the "Shabbat" *sheitlach* the Rebbe had spoken of so many years earlier. My Korean adventure was not a total loss as I did learn a great deal about the manufacturing of wigs, and I never forgot the Rebbe's blessings. So I set out to seek the most beautiful human hair for sale in that vast and unknown territory.

Believe me when I tell you, all kinds of doors opened for me. I literally saw the fulfillment of the Rebbe's blessing. It was not without difficulty, but today I employ 150 people in my wig factory in Dnepropetrovsk, Ukraine. My husband and children have joined me in the business, and wig salons from all over the world do indeed import the Freeda human hair wigs that so many women proudly wear on Shabbat.

The Definitive Conduit for Bracha

In the following letter, we sense the Rebbe's palpable joy upon hearing the news that a particular woman has purchased a *sheitel*.[68] In his signature style, the Rebbe reminds her of the great *brachot* this mitzvah elicits and encourages her to share her commitment to *kisui rosh* with others:

> **I was very pleased to receive your letter of Nov 3, in which you write the good news that you have ordered a sheitel during your recent visit in New York. The Almighty will surely fulfill His promise, as it is written in the holy Zohar, that it will bring hatzlacha to you, your husband, and children in good health and prosperity, especially in your case, where in addition to the deed itself there is also a Kiddush Hashem. I am sure you will wear it with joy, and as the Baal Shem Tov emphasized the importance of serving the Almighty with joy, G-d's blessings will be even greater.**
>
> **I want to add my prayerful wishes that the Almighty grant you the zechut to be instrumental in making your friends and acquaintances follow your good example, which you will support also by other forms of influence. Not only does the sheitel show the true Jewish spirit of adherence to our laws and customs, but it also shows strength of character and will and the power of conviction, not being swayed by external influences...**

The Rebbe constantly reminded all those with whom he corresponded that a woman's scrupulous adherence to this mitzvah served as a conduit for blessings in life. To an individual who wrote concerning difficulties with earning a living and had apparently acknowledged that his wife did not cover her hair, the Rebbe responded:

> **Why the surprise at the financial straits when the holy Zohar explains that when kisui harosh of the wife is in order, then "they shall be blessed with all blessings, blessings of above and blessings of below, with wealth, with children and grandchildren, etc." Our Torah is a "Torah of Life," instructing us how to live our lives, even on a daily basis.**[69]

---

68   Dated 19 Cheshvan 5715.

69   *Igrot Kodesh*, vol. 19, pp. 326-327.

Hide and Seek: The Mitzvah of Kisui Rosh

To another who asked the Rebbe for a *bracha* that his brother and sister in law be blessed with children, the Rebbe replied:

> **You should also find out from your brother whether his wife is careful to observe kisui harosh. For the Zoharic statement is known, that a woman's observance of tzniut and especially kisui harosh brings about "blessings of above and blessings of below, with wealth, with children and grandchildren, etc."[70]**

Easing the Impediments to the Observance of this Mitzvah

The Rebbe received a legendarily heavy volume of mail every day, including letters from women and men voicing hesitations about fulfillment of the mitzvah of *kisui rosh*. The concerns surrounding the Rebbe's call for women to wear *sheitels* ranged from anxiety about monetary costs to fears about physical discomfort, and from insecurities about the sociological implications to theological misgivings. In the sampling below, the Rebbe's responses are filled with compassion and an evident sense of urgency:

> **Because your wife has resolved to wear a sheitel, and to do so gladly, and will not be bothered by those who may scoff at her observance, her merit will be great. Specifically, [she will gain merit] as she is among the first in her neighborhood to return to this custom of modest Jewish women. It is well known how our Sages valued and praised the ability of an individual to teach many through example.**

> **It may be that in the interim it is difficult to commit to this because of the expenses involved. I want to inform you that there is here (administered through the Lubavitch office) a specific free loan fund for this purpose, which can be repaid over a lengthy period of time, in order to facilitate these purchases by anyone. It is not a good idea to delay this matter. As soon as you get this letter, write me with the name and necessary amount to issue a check; it will be sent out immediately and may Hashem grant you success.[71]**

---

70 *Igrot Kodesh*, vol. 7, p. 259.

71 *Igrot Kodesh*, vol. 8, p. 192, dated 25 Shevat, 1954.

As was his way, the Rebbe urged those committed to the observance of this practice to encourage their friends to act in kind:

> **You should also see to it that others act in like manner, explaining to them that this is the path and segulah to health, sustenance, and true nachat from children. And Hashem should help that you report good tidings in this regard.**[72]

The following is excerpted from the Rebbe's reply to a woman who wrote that wearing a wig caused her headaches. That the Rebbe follows up his theological points with an eminently practical suggestion is absolutely striking and suggests that, for the Rebbe, no concern proved too trivial when it came to this mitzvah:

> **With regard to your writing about covering your hair there is absolutely no question regarding this matter: Since G-d clearly said that for the benefit of the wife, her husband and their children, the hair should not be revealed, surely it is so. Thus it is impossible that by keeping G-d's commandments the head should hurt, etc.**
>
> **For example, when you write that wearing a sheitel makes your head hurt, it is possible that: A) This is a falsehood of the evil inclination who does not want mitzvot to be performed and does not want Jews to be showered with blessings. B) If indeed it is true, then this proves that you should cut your hair short. Then it surely won't hurt when you wear a sheitel.**[73]

For the following correspondent, the problem is less pragmatic and more theological in nature. Interestingly, the Rebbe did not counter her challenge with philosophical or mystical arguments. For many women (and men), no reason for *kisui rosh* will ever prove compelling enough. Rather, the Rebbe stressed that observance of all *mitzvot*, including hair covering, is predicated on one's subservience to Hashem's will. The Rebbe concluded his response with reference to the abundant *brachot* accrued through care with this mitzvah:

> **In response to your letter of the 13th of Iyar in which you ask how one is to explain the necessity of hair covering (for a married woman): One wonders at the very question, especially since we**

---

72 *Igrot Kodesh*, vol. 8, p. 217, dated 11 Adar, 1954.

73 *Likkutei Sichot*, vol. 33, p. 264.

now find ourselves in the days of preparation for receiving the Torah, which was only received by the Jewish people through their prefacing naaseh, we will do, to nishma, we will hear and we will learn.

It is self-understood and plain that man's belief in Hashem forces him to intellectually accept Hashem's commandments without seeking reasons for them in human intellect. For even simple common sense, if it is but healthy and sound, understands that it is impossible for a finite being to comprehend the infinite.

Indeed, it is a principle of faith among all the Jewish people, believers, children of believers, that Hashem and His understanding and will, are truly one and infinite, while man is finite in all aspects of his being.

In addition to the above, when one takes into account the explicit reward received for hair covering (Zohar), then even if one were to be extremely doubtful of this, chas v'shalom, it would still be worth covering the hair. This is most assuredly so, as the words of the Zohar – as part of our Torah of Truth – are completely true, perpetual and everlasting in all places and all times.[74]

Covering All of Your Hair: A Great Merit for Your Children

By the late 1960s, the Rebbe's ardent promotion of *sheitlach* had made wearing a *sheitel* the norm in most *frum* circles. But the Rebbe did not rest. He continued to teach the importance of a woman carefully covering all of her hair, even in the privacy of her home, in accordance with various *piskei halacha*, and specifically, the ruling of the Tzemach Tzedek. The Rebbe often referenced the scrupulous behavior modeled by Kimchit and other women of her generation: As cited in the Gemara, the walls of these women's homes never saw their hair, which means that their hair was never exposed.

On Chai Elul 5742, September 6, 1982, during a *farbrengen*, the Rebbe delivered the following impassioned words:

> **Torah, the "Torah of Truth," declares that as soon as a baby is born it is affected by all that transpires around it. Surely, the**

[74] *Igrot Kodesh*, vol. 13, pp. 102–103, dated 25 Iyar, 1956.

conduct of the infant's parents has a profound impact on the child, even when it is extremely young.

Moreover, even the conduct of the parents during the nine months that precede the infant's birth have a profound influence on the child.

Thus the Gemara[75] relates that "Kimchit had seven sons, all of whom merited to serve as Kohanim Gedolim, High Priests. The Sages asked her, 'What have you done to merit this?' She answered them: 'The rafters of my house have never seen the plaits of my hair.'"

In other words, her profound conduct of tzniut – to the extent that even when she was alone in the house "the rafters of her house never saw the plaits of her hair" – affected her sons to such an extent that they all merited to become Kohanim Gedolim.

Her behavior thus had an effect many, many years after she conducted herself in this manner – after her children had already become bar mitzvah and after they had reached the age of twenty, when they became fit to become Kohanim Gedolim.

Moreover, her conduct also had an influence on her grandchildren and great-grandchildren, for the son of a Kohen Gadol inherits his father's position.

At a *farbrengen* twenty five years earlier, the Rebbe had already replied to a question that might arise in women's minds:[76]

One should not think: Must I act with such a tremendous degree of tzniut that my children will become Kohanim Gedolim? Why should I care if my children grow up to be only regular priests? Furthermore, all Jews are intrinsically holy!

Herein is the lesson from the lighting of the menorah, which was to be done specifically in the Beit Hamikdash. This teaches us that, if at all possible, we are to increase the amount of illumination even in those places that are already most holy.

---

75 *Yoma* 47a. If the high priesthood is inherited through death, how is it considered a merit that Kimchit had seven sons, each of whom served in that capacity? Her son, Rabbi Yishmael, the regular High Priest, was temporarily ineligible to serve due to ritual impurity. Over time, each of his brothers had the opportunity to substitute him as High Priest. She did not, G-d forbid, bury her sons (*Tosafot Yeshanim*, ad loc.).

76 *Sichot Kodesh* 5717, pp. 337-338. *Likkutei Sichot*, vol. 2, pp. 319-320.

Here as well: If a woman is granted the ability to train her sons that they grow into Kohanim Gedolim, [i.e., that they achieve the maximum of their spiritual potential,] it indicates that this is her task; should she not do this, she is not carrying out her obligation and is not fulfilling G-d's desire.

In effect, the Rebbe asked: Which mother would consciously deny her child every possible advantage in life, especially if it hinges on her choice?

It is indeed fascinating that while *kehunah* always passes via the patrilineal line, *kehunah gedolah*, perhaps the most exclusive privilege of all, was affected by the mother and specifically, through her degree of care in the mitzvah of *kisui rosh*.

The Rebbe went on to underscore the impact of a mother's *kisui rosh* on her children's spiritual success via analysis of a seemingly puzzling *passuk*. As the Rebbe asks, why does the Torah state, דבר אל אהרן...בהעלותך את הנרות?[77] Why was the directive concerning lighting the *menorah* in the *Beit Hamikdash* given specifically to Aharon, the *Kohen Gadol*, when a *Kohen Hedyot*, a "regular" *Kohen*, could do this service and, in actuality, did so most of the time?[78] The Rebbe's answer to this question hinges on the *Kohen Gadol*'s unique connection to the Torah and draws on a chassidic teaching that symbolically equates lighting the *menorah* with sparking the Divine light in another Jew's soul.

While, indeed, the *avodah* of lighting the literal *menorah* in the *Mikdash* was usually carried out by *Kohanim Hedyotim*, the mitzvah's symbolic implication of igniting the *neshamah* of another Jew is work so delicate that it must be done by the *Kohen Gadol*, the one person in the world to enter the *Kodesh Hakodashim*.[79] Significantly, only the *Kohen Gadol* beheld the *aron Hashem*, which housed the *luchot*, upon which were engraved the *Aseret Hadibrot*. The superlative advantage of *otiyot chakikah*, engraved letters, the Rebbe reminded us, is that they cannot be separated from the stone, unlike ink, which can be rubbed off of parchment and, even at the outset, is merely superimposed. Thus, the engraved letters symbolize the *Kohen Gadol*'s immutable oneness with the Torah. And it is only with this type of passionate attachment to Torah, the Rebbe taught, that each one of us, as figurative *Kohanim Gedolim*, can "light the *menorah*" of our own

---

[77] *Bamidbar* 8:2.

[78] If the *menorah* was brought outside, even a non-Kohen could light it. As the Rambam writes, *Hadlakah kesheirah bezar* (Rambam, *Beit Hamikdash* 9:7).

[79] *Likkutei Sichot*, vol. 2, p. 314. The seven lamps of the *menorah* represent the seven soul types, each one rooted in one of the seven emotional attributes. In addition, as Shlomo Hamelech writes, נר ה' נשמת אדם. The soul of man is the candle of Hashem (*Mishlei* 20:27).

neshamah and the *neshamot* of those we encounter. It takes inspired oneness with the Torah on our part to inspire another.

The Rebbe then proclaimed that women, in particular, who raise children and set the tone of their homes, are called upon by Hashem to serve as the primary lamplighters of their children's souls. And to successfully kindle her children's *neshamot*, a mother must embody this *chakikah* fervor, the *Kohen Gadol*'s single-minded devotion to and fiery oneness with the Torah. Our commitment to this holy work directly shapes the spiritual experiences of our children. And remarkably, the Rebbe emphasized, just like Kimchit who was scrupulous with her hair covering and merited to see seven sons as *Kohanim Gedolim*, so too we can pass down to our children an immutable attachment to the Torah as personified by the *Kohen Gadol*.

The Rebbe completed this talk with a reminder that a mother's care and precision in her *tzniut* in general, and her *kisui rosh* in particular, mitigates difficulties in the lives of her children and draws blessings of children, good health and abundance in *parnassah* into her life and those of her household, in a literal way.[80]

The Gift that Keeps Giving

Often, people doubt the premise of reward and punishment in light of their own or others' seemingly unwarranted difficulties and/or successes.

During a *farbrengen* on Rosh Chodesh Elul, 1954, the Rebbe stated:[81]

> **Wearing a sheitel has a beneficial impact on children and grandchildren, livelihood and health, as the Zohar states.[82]**
>
> **…One should not ask: I know of a woman who does not wear a wig and still things go well for her regarding children, health and livelihood, as well as life in general.**
>
> **First of all, we do not know what transpires in the life of another, what types of travails he or she is undergoing; no one tells the other about all that takes place in one's life. Second of all, we are not to look at what is transpiring in others' [lives]; we are to do that which G-d commanded us to do.**

---

80   *Likkutei Sichot*, vol. 2, *Parshas Behaalotcha, ot hei* and onward.

81   *Likkutei Sichot*, vol. 13, p. 188.

82   *Zohar* III, 126a.

> **We are a minority among the nations. Should we also draw the corollary that since there are more gentiles than Jews in the world, and things are going well for them, that we are to imitate their ways? Were we to act in such a manner, the Jewish people would have ceased to exist, G-d forbid, a long time ago…**
>
> **Additionally, we must acknowledge the limited scope of our vision. Our Rebbeim taught:** חזקה לתעמולה שאינה חוזרת ריקם, **a positive overture will always yield a positive result.**[83] **The Frierdiker Rebbe added,** דער אויבערשטער בלייבט ניט קיין בעל חוב, **Hashem never remains indebted.**[84]

We may not perceive the *brachot* that flow into our lives as a result of careful observance of the mitzvah of *kisui rosh*. These blessings may come to fruition only a generation later or even after our own sojourn in this world, taking the form of a *bracha* enjoyed by our offspring down the line. That itself is a remarkable testament to the ripple effects of this mitzvah. As noted, Kimchit's care in covering her hair caused her sons to be *Kohanim Gedolim*, which also put her grandchildren, the subsequent generation, on the inner track to inherit the High Priesthood, should they prove worthy. In any case, Hashem will not remain in debt. The *brachot* will most certainly come to fruition.

The Rebbe Maharash revealed one particularly powerful example of a *bracha* that stemmed from *kisui rosh* which also manifested at a later time. In 1854, Czar Nicholas I of Russia instituted a decree against women covering their heads with a type of hat referred to as a "*knofin*." The despot famous for his anti-semitic laws clearly aimed this ban at Jewish women given to wearing this type of covering in fulfilment of the mitzvah of *kisui rosh*. Some defied Czar Nicholas and continued to cover their heads properly at great personal risk. Nearly twenty years later, all young Jewish men were ordered to conscript into the Soviet army. The Rebbe Maharash stated that despite this all-inclusive decree, miraculously, none of the sons of the women who had stood firm against the *gezeirah* of *knofin* were drafted. The sons of these women were spared that plight and pain in the *zechut* of their mothers' *mesirat nefesh* for the mitzvah of *kisui rosh*.[85]

---

[83] *Hayom Yom*, entry for 12 Tishrei.

[84] *Hayom Yom*, entry for 28 Elul.

[85] *Shmuot V'sippurim*, vol. 1, p. 74.

Seldom, throughout the years of his leadership, did the Rebbe veer from his positive focus on the wonderful effects of this mitzvah. In the letter cited below, however, one senses the Rebbe's exasperation with a man who could not find it in himself to allow his wife to cover her hair in accordance with *halacha* and seemed oblivious to the harm this could portend for his family.

> **Should one say that it is impossible for him to give in that his wife should observe kisui harosh with a kerchief or a sheitel (wig), and it makes no difference to him that by doing so he is placing in jeopardy his fortune and the fortune of his partner in a life partnership of many decades, then this person lacks any feeling of responsibility, duty and obligation.**
>
> **Nor does this person possess the proper measure and knowledge of the meaning of a shared life, and how much it is worthwhile foregoing even more important matters, as long as it leads to a united, fortunate and happy life.**
>
> **And as stated above, such a life is impossible to achieve for a Jewish man and woman unless it is lived in accordance with the Torah and mitzvot.**[86]

In the final analysis, it is hair covering as a *segulah*, a source of *bracha*, that was the hallmark of the Rebbe's approach. In each of the aforementioned examples, and in numerous instances not cited here, the Rebbe underscored the unique way this particular mitzvah channels Hashem's blessings into one's home and family.

The Rebbe never tired of quoting the words of the *Zohar*, words most of us might never have otherwise seen or heard! It was as if the Rebbe was presenting us with keys that unlocked a vault filled with treasures that he desperately wanted each Jewish woman to share with her family.

May we recognize and cherish our great merit to serve as conduits for these *brachot* and open ourselves up to receive this outpouring of goodness into our lives, the lives of our husbands, and the lives of all our offspring until the end of time.

---

[86] Excerpt from *Igrot Kodesh*, vol. 9, p. 112.

chapter nine

Fruitful:
THE MITZVAH OF PRU U'RVU

There is nothing in life more all-encompassing, no decision more freighted with lifetime ramifications, than the choices we make surrounding our fertility. Like twins who share space in utero – sometimes with less comfort and ease than optimal – most of us approach this issue with dueling sensitivities.

On the one hand for most women, bearing children is a primal desire. Our physiology includes numerous inner and outer organs that support conception, gestation, and lactation. These systems begin to assert their presence at approximately age twelve. Our psychology seems similarly aligned. After decades of a lower birth rate, with contraceptives so widely available, with societal pressure to have children lessened, data indicates that a larger percentage of women are having children compared to previous decades albeit, later in life.[1] The same study revealed that more than half of women in their early forties who have never married have given birth.

On the other hand, since the rupture in Gan Eden, conception, gestation, parturition, and child rearing have presented some of life's greatest challenges, certainly for women. No matter the historic era, sociological truths, and geographic location, every aspect of child bearing and rearing presents credible trials.

---

[1] "They're Waiting Longer, but U.S. Women Today More Likely to Have Children Than a Decade Ago." Pew Research Center, Washington, D.C. (January 2018).

While few things in the universe can compare to the wonder and thrill of feeling the first stirrings of a child within you, the nausea and/or varicose veins, the incessant fatigue, the weight gain and overall heaviness, can be next to impossible to bear. The awe of pushing a child out of your body, the joy of holding that flesh of your flesh for the first time, is unparalleled. But for just as many women, the thought of delivering a child fills them with dread and fear.

And then there is raising a child which is essentially the arduous, humbling process of raising ourselves. It typically begins with feeding and tending to the needs of a life completely reliant on you for everything, and never really ends until the day the parent(s) leave this world. Our children are the nexus where our greatest joys converge with our most profound worry, sadness and angst. The old saw about a parent being only as happy as the least happy of their children will always be true. Chazal succinctly referred to this truth as *tzaar gidul banim,* the pain of raising children.

This is all to say that for a woman, much more so than for even the most involved father, having children is about being all in. There is no aspect of life that remains untouched by this decision. Which makes it exceedingly counterintuitive that the mitzvah of *pru u'rvu* is not incumbent upon a woman. While it is a great mitzvah for her to bear children, if she should decide not to, she would not be in violation of a mitzvah *d'orayta* as would be a male who makes the same decision. Among the reasons given for this is the fact that the Torah's ways are ways of pleasantness and peace and therefore cannot obligate a person to endure the pain and travail of pregnancy and parturition.[2] Another reason is that it is unnecessary to legislate what is an inherent desire in most women. These explanations, paradoxical as they might seem, complement each other and reveal a startling truth about a woman's relationship with child bearing. While thankfully this is not the case today, for much of human history through the twentieth century, childbearing carried a frightfully high mortality rate. And yet, women willingly submitted themselves to this process. Motherhood is the quintessential act of *mesirat nefesh.*

While conditions are vastly different today, many of us still approach this area of life with trepidation, often with sparring voices in our head. We recognize the great *zechut* and privilege of bringing another *neshamah* into this world. We cherish the possibility of making a singular contribution to *Klal Yisrael,* both in the present and future. We seek that sense of unique fulfillment that comes from mothering. But, depending on variables in our life, we might also struggle with physical or psychological challenges, a less than able spouse and partner, or something as pedestrian as our need to breathe

---

[2] Rabbi Meir Simcha of Dvinsk. *Meshech Chochma, Bereshit* 9:7.

Fruitful: The Mitzvah of Pru U'rvu

(read: go to the bathroom by ourselves and without someone knocking on the door every two minutes with an emergency). We might also want to delay beginning a family for some time after marriage. That is, after all, the logical and near universal thing to do.

For women with sensitively developed spiritual personas this inner conflict is heightened; do my concerns originate with the *nefesh habehamit*, the animal soul, or the *nefesh elokit,* the Divine soul? It can be hard to find the line between self-care and self-absorption, just as it might, for some, be impossible to discern when pushing oneself to do more becomes downright dangerous and wrong. It can induce guilt and shame when a woman feels that she is not doing all that she can or as much as she should.

In no area of life is balance as important as in this one which interfaces with *shalom bayit*, personal health, the health of the larger family unit, and so much more. Which is why in the section below we highlight the role of a *mashpia*, an objective, experienced, sensitive to the specific variables at hand, spiritual mentor or coach.

In the below survey of the Rebbe's words on this topic, we find a recurring theme: his pushback against a society that increasingly puts the self front and center. Over the span of decades, the Rebbe consistently but lovingly reminded us that we are part of a vast plan orchestrated by the Creator and Sustainer of the universe, a plan much larger than our personal considerations. At the same time, the Rebbe recognized and honored the myriad ways in which each one of us is different and held space for that most important variable in the equation.

May Hashem help each one of us to merit bringing *neshamot* vested in healthy *gufim* into this world with ease and joy, and in good health. May those who have not yet been blessed with children and those who are challenged with secondary infertility, experience the joy of their own miracles very soon.[3] In the interim it behooves us all to be sensitive to the pain and angst of those for whom the fulfillment of this mitzvah is not a choice but rather a most difficult challenge. And of course, include them in our *tefillot*.

---

3 See Part IV, essay six "The Dream that Was" by Aimee Baron, MD for practical guidance on this matter.

Top Five Questions About Pru U'rvu:

Authors' note: We are aware of and respect the varied positions and *halachic* rulings regarding this most important mitzvah. What we present below is in consonance with the Rebbe's view which is the accepted *hanhaga* among Chabad Chassidim. The Rebbe's wisdom and blessings are relevant to all and have much to contribute, even to those who observe differently. We recommend that each woman consult with her rabbinic authority for practical applications of the *halacha*.

1. My husband and I want to get to know each other more fully before we start a family. We feel like we need some time to gel as a couple, and we also want to solidify our finances, travel a bit, and advance in our schooling. Can we take some time before bringing children into the mix?

All[4] of the above stated concerns are valid and important and completely reasonable. It seems eminently sensible to build your assets and squirrel away savings before beginning a family. The logical time to travel for recreation is when you are newlywed and least encumbered. And it is most certainly easier to complete a degree or engage in some other important venture without children in the mix. Above all, this would seem to be the time for a young couple to mesh, strengthen their union and solidify that foundation upon which they will continue to build out. And yet, barring extenuating circumstances, *halacha* bids us to approach this decision from a different perspective.

For *halacha*-observant Jews, having children is not a mere lifestyle choice, it is a mitzvah, indeed the very first mitzvah in the Torah and the base upon which all else stands. Without *neshamot* being brought down into this world, Hashem's ultimate desire and, indeed, His very purpose for creation, cannot come to fruition. Like with every mitzvah, there are details that define its proper observance, including the time frame.

Halachically, a man is obligated to get married and have children as soon as it is viable for him to do so. The *Mishnah* sets the age at eighteen and there are some communities who abide by this timeline.[5] Most communities, however, based on various codifiers of *halacha*, extend greater latitude to young men in this regard. Since one must find a suitable partner, marriage is not necessarily a process that can be precisely timed. What is more uniformly agreed upon is that the obligations of marriage and *pru u'rvu* begin

---

4 The authors thank JEM (Jewish Educational Media), TheDailySicha.com, and the Chassidishe Derher magazine for their compilation of source material from the Rebbe's talks and correspondence on this subject.

5 *Pirkei Avot* 5:22; presumably he was learning Torah until that time.

simultaneously. Just as a male infant[6] must enter into *brito shel Avraham Avinu* on day eight of his life, so does a Jewish man's obligation to fulfill the mitzvah of *pru u'rvu* begin as soon as he is married.

Halachically, *pru u'rvu* is the man's obligation. In getting married, however, a woman implicitly becomes her husband's partner in fulfilling this mitzvah *d'orayta*. In the words of the Ran: Even though she is not personally commanded concerning procreation, she performs a mitzvah in getting married because she thereby assists her husband in the fulfillment of his mitzvah of *pru u'rvu*.[7] The Rebbe points out, that it is the woman who makes it possible for her husband to fulfill this mitzvah, and it is only through her that conception, gestation and birth can occur.[8] The lack of legal obligation is because it is unnecessary, even redundant, in the face of a woman's inherent desire to bring this *shlichut* to fruition. A man, in contradistinction, must be commanded to do so. Furthermore, in commenting on the ruling of the Ran, the Rebbe explains that it is not simply via a wife's practical facilitation of her husband's mitzvah, that she, too, merits a mitzvah.[9] Rather, she holds a share in his actual mitzvah of *pru u'rvu*.

Therefore, with the exception of extenuating physiological or psychological health concerns, it is difficult to find *halachic* dispensation, also known as a *heter*, for the use of birth control before a man has fulfilled his basic Torah obligation of fathering two children.

The premise that newlyweds should take some time before beginning their families is eminently logical, but Torah has its own particular brand of logic. *Avraham Avinu* was called *ha'ivri* because his life was an exhibition of ideals that were *me'ever*, on the other side, completely antithetical to the norms of his time.[10] In a world awash with polytheism, he alone introduced the then unheard of notion of one G-d; a force that created nature and therefore transcends its constructs. As his children, we have from time immemorial carried this legacy of a distinct way of life, not necessarily correlated with the zeitgeist of any particular time nor limited by convention, otherwise referred to as "reality."

---

6   Barring health concerns that render this impossible.

7   *Chiddushei HaRan* to *Kiddushin* 41a.

8   *Likkutei Sichot*, vol. 26, p. 267-268.

9   *Likkutei Sichot*, vol. 14, p. 41-43.

10 *Midrash Rabbah Bereishit* 42:8

Based on the *passuk* פרו ורבו ומלאו את הארץ וכבשוה, increase and multiply, fill the earth and subdue it, the Mishnah teaches:[11]

> A man shall not abstain from the performance of the duty of the propagation of the race unless he already has children. [As to the number], Beit Shammai ruled: two males, and Beit Hillel ruled: A male and a female, as it is written, He created them male and female.[12]

This mitzvah *d'orayta* is minimally fulfilled by having two children. According to one opinion in Gemara, it is fulfilled by having four.[13] There are, in addition, two *mitzvot d'Rabanan*. The first is referred to as *lashevet*, to inhabit, based on the *passuk* in *Yeshayahu*, לא תהו בראה לשבת יצרה, not for void did He create the world, but for habitation did He form it.[14] The second mitzvah is called *la'erev*, in the evening. As Rabbi Yehoshua says in the Gemara:[15] "If one had children when he was young, he should continue to have children when he is old. As the verse from *Kohelet* states בבקר זרע את זרעך ולערב אל תנח ידך כי אינך יודע אי זה יכשר הזה או זה ואם שניהם כאחד טובים, in the morning, sow your seed, and in the evening, do not withhold your hand, for you know not which will succeed, this one or that one, or whether both of them will be equally good.[16]

The Rambam writes: Although a man has fulfilled the mitzvah of *pru u'rvu*, he is commanded by the Rabbis of the Talmud not to desist from procreation while he yet has strength.[17] Simply speaking, this mitzvah *d'Rabanan* has no expiration date or statute of limitation.

The Torah places a premium on *shalom bayit*, and on cultivating the fledgling marital relationship during the *shana rishonah*. Who more than Hashem would want *shalom* to reign in our homes? From the Torah perspective, all things being equal, beginning a family can offer a couple the best way to grow together. As one child and then another enters our lives, *b'ezrat Hashem*, we grow, we mature, we learn about

---

11   *Bereishit* 1:28.

12   *Yevamot* 6:6.

13   *Yevamot* 61b-62a. If a man had children and they died... R. Yochanan said: He has not fulfilled the duty of propagation because *lashevet* is required, which did not happen. Furthermore if his son is sterile or his daughter barren, he has not fulfilled his duty; whereas, on the other hand, grandchildren are like children, so that if a man had only one son but his son had a daughter, his own duty is thus discharged. (Ibid. 62a-b)

14   *Yeshayahu* 45:18.

15   *Yevamot* 62b.

16   *Kohelet* 11:6.

17   *Ishut* 15:16.

Fruitful: The Mitzvah of Pru U'rvu

ourselves and our spouses; parenthood elicits a new, less self absorbed version of ourselves. As we shed our childhood we bring to our union a new level of commitment and dedication.

The home of a Jew, the Rebbe taught, is considered a *Beit Hamikdash*, and each one of us is privileged to build our personal *mikdash me'at*. On that note, he cites the phrase from *Vayikra* ומקדשי תיראו, you shall fear my *Mikdash*.[18] The Rambam rules that these words include a *mitzvat asei* to fear or be in awe of He who commanded that the *Mikdash* be built.

In building our homes, we are essentially granted the exalted privilege of building Hashem's home. And as was true with the building of the *Batei Mikdash*, there is an awe for Hashem who charged us with this privilege that should suffuse our consciousness.

Regarding couples who considered waiting before beginning to build their families, their personal "*midkash*", the Rebbe noted the well known Talmudic adage: מצוה הבאה לידך אל תחמיצנה, when a mitzvah comes to your hand, do not delay its fulfillment.[19] In the case of this crucial mitzvah, we are bidden to allow the Senior partner in our marriage to make the decision.[20]

2. In the Rebbe's perspective on pru u'rvu is there ever room for contraception? What about in the case of illness, or if I feel completely overwhelmed and need some time? What is the proper protocol for seeking a psak from a Rav regarding the use of birth control?

For most of us, life is not without challenges. There are times when it is difficult to see the path forward beyond the various obstacles in our way. The one constant metric by which all scenarios must be assessed is *halacha*.

When all relevant practitioners agree that pregnancy and birth would be dangerous to a woman's health, *halacha* demands that she employ contraception even if and when she desperately wants to have (more) children. In such a case, when two *mitzvot* present a conflict, for instance, *pru u'rvu* vs *v'nishmartem m'od lenafshoteichem*, the injunction to guard our health, a Rabbinic *psak* must be sought. In the Rebbe's words:[21]

---

18 *Vayikra* 19:30.

19 *Mechilta Shemot*, 12:17.

20 *Torat Menachem* 5744, vol. 4, p. 2652.

21 24 Tevet, 5741.

> **... if, in fact, the situation calls for a heter, then it is the Torah itself that is directing the person to push off having children.**

When given the circumstances of our life – our own health, spousal and family dynamics, and/or other factors – we simply cannot have more children, we should embrace the truth that we are fulfilling Hashem's will for us at this exact moment in time. That knowledge gives us the peace of mind and *simchah* that flows from doing exactly what we are meant to be doing.

Many situations, however, are not as black and white, and call for careful attention to *halacha* and the Rebbe's words.

Few people can achieve absolute objectivity. This is certainly true regarding matters that concern ourselves and our lives. In the words of our *Chachamim*, אדם קרוב אצל עצמו, a person is [lit. close to] subjective concerning himself, especially when we are dealing with matters that elicit great emotion.[22] When a physician suggests birth control, it is necessary to seek out the proper guidance as to exactly which type of contraceptive would be best both medically and *halachically*,[23] rather than rely on one's doctor alone. In the response from the Rebbe below we find explicit directions to consult with a Chassidic *rav*.

> **...In this, it is difficult to outline general directives, because [the ruling] depends on the nature of the difficulty which giving birth could cause a mother and the type of birth control used.**
>
> **Therefore, I advise you that, after discussing the matter again with your doctor, [when] he instructs you which form of birth control he has in mind, you should consult a Chassidic Orthodox Rav and hear his opinion.**[24]

The medical field is not a monolith; there are a variety of positions and perspectives. Some practitioners lack religious sensitivity, and a fundamental understanding of the desire to have more children. With such practitioners, this lack can inform their medical advice regarding procedures that will impede a woman's ability to have more children in the future. While one doctor might take a more conservative approach, another might be more willing to employ newer therapies and creative strategies, which is why

---

22 *Sanhedrin* 9b.

23 It is important that the form of contraceptive be chosen with an eye towards mitigating the time you are *nidah* due to staining, etc. Tahareinu can be very helpful in this regard.

24 Excerpted from a letter from the Rebbe dated 17 Kislev, 5711.

it is often advised to get a second opinion and always a good idea to find a doctor who is sympathetic to the Torah's view. Additionally, the Rebbe often advised, consulting with a *rofei yedid*, a doctor that is a friend.

When a woman feels overwhelmed, she and her husband should actively set aside time to reflect on their situation. This should not be expected to resolve instantly or even in a series of conversations; it can take time. If they have brainstormed various solutions, and feel that they are still facing insurmountable obstacles, seeking *halachic* guidance regarding the temporary use of contraceptives would be the path forward.

Before doing so however, speaking to their *mashpiim* can be extremely helpful. Optimally, this should be a person who themselves has a family and understands the various challenges, but has the advantage of experience as well as hindsight. There is a life perspective that is hard – nigh impossible – to attain in the thick of things but comes only in retrospect. We often call this the long view. Just as importantly – especially for those committed to following the Rebbe's path – is the *mashpia*'s familiarity with the Rebbe's view on this important subject. And above all, the ability of the *mushpa*, mentee, to feel comfortable expressing herself honestly.

Regarding the pivotal role of a *mashpia* in our lives, the Rebbe told us:[25]

> **The way to draw blessings into our lives for all that we need – both physical and spiritual – is only through fulfilling the Torah's instructions. Among them is "asei lecha Rav" make for yourself a mentor."**

As a first step, a *mashpia* can help a woman articulate what, specifically, she is afraid of or anxious about. She can find out what kind of support system the woman has in place, if any, and what other variables are at play. Hopefully, the *mashpia* can differentiate between clinical anxiety and the pedestrian type of doubt and "nerves" that assail us when we ponder a "big move." Once that is clarified, she can further direct the woman to helpful resources and share practical advice, such as encouraging the woman to get more household assistance, as well as learn and put into place time management and organizational techniques.[26]

When necessary, the *mashpia* can help formulate the question to the *rav*. Indeed, many Rabbis will not issue a *psak* without ascertaining that the woman or couple

---

25   *Sefer Hasichot* 5749, vol. 1, p. 402.

26   The Nechoma Greisman Anthology: Wisdom from the Heart is a wonderful book filled with inspiration and practical tips for mothers of large families.

has consulted with a *mashpia*. If you don't have a *mashpia* at this time, the *rav* can sometimes assume that role for this purpose.

Once the question comes to the *rav*, we know that the *rav's* response is with *siyata d'shmaya*, with help from heaven, and therefore offers us the proper path forward. The woman can then proceed with *simchah*.

3. *I don't feel that it would be responsible for us to bring yet another child into our family; we are barely making ends meet as it is. I grew up with scant resources, and I don't want my children to feel deprived of the "better things" in life. Why is this not a good enough reason to limit the size of our family?*

It is normal and natural for us to experience anxiety in this realm. We want to be fiscally responsible; we want to give our children all the best this world has to offer. Thus, on a purely logical level, it would seem finances should figure prominently in our plans for family size.

Worries concerning *parnassah* have plagued humanity ever since Hashem decreed, בזעת אפיך תאכל לחם, by the sweat of your brow will you eat bread.[27] The challenge of making ends meet is one of the profound consequences of the *chet eitz hadaat*. Our current reality only exacerbates these worries with prices for just the basics constantly on the rise. The cost of school and camp tuition alone is overwhelming, and that is just the beginning.

The Rebbe, however, lovingly reminded us:

> **When you bring a child into the world, Hashem is the one who has the responsibility of sustaining him, and a new channel of parnassah is created for each child. Later on, this channel will go directly to him, but for the first part of his life, the parents have the merit to serve as Hashem's messengers to bring the parnassah—Hashem's money—to the child.[28]**

On multiple occasions, the Rebbe underscored the fallacy of allowing financial considerations to get in the way of having children:[29]

---

27 *Bereishit* 3:19.

28 17 Sivan, 5740.

29 17 Sivan, 5740.

Fruitful: The Mitzvah of Pru U'rvu

> **It is a fundamental part of our faith that Hashem is the one who provides our parnassah, as we say in bentching:** הזן את העולם כולו... בחן ובחסד וברחמים, **Hashem sustains the entire world with kindness and compassion. Hashem bears the responsibility to sustain all of the billions of human beings in the world, along with all animals, insects, and even vegetation, and he always comes through for each one.**[30]
>
> **True, the parents need to create a vessel to receive Hashem's parnassah, but that's all it is, a vessel. If you choose not to have children, and, consequently, the new channels of parnassah they come with, you're harming your own parnassah! This person has been working hard to make a living, and he only made this-and-this amount of money, which wouldn't be enough to support more children. So, he says, this proves that he was right [not to have more children] He was wrong! When Hashem partners with parents and gives them a child, Hashem's child, then He provides parnassah because of this child... The bracha of Hashem brings riches, not only bare necessities. So if you want riches – both physically and spiritually – you need to provide the vessels [through having children].**[31]

These are words to review constantly so that they ring in our ears each day, as we confront a world that broadcasts a message to the contrary and seeks to wear down our resolve.

It is important to seek out a friend group of like-minded individuals who appreciate the blessing of a larger family and can commiserate with you about the inevitable challenges and difficulties from a place of empathy rather than judgment or scorn. These are your people, who understand your values and priorities. Like you, they understand children to be our greatest assets rather than, *chas v'shalom,* liabilities. These are people with whom you can brainstorm about making a staycation enormously fun for the kids. They will share information, for example, about affordable attractions and Groupons that make pricey venues more reasonably priced.

Just as importantly, this is a group that can help nourish your spirit. People who share your life's view can help validate your decision to possibly leave or pause a very

---

[30] *Likkutei sichot,* vol. 25, p. 36.

[31] *Shabbat Parshat Yitro,* 5744.

lucrative career to spend your time raising children. Especially when things get tough. Unlike a business venture where one can often see immediate benefit or gain, the hard, day to day work of raising children does not always yield immediate, discernable results. Reminding each other why we made this choice – and that our choice notwithstanding, we also need to take care of ourselves – can be one of the greatest gifts women can give each other. This can be a group with whom to exercise, swap books and recipes, and generally "share life."

Barring extreme circumstances, the way children perceive their socioeconomic bracket largely depends on the attitude and level of contentment of their parents. When they realize how lucky and "rich" they are to have many siblings, the fact that they don't take exotic trips and destination vacations will not corrode their insides. If the home is a loving, happy place and their essential needs (taking into account that this is different for each child) are met – with the occasional gift and surprise splurge – they will ultimately recognize how fortunate they are even if their clothing is not graced by designer labels.

The Rebbe's words make clear that it's all in Hashem's hands; that we are sustained by a force much higher than ourselves. How exactly that will manifest is not always clear. Often, having a large family means asking for scholarships from schools and camps; it could mean taking out loans, accepting help before marrying off a child, etc. For many of us, it is distinctly uncomfortable to be on the receiving end in this fashion. That is understandable.

We need to be reminded, however, that Hashem created the entire world in the *mashpia/mekabel* binary. At any given moment, there is a provider and a recipient. The role we fill, however, is dynamic rather than static. We may need financial aid, but that is because we are contributing to our community and our people by parenting more children than some others might be able to. We might not possess great wealth, but we may be the teachers or *mashpiot* of children whose parents have financial resources but lack the gifts we can share.[32]

While concern with finances continues to be one of the biggest challenges in terms of growing a family, there is a fascinating case study that deserves recognition.

In early 2000 Rabbi Yitzchok Schochet, Rabbi of the Mill Hill Community synagogue in London (a United Synagogue under the auspices of the Chief Rabbi), began to actively encourage his congregants to consider having just one more child

---

[32] In the words of contemporary author and scholar Rabbi Tzvi Freeman: Our view of the world and its Creator's view are very different. From our perspective, there is always a giver and a taker. Whether the merchandise be knowledge, affection, or money—somebody always comes out on top and the other on the bottom. In the Creator's view, giver and taker are one. The taker is really giving and the giver, receiving. For without the opportunity to give, the giver would be forever imprisoned within his own self.

Fruitful: The Mitzvah of Pru U'rvu

than they had been planning for. Two decades later, the results are startlingly obvious. His synagogue membership (in excess of 1800 members with more than sixty percent under the age of forty) of varying observance levels, has the largest proportion of children under the age of 20 of any other individual community in Europe. While he concedes that finances are still a primary concern, he points to a community wide culture that supports young children, with two schools within a mile radius of the synagogue, a Sunday *Cheder,* and more. In his community, the average young family has 3.2 children, as opposed to the national average of 1.9. Because there is a lot of opportunity for children in the community, it is at that level, conducive to have and raise children in the immediate area. Families feel supported in their choice to have another child even if it means finances are more strained.[33]

The lesson regarding Hashem's sole guardianship of resources is poignantly expressed in *Sefer Vayikra.*[34]

When discussing the *mitzvot* related to leaving the land fallow, during *shemitah*, every seventh year, and *yovel,* every fiftieth year, the Torah anticipates a question: "What will we eat in the seventh year? We have not planted nor gathered our produce!"[35] In response, Hashem answers "I will command my blessing for you in the sixth year, and [your fields] will produce enough for three years."

The Rebbe emphasizes that Hashem's response is uniquely instructive. He does not simply proclaim, "I am the sustainer of the universe and you can rely on me." What He actually says is that if we trust Him and follow the *mitzvot*, He will transcend the laws of nature to provide for us. The crops from one year will prove ample, providing more sustenance than the Jewish people need to carry them over for three years.

However, receiving the blessing of supernatural bounty cloaked within natural bounds is all predicated on the Jewish people's strong resolve to keep the unique *mitzvot* of *shemitah* and *yovel*. The Torah states כי תבאו אל הארץ אשר אני נתן לכם, ושבתה הארץ שבת לה', when you will come to the land that I am giving you, the land shall rest – a Shabbat for Hashem.[36] Despite external appearances, nature bows to and is contingent on the command of Hashem.

In this vein, the Frierdiker Rebbe addressed the concerns of those worried that remaining steadfast to *halacha* would obviate making a living in America. He

---

33   *Shall We have Another?* Lubavitch.com. July 25, 2019.

34   *Motzei Lag B'omer,* 5740.

35   *Vayikra* 25:20.

36   *Vayikra* 25:2.

proclaimed, "*Machen a leben, macht der Aibershter,*" only G-d "makes" a living. Despite all our best and necessary efforts, our *parnassah* is provided by Hashem and, therefore, living in consonance with Hashem's desire is the only conduit for this *bracha*.[37]

There is no question that overcoming financial burden remains a strong *nisayon*, a test of our faith. Which is why we turn again and again to the words of our Rebbe to give us guidance and strength of conviction.

4. ***I am worried about how I will manage a large/r family because:***
   a) ***I did not grow up in a large family, and I lack strong female role models with whom I have a personal connection.***
   b) ***I am not patient or resilient, nor a great "balabuste."***
   c) ***I don't think I have the necessary parenting skills to raise emotionally healthy, happy children.***
   d) ***I am a baalat teshuvah. While my family has made peace with my lifestyle choice, they offer little in terms of support for our growing family. In fact, each time I am pregnant, I face disparaging comments and am made to feel irresponsible, or worse.***

No matter our personal background – whether an only child or one of many, *frum* from birth or *baal teshuva*, raised in a loving home or one more conflicted – parenting is humbling. And no matter how many children one has, each child is different. Children don't come with manuals, they don't perform on command, there are no algorithms to fall back on. We each make mistakes, we try our best, we grow with our children. No one really tells us how hard parenting can be, how messy life can get, and how elusive perfection is. No matter who we are, the realities of life as a parent is a great equalizer.

Remember, you are not in this alone. You and your husband can seek out role models; talk to couples who have been there and done that, so to say. If your biological family is unable to give you the necessary support and/or you are a *baalat teshuvah* and your lifestyle choices are difficult for your family to understand – yes, it **does** take a village! – nurture close relationships with friends who can become your second family. Connect with a family whose values and lifestyle you would like to replicate and don't be shy about asking for help and taking counsel. It is also helpful to nurture relationships with couples who are slightly older than you are so you can glean from

---

[37] See the Rebbe's words in chapter nine for more on the analogy of the Torah as the backend coding of the website while the surface world we experience, with all its natural laws, functions much like the user interface on the screen. Although not apparent to the naked eye, the coding (i.e. the Torah and adherence to its commands) serves as the sole determinant of the quality of the user's experience on the front end of the website.

their life experience and benefit from their hard earned wisdom. Additionally, there are many resources available to parents: a plethora of workshops, podcasts, and books on parenting, home management skills, time management etc that can be extremely helpful.

There is no question that raising children is the hardest job in the world. We sometimes need to be reminded that there is much that eludes our control. Hashem is the source of all blessings, and He dispenses blessings in accordance with His will.

Through his teachings, the Rebbe urged us to adjust our lens on this matter; he hoped to bring us to a place where we would welcome a new child like we might, for example, welcome winning the State Lottery (but with much more joy!). People don't win the lottery because of their capabilities. It's the luck of the draw or, in our world view, *hashgachah pratit*, Divine providence. Certainly, managing a windfall of millions of dollars brings new challenges, and necessitates that we make important decisions that stretch us beyond our comfort zone. Most of us lack the training and/or natural acuity for dealing intelligently with that kind of money. It might very well complicate our lives in ways we could never imagine, but it certainly opens up previously unimaginable opportunities and benefits. No one would turn down such a gift!

The Rebbe recognized, and spoke directly to these nagging doubts:[38]

The mitzvah of having children was entrusted to every single couple—whether or not their home environment is ideal; whether or not they are confident in their ability to raise good children; and whether or not they believe that they have the financial resources to continue having children.

The Rebbe urged us to leave the long-range planning and prognostics to our Senior partner, Hashem, who is always at our side, doing the heavy lifting. At the same time, the Rebbe was hardly giving us a pass in terms of our responsibilities to our children. Indeed, he was eminently practical in considering the necessary steps both wife and husband must take, as evidenced in the following story:

> **Sara**: For my mother, the children came quickly and closely spaced. She was expecting her fifth baby when her oldest was not yet four; she could hardly catch her breath. In fact, she was not managing very well, and my father convinced her to join him for a *yechidut* with the Rebbe granted on the occasion of his birthday.

---

[38] 17 Sivan, 5740.

In her words, this is what the Rebbe told her that night, on Tevet 19 5730 (January 1970):

> *Your occupation – עסק – is children. You have to make things easier for yourself... If you will get help and let them do their work, then you will have the menuchah, the calmness, to fulfill what you were created for. So, if you have a cleaning lady once a week, you should take her twice, and if you have her twice a week, you should take her three times. And you shouldn't check up in the corners after she leaves to see if she cleaned well enough.*

At a previous *yechidut* the Rebbe had urged my father not to worry about money for cleaning help (then he suggested two times per week instead of once). Hashem provides for all necessities, and this cleaning help is necessary.

On another occasion, the Rebbe told my mother to teach in the Bais Rivkah High school. We need to bring those *neshamot* into the world, but we don't need to do all the dishes, the floors, and the laundry all by ourselves. And we DO need to stimulate our minds and nourish our spirits.

Regarding another reality of parenting, the guilt, the feelings of inadequacy, and the sense that we can never do enough, the Rebbe offered a parallel to the *halachic* constructs of borrowed items.[39] Generally speaking, a borrower assumes responsibility to return in good condition what has been loaned to him by the owner. One exception to this rule concerns the scenario in which the object's owner is present. If the borrowed item gets damaged in the presence of its owner, the borrower does not carry the responsibility.

Each child, the Rebbe gently but firmly reminded us, is a *pikadon,* a deposit, given to us by Hashem for us to watch over and protect to the best of our ability. Hashem, the true "owner," is always there; He plans a family's journey. If you let Him be a partner, then you inevitably have to let go of control – and that's okay. Life might bring things our way that are bigger than we are despite our best efforts. Since Hashem is right there with you caring for this beloved child, we never assume ultimate liability for mishaps.

Remarkably, while the Rebbe and Rebbetzin did not themselves have biological children, the Rebbe was keenly understanding of the difficulties and the immense responsibility inherent in child bearing and rearing. Along with offering pragmatic advice, he encouraged us to understand how blessed and privileged we were to be entrusted with this mission and to be patient in all aspects of this great mitzvah.

---

39 13 Tishrei, 5744.

The Rebbe once described the process of nurturing a child as:[40]

> **Taking care of Hashem's neshamah; in this little infant the Shechinah rests, it's worth all the 'trouble' in the world!**

To a parent who wrote to him concerning difficulties with childbearing, the Rebbe replied:[41]

> **When one plants a beautiful fruit tree fit to be served to a king, and especially a great king, this requires great effort,...and sometimes even at night. And certainly it isn't expected for the fruit to appear on the day of his toil.**
>
> **Indeed planting potatoes is incomparably easier, and the wait is incomparably shorter, etc.**
>
> **And yet, someone who was chosen by the king to grow his royal vineyard or orchard would never request to switch places with the potato grower, but will actually take pride in the fact that he was chosen and entrusted by the great king for this [intense] job.**
>
> **What do you think – is he correct?**
>
> **Azkir al hatziyon (loosely translated as I will pray for you at the resting place of the Previous Rebbe).**

If you are feeling overwhelmed and believe that having another child is simply impossible for you at this point, or ever, do not allow this issue to consume you. Remember, each family is different. The Rebbe wanted each one of us to do more than we thought we could, but by no means does this translate into a uniform equation for each couple.

5. *I take my leadership roles and responsibilities to the community very seriously, and I truly believe that what I am doing is bringing Mashiach closer. Should I not be concerned that having more children will detract from my ability to be effective outside of the home? No one else can/will do for my/our organization what I can; I feel terribly conflicted!*

Many of us are not cut out to stay home and bake chocolate chip cookies. We love our children to the moon and back, but we need other means towards self fulfillment as well. Sometimes, it is easier to take care of other people's children and problems than

---

40   16 Adar, 5747.

41   Tishrei 5742.

to address our own. For many of us, however, working outside of our homes is not just a personal choice or financial imperative; it is our *shlichut* in life and that makes the question all the more confusing.

The Rebbe encouraged and empowered both women and men to do their utmost in terms of *hafatzat hayahadut*, promulgating Judaism, in all of its varied forms. He encouraged women to lead, to teach, to write, and to bring their various strengths and gifts to bear in affecting the global project of *dirah betachtonim*. The Rebbe believed that we are all capable of much more than we realize, and he pressed us to bring our capabilities to the fore. And yet, when engaging in this holy work presented an impediment to having more children, the Rebbe was unequivocal in his position:

> **The Midrash tells us that "the concept of Torah" came before the creation of the world, but "the concept of Jews" came before everything, including Torah. The birth of another Jewish child comes before everything, even "the concept of Torah!"**[42]

Regarding the argument that having more children would negatively impact the quality and quantity of their work in the public realm, for instance, in regard to moving forward with *mivtza'im*, mitzvah campaigns, the Rebbe responded:

> **If Hashem chooses to bless you with a child, then he obviously believes that this is more important – much more important – than mivtza'im. As discussed above, having children is the single most important thing that a person can do – "the concept of the Yidden preceded the Torah!"**[43]

Ultimately, the Rebbe encouraged couples to take a longer view, suggesting the very thing they fear as an impediment will increase their effectiveness:

> **In the long run, the mivtza'im work itself will likely benefit. When you have a child, that child can go on to accomplish tremendous things in mivtza'im, possibly even more than you. So, in effect, having another child is better for the mivtza'im work, too.**

---

[42] Rosh Chodesh Shevat, 5741.

[43] Rosh Chodesh Shevat, 5741.

Fruitful: The Mitzvah of Pru U'rvu

Furthermore, the Rebbe spoke of *hatzlacha b'zman,* added success in the use of one's time, as another blessing that flowed from having children.[44]

Similarly, in writing to a school teacher who was struggling to balance her home duties and her work responsibilities.[45], [46] He reiterated how important it is that a woman hire the help she needs at home to ensure she can strike the proper life balance.

> **Every effort, even intense effort, that can be made in the field of youth education is worthwhile. This is because any improvement, even improvements that seem minor in the moment, can result in fundamental and lifelong [character] improvements that are verily visible.**
>
> **I am confident that you organized your home life, especially as it pertains to your children, may they live, in a manner that ensures that your sacred pedagogical work with the students at school doesn't conflict with your sacred task of raising your children at home. [After all], a mitzvah facilitates another mitzvah, and not the opposite.**
>
> **Certainly, since G-d repays measure for measure, and many times over, you will see increased blessing and success with your children—that they will be faithful to G-d, to His Torah, and to His commandments. You together with your husband, the Rabbi may he live, should derive true nachat, that is chassidishe nachat, in abundance, with peace of mind and proper health.**

We can discern a pattern; the Rebbe did not, in most cases, embrace the stark binary that pits family life against other responsibilities or concerns. Instead, he viewed both as being of one cloth; our life's *shlichut* comprised of various aspects. At some points in time, however, some aspect thereof might temporarily have to yield to the other.

---

[44] Rosh Chodesh Shevat, 5741.

[45] *Igrot Kodesh*, vol. 12, p. 247.

[46] Similarly, in 1970, after hearing the Rebbe speak vehemently about the importance of growing and raising one's family, a group of teachers at Beis Rivkah, the flagship Lubavitch girl's school, wrote to ask the Rebbe if they should indeed continue working outside of the home. The Rebbe replied that the *zechut* of working in his father in law's *mossad*, institution, will stand them in good stead. (Based on a conversation with Mrs. Chanah Gorovitz, dean of Beis Rivkah Schools.)

Rivkah: Relatively early in my pregnancy with our fifth child, the doctor announced that I had to go on complete bed rest. The pains I had been feeling were due to my uterus contracting prematurely, which could lead to a dangerously early delivery. When my beloved doctor pronounced her recommendation, I looked at her in total disbelief. There was just no way I could suspend all of my activities for so long! She saw that I was having a hard time processing the information, and she firmly repeated: Rivkah, this is no joke. If you don't promise to adhere to my recommendations, I will have to ask that you leave my practice; I simply cannot take responsibility for what might ensue...

As we are close in age and similarly hard driven, I looked into her eyes and asked her: Dr. Amin, please tell me the truth: if our roles were reversed, would you close your bustling solo practice?

Without batting an eye, she replied emphatically: Of course, do you think I am crazy?

I now understood the gravity of the situation, but still, I was used to "being crazy," and besides, *shlichut* is not equivalent to any other position. My husband and parents asked me to stop being ridiculous and grow up already. Quickly.

Once safely ensconced in bed (pre- personal computer and cell phone days) the real difficulties ensued.

We had to make many practical arrangements: childcare for all the hours the babysitter could not be with us, meals, laundry, and the list went on and on. And of course for the Chabad House: events, Shabbat, Yom Tov, the day to day administration, and the classes... Luckily I was still able to give classes (our second floor was never cleaner, as people were coming up to learn in my bedroom) but the rest of the time I was mentally climbing the walls!

My poor husband, who was now ably juggling everything alone, had to deal with my despondency as well.

Every single day, my dear father would call me to see how I was doing, and every single day, he would repeat: you are engaged in this single most important *shlichut*: you are bringing another *neshamah* into this world...

All these years later I can still hear the love in his voice. The profound truth of the lesson he was trying to impart to me then only becomes more clear with the passage of time.

The above vignette is the experience of just one woman. Yet again, we urge each woman and her husband to take counsel with their respective *mashpiim* and with a *rav* with whom they have shared all of the factors that need to be taken into account. Only then can he advise them as to how to proceed with the mitzvah of *pru u'rvu* based on the reality of their life – distinctively – to the exclusion of all others. May Hashem grant that each one of us merit to fulfill our personal *avodah* – in whatever form that takes – with *menuchat hanefesh,* calm and equanimity, and great joy.

The View From On High:
The Rebbe's Words on Pru U'rvu

The gift of sight allows us to see the world around us. Vision is the capacity to think about or plan the future using our wisdom and imagination. Understandably, those on a higher plane – both literally or figuratively – can see further ahead than those at a lower elevation. And then there are the higher levels of perception we refer to as *Ruach Hakodesh,* divine inspiration and *nevuah,* prophecy.

The Rebbe's public addresses and private correspondence about *pru u'rvu*, all give the impression of the Rebbe lovingly bidding us to view things not as we might conventionally, but from a heavenly perspective.

The Rebbe famously insisted that each person is brought into this world to fulfill a *shlichut*, a specific mission. For us women, most generally speaking, our paramount *shlichut* consists of being the *akeret habayit*, the mainstay and anchor of our homes. Regardless of what else we might be involved in – and as is well known, the Rebbe fully believed in our powers to be the anchors of our communities and institutions – we were tasked by Hashem with bringing *neshamot* into this world and with raising them, physically and spiritually.

When we encounter difficulties in this mission, we might remember that our Creator has endowed us with the necessary resources to fulfill our mandate. Furthermore, the Rebbe emphatically asserted, if the Torah prescribes a way of life, undoubtedly, that pathway is best for us.

One of the Rebbe's greatest *chiddushim*, most novel teachings, was his insistence that *gashmiyut*, the material aspects of this world, cannot be separated from *ruchniyut*, their spiritual antecedents. As the *Zohar* teaches, אסתכל באורייתא וברא עלמא, Hashem looked into the Torah and created the world.[47] The most well known reading of this verse explains that the Torah serves as the blueprint for the creation of the universe, and that the world's material aspects are a manifestation of a spiritual reality rooted in the Torah.

In the Rebbe's novel approach, the Torah functions less like a blueprint and more like a website's backend.[48] When an architect creates blueprints for a project, there is

---

47 *Zohar* II 161a.

48 This analogy is taken from the JLI course titled Paradigm Shift: Transformational Life Teachings of the Lubavitcher Rebbe written by Rabbis Mordechai Dinerman and Naftali Silberberg.

still room for the project to evolve. Sometimes, their building looks very different from the final specs.

On the other hand, a computer is powered by backend coding. To a novice, this code can look like gibberish; but, in actuality, this series of letters and numbers controls the entire page. Everything that happens on a webpage is controlled by the code. The Rebbe taught that the Torah is the coding of our world. In every age, the world flows out of the truths of the Torah.

Because the world is inextricably bound in the Torah, when we fulfill the most important *shlichut* the Torah has bestowed on us we experience the greatest happiness and peace. While bearing and raising children may be hard, this unique mitzvah grants us a life of meaning and fulfillment.

In the Rebbe's words:[49]

> **The Torah reveals the true nature and function of everything… Practically, this means that when we use an object as per the Torah's directives, our usage is consistent with the true nature of that object. If, G-d forbid, we do not do so, we are not only contravening the Torah's instructions and G-d's will; we are also in conflict with the object itself by using it in a manner that is contrary to its own nature and existence.**

The above truths notwithstanding, for many, *pru u'rvu* is a difficult mitzvah to perform. While the pregnancy and birthing process proves different for each woman, everyone experiences some measure of difficulty and pain. More often than not, it is the complexity of raising children that causes women to think twice about having another, and another.

The Rebbe's office was the address to which much of world Jewry sent news of its hardships. Its walls absorbed thousands and thousands of lamentable stories. The Rebbe was privy to the difficulties parents might encounter, including compromised health, a dearth of financial resources, and even, lack of patience. Still, he consistently prodded our embrace of the truth that children, as many as Hashem blesses us with, are the source of ultimate *bracha* in our lives.

Broadly speaking, the Rebbe did not tell us **what** to think, but he most certainly taught us **how** to think. He pushed us to widen our scope, to probe more deeply beneath the surface, and to imagine what seemed to most to be utterly impossible.

---

49   *Sefer Hasichot* 5748, vol. 2, p. 590, fn.10.

You might say that the Rebbe fully believed we were super women: possessed of infinite powers because we carried infinity within us. He begged us to believe in ourselves and not underestimate our capacities; to firmly anchor ourselves to the *Ein Sof*, the endless energy of Hashem, and expand ourselves to receive the blessings and the light.

It has been noted that more than people believed in the Rebbe, the Rebbe believed in us. In the words of Rabbi Adin Steinsaltz:[50]

> Through all the years of his leadership, it was plain to see that the Rebbe was set on an objective. What do you think the Rebbe was agitating to achieve?
>
> The Rebbe wanted to do something that was more far-reaching than any revolution... he wanted to change human nature...to change the whole world. In the Talmud, we have Hillel and Shammai, the latter characteristically unforgiving of human limitations, and the former in resigned acceptance of reality. The Rebbe offered another alternative. He said, "let us change human nature."
>
> In physics, something happens under conditions of great pressure. The molecules collapse and the very nature of the object changes. The Rebbe believed that the impossible was possible. He believed that when we do not only what we can do, but also what we cannot do, and that even though there are only 24 hours in the day, we somehow work more than that, we pass into the world of impossibilities, into the era of Mashiach. It is removing human limitations and becoming transformed into an entirely different existence. It was as if he told us, "Run! Run! And if you cannot run, walk! And if you cannot walk—crawl! But always advance, always take at least one step forward." The Rebbe wanted to bring Mashiach now. That is revolutionary.

One example of this is evident in the following story:

> **Bat Sheva Deren relates**: My mother in law, Kenny Deren a"h, was principal of the Yeshiva School girls High School in Pittsburgh. At a certain point, after suffering a setback in her health, she notified the Rebbe that she planned to promote me to the post of principal while she would continue as a teacher. The Rebbe gave his blessings and consent. Upon hearing about this, however, I was perturbed. I was at that point a mother of seven young children and I was concerned with how I would manage to successfully fulfill what seemed to me to be towering and dueling responsibilities. I wrote to the Rebbe with my concerns and received the following reply:

---

[50] From an interview with Rabbi Adin Steinsaltz by Baila Olidort of Lubavitch.com published February 3, 2020.

> הקב״ה הוא בעל הכח ובעל היכולת ובלתי בעל גבול ותוספתו מרובה. וכל המוסיף מוסיפים לו.
>
> Hashem is the Master of power and ability. He has no constraints, and His blessings are of immense proportions. The more you will do, the more you will receive.
>
> I have kept a copy of this reply both in my school office and at home as a constant reminder that when one takes care of Hashem's children, we access higher and deeper energy from Hashem's boundless treasures.

As you read this you might think that you don't fall in that category at all! That you are completely overwhelmed at the idea of getting pregnant again. In fact, you might even feel guilty because when you find out you are pregnant, anxiety grips you.

If that is the case, know that you are not alone.

In the following letter we see how the Rebbe, in his characteristically encouraging fashion, replies to a woman who wrote that she was beset by despondency, compounded by disappointment in her lack of happiness about her pregnancy. In this reply, the Rebbe is exquisitely attentive to the mood swings and irritability that often come with pregnancy and offers a new framework to make peace with those feelings:

> **You wonder and are shocked at your reaction.**
>
> **But surely you know from your own previous experience when G-d had blessed you and you were in a similar condition, that it is natural, in a state of pregnancy, to have certain reactions, reactions that have nothing to do with the blessing itself.**
>
> **Just as there are certain physical reactions during pregnancy, such as, for example, a craving for or dislike of certain foods, so, too, can there be a certain moodiness, irritability and the like. At any rate, there is no basis at all to feel depressed or discouraged when such feelings occasionally appear.**
>
> **I am therefore confident that this letter will find you in a much improved state of mind and in full appreciation of this great Divine blessing with which you and your husband and family have been blessed.**

May G-d grant that you have an easy and normal pregnancy, giving birth to a healthy child at the proper time, and that, together with your husband, you should raise all your children to a life of Torah, chuppah, and good deeds[51].

The First and Greatest Mitzvah of All

Chazal taught, and the Rebbe often and vehemently underscored, the primacy of the mitzvah *rabbah,* the great mitzvah of *pru u'rvu*.[52]

In yet another letter on the topic the Rebbe writes:[53]

> **...Surely you realize that children are the greatest of all Divine blessings. Indeed, it is the first commandment in the Torah – "Be fruitful and multiply." Moreover, the fact that this is the first commandment and blessing in the Torah demonstrates how very significant and important this commandment is. Thus, the news of the expected addition in the family should have brought you considerable joy.**

In fact, the Rebbe asserted, *pru u'rvu* is the first mitzvah and *bracha* in the Torah, for it is the greatest *bracha* with which one can be blessed..[54] The fact that this mitzvah precedes even the words "I am Hashem your G-d" indicates just how important it is.[55]

He further made clear that the fulfillment of this mitzvah forms the bedrock of our people:

> **Every individual child is an olam malei, an entire world. When you bring a child into the world, you are bringing an entire world, and you are creating an infinite lineage of people that will come from that child. When you choose not to have another child, that is spiritually eliminating an entire lineage of people that could have resulted from this child.**

---

51 From a letter of the Rebbe, dated 20 Kislev, 5732.

52 *Tosafot* to Shabbat 4a and to Gittin 41b.

53 From a letter of the Rebbe, dated 20 Kislev, 5732.

54 17 Sivan, 5740.

55 *Shabbat Parshat Behar-Bechukotai,* 5731.

> Throughout all the generations—in Eretz Yisrael, as well as during all times of galut— Jews always considered it to be the greatest bracha to have many children. This goes back to the earliest history of the Jewish people. The Imahot whilst very different from one another all shared this one thing: a yearning and striving to have children. "Sara hut eingeleigt di velt!" (loosely translated: 'She gave it her all'). She came with complaints to Avraham Avinu, and she didn't allow him to rest: she needed to have children! The same was true with Rivka and Rochel. Even Leah, who merited to have children immediately after her marriage, did everything in her power to have more.[56]

Along with establishing the primacy of this mitzvah, the Rebbe stressed the importance of bringing as many children into the world as possible:

> One cannot argue that it suffices to have two children, a boy and a girl, for they are leaving a replacement for themselves and not reducing the amount of people in the world – because you weren't created only to desist from causing damage; you were created to build worlds through having children and grandchildren, thereby becoming a partner with Hashem in creation.[57]

The Rebbe often referenced the difficulties of life in Egypt and noted how, through *emunah* and *bitachon*, the Jewish people overcame seemingly insurmountable impediments to growing their families. Ultimately, this unshakable commitment to bringing more Jewish children into the world paved the way for *geulah*:[58]

> When Pharaoh decreed that every newborn boy should be drowned in the Nile, Amram, the leader of the generation, said: Should we toil in vain? Why should we continue having children when they will be immediately thrown into the river? He proceeded to divorce his wife Yocheved, and he was followed by the rest of the Jewish people.

---

[56] *Rosh Chodesh* Shevat, 5741.

[57] *Shabbat Parshat Tzav*, 5744.

[58] כמו שנגאלו ישראל ממצרים בזכות שהיו פרים ורבים. כמו כן יגאלו לעתיד בזכות שהם פרים ורבים. Just like the Jews were redeemed from Egypt in the merit of their having children, so too they will be redeemed in the future in the merit of having children. *Tana Devei Eliyahu Zuta* 14.

> His young daughter [Miriam] told him that he was making a mistake. Hashem told us to have children, so how can you consider what Pharaoh says?! He immediately listened to his daughter and reunited with his wife.
>
> Now, his calculation seems to have been eminently logical…
>
> What happened as a result of the fact that Amram ignored the odds and reunited with his wife? Moshe, the savior of the entire Jewish nation, was born. Not only was he not drowned, but his birth brought about a swift end to the decree against baby boys, and ultimately he was the one who brought redemption for the entire nation!
>
> Today, the considerations are much less substantial than they were then. And when someone considers pushing off children for considerations of parnassah and so forth, they must know that they are holding up the geulah! אין בן דוד בא עד שיכלו כל הנשמות שבגוף, Mashiach will only come when all the neshamot that were destined to be born in galut are born.[59]

Each Child Opens a New Channel of Bracha

For most couples, the birth of their first child brings an unsurpassed thrill. The birth of their subsequent children deepens the joy, provides their children with the singular gift of filial connections, and completes the picture they had in mind when imagining their perfect family. But what about the mandate to have more than the number the couple imagines is perfect?

This charge is hardly a sacrifice, the Rebbe would say, because each and every child is a conduit for a new and distinctive *bracha* in the lives of their parents. Furthermore, each additional child opens up new channels of *bracha* for all the members of the family.[60]

Aside from children providing *brachot* in the material realm, the Rebbe spoke of the greatest gift offspring bring their parents: *nachat*. Sociologists have long taught that the least translatable words in a civilization's language teach us most about that culture. The one Yiddish word *nachat*, necessitates many words to define it in any

---

59 25 Iyar, 5743.

60 *Shabbat Parshat Yitro,* 5744.

Fruitful: The Mitzvah of Pru U'rvu

other language: the singular happiness and pleasure derived from the accomplishments and achievements of loved ones, especially children and grandchildren. Expressing the wish that someone experience great *nachat* has long served as the gold standard in blessing Jewish parents. In the Rebbe's words:

> **It is impossible to receive this same nachat from a single child, for with every additional child comes a new world of nachat, each in their own unique way: One child gives nachat in the arena of Torah, another in avodah, and a third in gemilut chassadim.**[61]

The Rebbe, further urged us to think into the future, even conjuring the realities of empty nesters:

> **When children grow up and move away to build their own families, the parents want to visit their children and grandchildren, and even great-grandchildren. But if they have only one or two children, they can only visit every half a year or so…The parents can't sit in their children's homes all the time. Between trips, they are forced to be alone, without having someone to open themselves up to. Whereas parents who have many children can visit one child, stay for a while and then move on to the next child. Similarly, the children and grandchildren come to visit their parents and grandparents from time to time, and everyone sits together – a minyan at the table, ושמחת לפני ה', אלוקיך אתה ובניך ובנותיך, and the grandfathers and grandmothers receive much nachat from their children and grandchildren.**[62]

A Brief History of the Rebbe's Focus on this Mitzvah

It was 1968 when Stanford biologist Paul Ehrlich published his best-selling book *The Population Bomb*.[63] In it he predicted that "in the 1970's, hundreds of millions of people will starve to death" because of overpopulation. Later editions modified the sentence to read "In the 1980's."

---

61 *Shabbat Parshat Nasso*, 5740.

62 *Shabbat Parshat Nasso*, 5740.

63 On the cover of this book which sold millions of copies, under the complete title: Population Control or Race to Oblivion THE POPULATION BOMB the following words were highlighted by a yellow background: While you are reading these words four people will have died from starvation, most of them children.

Demographers, futurists, and fiction writers all joined in his chorus predicting an apocalypse. In 1960, the world population had hit 3 billion. In 1975 it was estimated to hit 4 billion, and the powers that be were frantic with worry about sustainability. Zero Population Growth became the *cri du jour*, cry of the day. Decades later, we live in a world populated by 8 billion, and the horrors of overpopulation were never realized.

Living in a country culturally saturated with hysterical doomsday predictions, the Rebbe adopted a decidedly positive world view. As the twentieth anniversary of his *nesiut*, leadership approached, the Rebbe announced that "*Mashiach*'s Sefer Torah," a Sefer Torah that had been written but not completed during the lifetime of the Frierdiker Rebbe, would finally be completed.[64]

There was palpable excitement and tremendous anticipation in the air, and chassidim flew in from all over the world to be present.

On *Motzei Shabbat*, the Rebbe led a *farbrengen*, and spoke of a critical and practical step that could and should be taken to bring the arrival of *Mashiach* closer:

> **The Gemara states, אין בן דוד בא עד שיכלו כל הנשמות שבגוף, Ben David [Mashiach] will not come until all souls in [the treasury of souls called] 'guf' will be finished...**
>
> **There are those who are mistaken and want to debate about birth control and so on – but they are misinterpreting the Torah. Having children is not only a personal obligation to fulfill the first mitzvah of the Torah to "fill the world and conquer it," but it is a matter that affects everyone – the geulah of the entire Jewish nation depends on it. This is a special shlichut that depends especially on women and girls, wherever they may be; how much more so regarding those who are already aware of the teachings, directives, and guidance of the [Frierdiker] Rebbe...[65]**

The Rebbe's words galvanized his chassidim, but the Rebbe had a much broader target audience in mind. Ten years later, on 17 Sivan 5740, addressing the annual N'shei U'Bnot Chabad Convention, the Rebbe charged the women of Lubavitch with strengthening the campaign to promote the practice of *taharat hamishpachah*, family purity. Additionally, he asked the women to include emphasis on bearing larger families

---

64 10 Shvat 5730 (1970) referred to by chassidim as *"Yud Shevat Hagadol."*

65 *Motzei Yud Shevat*, 5730.

Fruitful: The Mitzvah of Pru U'rvu

in contradistinction to the prevalent zeitgeist that looked askance at a family of more than the responsible to the environment magical number of two children.

The Rebbe continued to touch on this theme at *farbrengens* over the ensuing years, encouraging people to open themselves up to the blessings of a large family.

It is important to note that, while the Rebbe spoke on this topic very publicly, he was also speaking privately to individuals, giving them tools as to how this could be achieved in practice.

One such example concerns Rabbi Shmuel Lew, who relates:

> I merited to be in New York for Yud Shevat "Hagadol" in the year 5730; Mashiach's Sefer Torah was completed! What an awesome Mashiach'dike feeling encompassed our very beings.
>
> An especially uplifting Shabbat *farbrengen* was followed by a Motzei Shabbat *farbrengen*. Sunday night at 2 a.m. I was *zocheh* to go into *yechidut*, a private audience with the Rebbe, and I was flying high with the Mashiach spirit.
>
> The Rebbe asked me: "How is your wife managing with running the home?"
>
> (At that time we had 5 children under the age of 6.)
>
> I was stunned and answered "*Baruch Hashem*!"
>
> The Rebbe asked: "Does she have help in the house?"
>
> To which I replied, "three times a week she has a lady coming to help out with housework."
>
> The Rebbe then asked: "Why not more often? Is it due to financial constraints or there is no one available?" (At that time, even wealthy people had household help only once or twice a week…I just kept quiet…)
>
> When I got home I told my wife to add one more day of household help.

Sharing information about a mitzvah like *taharat hamishpachah* with less or non observant Jews was a much taller task than the previous *mivtza'im*, mitzvah campaigns, such as encouraging the donning of *tefillin*, the affixing of *mezuzot*, lighting Shabbat and Yom Tov candles, all of which necessitated a relatively small commitment. But speaking out against family planning seemed, even to the Rebbe's staunchest female soldiers, too far a reach.

During that era, Rabbi Nachman Bernhard, a prominent *rav* in Johannesburg, South Africa, had occasion to visit in NY. He was asked to address a group of Lubavitcher women active in promoting the Rebbe's *mivtza'im*. He was tasked with lecturing on the challenging topic: "How to Present the Mitzvah of *Pru Urvu* and *Taharat Hamishpachah* to the Uncommitted." Before his scheduled talk, he wrote to the Rebbe for guidance:

...One of the young women active in this field told me that she, as well as all of her colleagues (both contemporaries and older), are having great difficulty in convincingly presenting one particular aspect of... family planning. Many people are willing to accept all the points about the ongoing obligation of *piriah v'riviah*, as well as the observance of *taharat hamishpachah*, but nevertheless they (and this includes very many *frum* couples) tend to indulge in a limited degree and kind of 'family planning' by 'spacing' or spreading out their children over several years, instead of having one right after the other without a break...

The Rebbe responded to each argument:

> **"Regarding "Spacing etc."**
>
> **[Such logic] can only be applied to something that is a person's choice. But a person can only choose not to get pregnant – it is up to only Hashem as to whether a person will actually get pregnant and whether the infant will be completely healthy. It's possible that "if not now, then when?"**
>
> **According to everyone (in the natural order), the younger a woman is, the healthier the baby will be...**
>
> **The main [subconscious] reason – based on the founding principle and beginning of the entire Shulchan Aruch – is that people will scoff at them!**
>
> **When you explain to them that this is the true obstacle—then they will joyfully hand over the decision of the best time to have more children to Hashem...**

N'shei Chabad did indeed promote the Rebbe's view on this important issue, even placing full page ads in the New York Times and other periodicals, hoping to reach the widest audience, inclusive of *bnei Noach*. In several *sichot,* the Rebbe mentioned that all *bnei Noach* are included in the commandment of *lashevet*, to populate the world with children that will be taught about Hashem and build societies based on that belief.[66], [67]

---

66   Shabbat Parshat Shlach and Korach, 5740.

67   He was also concerned with the negative effects of family planning and the use of contraceptives, going as far as urging the FDA for a review of their safety.

Fruitful: The Mitzvah of Pru U'rvu

Fascinatingly, the Rebbe requested that Rabbi Moshe Feller, head *shliach* to Minnesota, have Minnesota state senator Rudy Boschwitz read one of his *sichot* on this subject into the Congressional record.[68] It appears that the Rebbe wanted these ideas to break through societal resistance, and he used every possible medium at his disposal. Simultaneously, the Rebbe worked with Israeli politicians, encouraging them to take practical steps towards raising the Jewish birthrate in the Holy Land.[69]

As we know, the dire predictions concerning a dystopian world in which too many people scramble for non-existent resources never came to pass. Technological innovations have made it possible for us to grow more food than we can possibly use and have helped us efficiently transport necessary resources around the globe.

Ironically, since, medical advances have made life safer and longer, lower mortality rates no longer necessitate that couples have more children. Coupled with the fact that most no longer live an agrarian lifestyle which necessitates more hands to work the land, this has led to population decline. Additionally, women entering the halls of academia and the workforce en masse, and more sophisticated contraception have further contributed to shrinking families. To date, (with the exception of Africa) countries on all continents face worries over depopulation.

Birth Control is a Misnomer

The Rebbe taught that words have weight and potency and should be used with care and precision. He decried the arrogance inherent in the term birth control and on more than one occasion revealed the fallacy therein.

On *Vov* Tishrei 5741 the Rebbe asserted:

> **There are three partners in the creation of every child: the father, the mother, and Hashem. The father and mother can only control that they definitely won't have children, but anything past that, in fact everything else— that the mother will become pregnant, that the child will be healthy, and how the child's life**

---

[68] Boschwitz served as an Independent-Republic in the Senate from December 1978-January 1991. He also served as United States Ambassador to the United Nations Commission on Human Rights.

[69] For an example, see letters from the Rebbe (*Igrot Kodesh*, vol. 25, pp. 204-205 and vol. 26, p. 145) to MK and activist Geula Cohen.

will turn out—is controlled completely by the third partner, Hashem. And Hashem gave his opinion as to whether or not a person should try having children; He said pru u'rvu, be fruitful and multiply—without exceptions or quotas.[70]

At a *farbrengen* on Rosh Chodesh Shevat 5741, the Rebbe returned to the same theme:

> **Just a few generations ago, parents would never have considered interfering with Hashem's business, especially when it comes to something as important as having children. Now, because parents do have a small say in the matter, this was misinterpreted (in recent times) as an invitation to mix into Hashem's affairs. It was forgotten that Hashem gives the parents the choice only to prevent themselves from becoming pregnant—but to become pregnant, and to have healthy children, depends only on Hashem, and He will surely choose the best time for the mother and father.[71]**

Beyond pointing out that the very term family planning was a misnomer, the Rebbe saw inherent danger in the accepted practice of family planning defined as the ability of individuals and couples to anticipate and attain, through the use of contraception, their desired number of children, and the spacing and timing of their births. On the surface, the Rebbe said, family planning may sound like a sensible idea: If you plan everything else in your life, how much more so should you be organized in an endeavor as significant as child-bearing, ensuring that the children come at the appropriate time and under ideal circumstances.

In reality it is a dangerous plan, concealed in a silk *kapote*, in holy clothing; it might have a fancy, politically correct name, but really it's a deceptive term for disrupting Hashem's natural order, the natural functions of our bodies.[72]

---

70 *Rosh Chodesh* Shevat, 5741.

71 *Rosh Chodesh* Shevat, 5741.

72 17 Sivan, 5740. *Rosh Chodesh* Shevat, 5741.

Fruitful: The Mitzvah of Pru U'rvu

On Hashem's Timetable

The Rebbe encouraged us to let Hashem run the world and reminded us that *brachot* do not just flow when we decide to accept them:

> The Torah tells us that, when Moshe Rabbeinu was on the mountain, he made a request of Hashem: "Show me Your face." Hashem responded, "You will see My back, but My face must not be seen." The Gemara explains[73] Hashem's message to Moshe: When I wanted [to show you My glory at the burning bush], you did not want [to see it, as it is stated: "And Moshe concealed his face, fearing to gaze upon Hashem"]. But now that you want, I do not want [to show it to you]."
>
> This teaches us a lesson. Obviously, Hashem wasn't getting "even" with Moshe Rabbeinu. But when Hashem gives us a bracha, He doesn't want it to be free and underserved; He wants us to be partners with Him.
>
> How can we be good partners with Hashem? By letting Him run the world—by depending on Him fully as a partner and letting Him determine the best time to have a child. When the decision is left up to Hashem, it happens at the best time for all parties involved. But as soon as the person gets involved, and he doesn't allow Hashem to make the decision—he doesn't allow it when Hashem wanted it—then even when the person decides that, according to his calculations, he is ready—you want—he lacks the vessel that brings Hashem's brachot.
>
> (The Rebbe added that certainly Hashem is maarich af [slow to anger], especially since these people have good intentions, and added that, "I don't want to scare people, but simply to give over what it says in the Torah.")
>
> Furthermore: the timing of a child's conception, birth, and growth is pivotal, and impacts his entire life. Not only does it affect the child himself, but all the future generations that will come from him. When a parent considers the best time for the child to be born, the calculation is bound to be limited to their

---

[73] *Brachot* 7a.

foresight. Whereas the parents are thinking a few months ahead, Hashem is planning decades and generations ahead. Only He knows the future generations and the unlimited factors that must go into such a decision—so such a decision must be left up to Him, and He will decide when it is best.[74]

The above words give us strength to embrace Hashem's *brachot* when they come our way and to recognize them as the great gifts that they are.

What Does My Soul Say?

The Rebbe, ever empathetic to the challenges of building a large family, encouraged us to think more deeply about our motivations and see the unsurpassed rewards accessible only through rearing additional children:

> This nachat doesn't come without effort; rather, it involves the challenge of raising sons and daughters. But "According to the pain is the reward": the nachat is even deeper, broader, and richer than something received without effort, without doubts and difficulties. This includes the difficulty: "What will my neighbor across the street say? Will she say that this behavior is in style, or not?"
>
> ...The Jew must ask: "What does my G-dly soul think?" – and automatically he conquers his materialistic inclination. And G-d's promise, "Be fruitful and multiply and fill the earth, and conquer it," will be fulfilled literally: when he conquers the material world utilizing it in the service of G-d, then if he needs more money, G-d gives him more money; if he needs a bigger house, because another son or daughter was born, G-d gives him a bigger house; if he needs more clothes – beautiful clothes, because a beautiful child requires beautiful clothing, G-d gives him the means to buy beautiful clothes. And most importantly, children are born, who grow to "find favor in the eyes of G-d and man.[75]

---

74   *Rosh Chodesh* Shevat, 5741.

75   24 Tevet, 5741.

Finally, the Rebbe spoke to a mother's most fervent hope and desire, and promised us:[76]

> **Ultimately, after a number of years have passed, and the children grow up, Hashem sends success and we get to see the fruits. 'Your Olam Haba you will see during your lifetime,' you literally see the world-to-come in this world—through true everlasting nachat from children and grandchildren. The nachat is so clear and indisputable, that even the neighbor and 'peer' must admit that she followed in the path of true bracha begashmiyut u'beruchniyut, physically and spiritually.**

Sara: In the 1980's I was in high school when the Rebbe spoke often and vehemently about family planning. I heard those *sichot* (and many others) through a telephone hook up in my city of origin, Montreal, Canada. I would watch my mother's eyes and face light up with joy while listening to the Rebbe's encouraging words on this subject. I, on the other hand, did not really connect to the message, or so I thought... My mother was the one giving birth to children, not me.

Fast forward five years - I was in labor with my second child. I was very petite and looked even younger than my age. The nurse in the birthing ward in the hospital looked at me in disdain while she took my vitals. Then, in a mocking tone, she asked, "Was this a planned pregnancy?" implying, another teen pregnancy!?

"Yes, it was!" was my instant emphatic reply. "Planned by G-d!" I insisted that she write those words down on my chart. After my outburst declaring my confidence in my (G-d's) choice, she changed her tone completely. With great respect and admiration, she proceeded with the intake. At that moment, I realized that the Rebbe's words had indeed seeped into my subconscious; when it counted, I knew the truth.

More than a decade later, I was challenged once more.

It was a bleak, rainy Shabbat morning, and I was unsuccessfully trying to console a very colicky newborn while simultaneously attempting to entertain a toddler. My husband was late coming home from *shul* with my older boys. I was tired, hungry and a real *kvetch*. He walked in the door together with my three children, who had been fighting...not a pretty scene.

At that moment, a guest happened to pop in. Engaged to be married at the time, the young man surveyed the scene and exclaimed, "This is insane. When I get married, I plan to have one, maybe two children, that's it!"

[76] *Rosh Chodesh* Shevat, 5741.

> I was furious with him, but after a moment, I shifted the focus of my upset to myself. That *he* should harbor such ideas was predictable; given his background, that was the norm. But me – why was I tongue tied? Why did I not have the conviction to speak the truth? Was I questioning Hashem's plan for my family?
>
> *Boruch Hashem* for children. In a split second, my then twelve year old child got up and faced him squarely – "you are talking like this because you do not have a child yet. I promise you that when you have one child, you will beg Hashem to bless you with double the amount of children that are sitting around this table!" Now, this guest was utterly shocked that the child had this response. In that moment of silence, my husband quickly made *kiddush,* and within a few minutes, we were all happily enjoying ourselves.
>
> On that Shabbat, I made a decision that I would research and learn all of the Rebbe's talks on this subject and make them available for anyone who needs to strengthen their conviction. With the help of my brother, Rabbi Tzvi Hirsh Gurary, we got the job done.[77]
>
> Years later, I was once again challenged. Raising children in our postmodern world was daunting, and I questioned my capabilities as a mother. I believed that Hashem must have made a mistake by putting his most precious *neshamot* into my hands... Were these thoughts coming from my *yetzer tov* or the opposite?
>
> I began to listen to the Rebbe's talks on this subject. I did so over and over again until, *Baruch Hashem*, I realigned my thoughts with those of Torah and chassidut.
>
> Of course, I avail myself of current research and practical advice in helping me raise these precious gifts with *simchah*! The Rebbe's words, however, are timeless and timely; they provide a sense of security and confidence in our mission as Jewish mothers.

The Rebbe's enduring message was a wake up call to a world increasingly fueled by a narrow minded concern with self and too often, a jaundiced outlook on life both present and the future. The Rebbe constantly led us in the opposite direction; he rallied us to actively work towards and welcome *Yemot HaMashiach*, a perfected and redeemed world. He reminded us that children are not brought into this world for utilitarian purposes, nor solely to fill an emotional vacuum, grant us enduring legacy or provide us with joy. Bringing children into this world is our most sacred responsibility and greatest privilege. Finally, the Rebbe reminded us that there were *neshamot* waiting since *Matan Torah* to come into this world and fulfill their mission and that only

---

[77] Visit thedailysicha.com. *pru u'rvu* section to access the *sichot* in the original Yiddish and in Hebrew and English translation. and mikvah.org/audio for lectures on this topic.

after the descent of every last *neshamah* that is destined to come into the world, could *Mashiach* finally arrive.[78]

May that be speedily in our days. Amen.

---

78 15 Shevat, 5741.

Frequently Asked Questions

ADDRESSED IN THIS BOOK

- » Why an emphasis on being intimate at night and specifically, in the dark? (page 16)

- » Are there limitations on touching, caressing, kissing, and cuddling outside of the framework of sexual intimacy? (page 17)

- » Does a wife have an obligation to give her husband pleasure? (page 27)

- » What if I am not in the mood and I can tell my husband wants us to be together, or I am in the mood but he seems out of it? (page 28)

- » Is PDA, otherwise known as public displays of affection, okay? (page 35)

- » If our children never see us hugging and kissing our spouses, how will they know we love each other, and how will they develop an understanding of healthy touch? (page 38)

- » I have learned that the thoughts of the parents during intimacy impact the children who will be conceived. Practically speaking, how can I channel my thoughts correctly? (page 43)

- » I have heard something about waiting until after midnight to have relations. And, is it true that intimacy on Friday night is a mitzvah? (page 45)

- » I hear that sometimes couples watch a range of sexually explicit materials together as a form of arousal or just for fun. Is that okay? (page 52)

- » Can we talk about female masturbation? (page 55)

- » Why are there so many *hanhagot*, suggested behaviors, concerning what a couple does in the bedroom? Isn't sexuality all about uninhibited expression? (page 67)

- » What about lingerie and sex toys? (page 73)

- » I have not always followed the rules, but I truly want to do things correctly going forward. How can I build my marriage on a foundation of purity and wholesomeness? Is that possible for me/us? (page 79)

- » When people refer to intimacy as "the mitzvah," it grates on my nerves; can't we just enjoy ourselves? (page 81)

- » I am having a very hard time with being Shomer Negiah; where does the concept come from and how important is it really? (page 95)

- » I am engaged to be married and my *chatan* wants us to touch "a bit." This makes me uncomfortable but I don't want to cause problems in our relationship. What should I do? (page 103)

- » After a day at work, I like to relax on Instagram. Is there a problem with that? (page 109)

- » I'm worried about getting my period on or before my wedding day. Is there anything I can do? (page 120)

- » How can I best prepare for "The First Night?" (page 121)

- » How can I/we go from 0 to 100 so suddenly? (page 127)

- » Being in *nidah* is extremely difficult for me; I am moody, lonely, and resentful. Do you have any practical suggestions? (page 142)

Frequently Asked Questions

» I heard that a married woman covers her hair to "reserve it" specifically for her husband. Is that the reason for the mitzvah of *kisui rosh*? (page 150)

» If a *sheitel* looks just as good or better than your hair, especially with the newest *sheitlach* looking like they are 'growing out of your scalp,' what is the point of a *sheitel*? (page 150)

» What about *marit ayin*, people mistakenly thinking that my hair is uncovered? Wouldn't a hat or *tichel* be a better option for obviating this concern? (page 152)

» I have heard that it is not, strictly speaking, necessary to cover one's hair while at home, and that when out and about, some hair can be exposed. Can you help me understand the differing opinions on these two matters? (page 155)

» I have heard that the *Zohar* emphasizes the importance of a married woman's hair being completely covered, and teaches that abundant blessings flow to the woman, her husband, and her children in this merit. Which Kabbalistic teachings can help me understand the importance of this mitzvah? (page 157)

» My husband and I want to get to know each other more fully – we feel like we need some time to gel as a couple – we also want to solidify our finances, travel, and advance our schooling. Can we take some time before bringing children into the mix? (page 180)

» In the Rebbe's perspective on *pru u'rvu* is there ever room for contraception? What about in the case of illness – physiological or psychological – or if I feel completely overwhelmed and need some time? What is the proper protocol for seeking a *psak* from a *rav* regarding the use of birth control? (page 183)

» I don't feel that it would be responsible for us to bring yet another child into our family; we are barely making ends meet as it is. I grew up with scant resources, and I don't want my children to feel deprived of the "better things" in life. Why is this not a good enough reason to limit the size of our family? (page 186)

- I am worried about how I will manage a large/er family because: (page 190)

  - I did not grow up in a large family; I have no personal experience to pull on, and I lack strong female role models with whom I have a personal connection.

  - I am not naturally patient or resilient, not to mention, I am not a great "balabuste".

  - I don't have the necessary parenting skills to raise emotionally healthy, happy children.

  - I am a *baalat teshuvah*. While my family has made peace with my lifestyle choice, they offer little in terms of support for our growing family. In fact, each time I am pregnant, I face disparaging comments and am made to feel irresponsible, or worse.

- I take my leadership roles and responsibilities to the community very seriously, and I truly believe that what I am doing is bringing Mashiach closer. Should I not be concerned that having more children will detract from my ability to be effective outside of the home? No one else can/will do for my/our organization what I can; I feel terribly conflicted. (page 193)

Part Four
Readings

Rivky Boyarsky, APRN, CNM

Appreciating Our Bodies:
INSIDE AND OUT

Some of us grow up with a lot of knowledge about our body and how it works, and some without the basic knowledge of our female anatomy, or even with shame associated with it. However, it is a fallacy to assume that *Yiddishkeit* shies away from talking about our body, especially in ways we can use it to serve Hashem and reach our full potential. While the Torah does not shy away from talking factually about our bodies and our sensuality, the Torah is very careful to use *Lashon Nekiah*, an elevated form of language. For clarity sake, I will be using colloquial English terms in this chapter.

We begin with our external anatomy in the genital area. Our vulva is often referred to as *Oto Makom* in Torah sources, "that space," a designation that highlights both its value and its inherent privacy. Within the vulva are the labia majora and labia minora, which conceal the internal portions of the vulva much like the lips do for the mouth. In fact, they are called *Sefatayim*, "lips," as their function is similar. Within the labia majora and labia minora are three areas. On the top is a small nub called the clitoris that is made up of erectile tissue (much like its counterpart in a male) and is the source of pleasure for a woman. Any direct or indirect touch can create pleasure, or if the area is too sensitive may cause a bit of pain. There is more clitoral tissue along the undersides of the labia but that is not something you can see from the outside. If we continue downward in a straight line, you have a small opening called the urethra. The urethra may not be very noticeable, but it is the space from which urine is released. Following further down towards the anus is one more opening called the vagina. The vagina is the opening from which period blood comes out, a baby is birthed, and in which physical intimacy takes place.

I would encourage anyone who isn't too familiar with their external genitalia to take the time to go to the bathroom and use a mirror to find the landmarks we just discussed. As a woman, it is important for you to know where everything is and how it works. When you are comfortable with your body you can better fulfill the mitzvah of *taharat hamishpachah*, have a more satisfying intimate life with your husband, and take better care of your health.

Now that we're comfortable with our external anatomy, let's explore internal anatomy and our menstrual cycle. Your reproductive organs consist of:

Your uterus: This is the place in which a baby grows after an egg is fertilized. It is also where your endometrial lining thickens and sheds from (what your period blood consists of).

Your fallopian tubes: These connect the ovaries to the uterus. They are like the highway connecting two cities.

Your ovaries: These are on either side of your uterus and are where all your eggs are stored, developed, and released.

Your cervix: This is at the bottom of your uterus and is the "boundary" between your uterus and your vagina. Your cervix opens when it is time to birth a baby; other than that it is usually not open.

Your vagina: This is the external opening to your internal organs. Your vagina has angles, hills, and valleys and is lubricated. Every vagina has its own form and its own level of lubrication and this will change with time, reproductive stage, medications, and births.

The menstrual cycle consists of different stages as our body prepares for the possibility of a pregnancy. Each stage is controlled by hormones and a shift in our hormonal levels will shift how the cycles feel and what they look like. Each menstrual cycle is counted from day one of your period to day one of the following period. In the first half of your menstrual cycle a hormone called estrogen is the main player as its level rises. This causes the uterine lining to thicken and an egg to be released as your body ovulates. During the second portion of the cycle a hormone called progesterone is the important player as its level rises to cause the uterus to prepare for a pregnancy.

Progesterone is also the hormone of pregnancy as it supports the needs of a growing uterus and fetus. When both estrogen and progesterone levels drop off, the uterine lining sheds and you get what we call your period.

Most women get their first menstrual period between 8-16 years old with the average age being 12 years old.

The normal range for a menstrual cycle is 21-35 days in length, with 28 being average.

The normal range for a period is between 2-7 days of active bleeding, with 5 days being average.

The normal range for the amount of blood lost during a period is approximately 2 ounces. For perspective, this is about a shot glass and a half. The amount of blood lost may seem like more than it actually is due to other secretions.

Typically (although not always and not for every woman), ovulation occurs fourteen days before day one of your next period.

Factors that can change your normal cycle:

- Hormonal contraceptives
- Pregnancy and Birth
- Breastfeeding and any other change in prolactin levels
- Medications
- Extreme dieting and weight loss
- Extreme weight gain
- Stress
- Traveling
- Menopause
- PCOS
- Fibroids or uterine growths
- Pelvic Inflammatory Disease
- Extreme infection and/or inflammatory processes such as COVID
- Thyroid conditions

See a provider if:

- You haven't had a period in 90 days and are not pregnant.
- You bleed for more than 8 days (excluding brown staining).
- Your cycle changes dramatically in length, intensity of pain, or amount of blood lost.
- You are having breakthrough bleeding or spotting.
- You saturate a pad/tampon every hour or two.
- You stop having regular periods after having a set cycle (and you are not postpartum).
- You develop fever or flu-like symptoms after using tampons. (Toxic Shock Syndrome)
- Your period is causing you so much pain or bleeding that you are missing school, work, or general life responsibilities.
- Your PMS (Premenstrual Syndrome) is so intense it is disrupting your relationship with yourself or others.

Married women are already keeping track of menstrual cycles for *taharat hamishpachah* purposes. If you're single it is a good idea to keep track of your cycle with a period app so that you can get a sense of what is normal and address any concerns that may come up in a timely manner. Keeping track will also help you choose an appropriate wedding date when the time comes.

General Health and Hygiene

When I was in high school, my class went on a Shabbaton. We all took turns jotting down questions on a small piece of paper and having someone else open it and answer in front of the group. The question I got was "How often do you use Q-tips?" Simple enough, right? Nope. Being an overthinker, I seriously did a double take. I started thinking *when was the last time I used one? Am I supposed to use one daily/weekly/monthly? Will I seem less than clean if I give the wrong answer?* So, erring on the side of caution, I said every day. These are not things we discuss after our parents are assured of our general hygiene, but here is the perfect place to discuss them.

Keeping general hygiene standards reduces the space for infections and improves general health outcomes. This includes dental health. In fact, keeping our teeth and gums healthy has been linked to better heart health and better pregnancy outcomes.

A general dental exam with cleaning should be done every six months and sooner if you're experiencing pain or any change. Brushing teeth should be done twice daily and should take 2 minutes, making sure to brush all the surfaces of your teeth and your tongue. Use fluoride toothpaste and a soft toothbrush. Replace the toothbrush every three months. Use floss every night after brushing your teeth. Adding an electric toothbrush and a Waterpik to your routine is recommended.

Working as a nurse for 10 years, I can attest to the power of handwashing. In any facility I worked in, the number one thing that was stressed is handwashing. It sounds so simple and easy that it almost doesn't seem powerful. However, it is the single most powerful tool we have to reduce infection risk. Washing your hands with soap when you come in and out of the house, and before and after you touch food or interact with others, is always a good idea. I do an experiment with the preschoolers when I go in for "Community Helper Day," in which one person touches glitter and then the next person touches that person, and so on. Suffice it to say that in a class of 20-25 children, the last one always has glitter on them. Bacteria spreads in a similar fashion, and hand washing is the best prevention against its progression. If you are unable to use soap and water, you can use an alcohol based cleaner, but it is important to use one that has a high alcohol content and to let it dry on the skin.

Bathing or showering daily is important as it will wash away any dead skin, oils, bacteria or dirt from the surface of our body. The sweatiest areas of the body – underarms, groin area, and feet – require the most attention. When those areas are fully dry you can apply deodorant or powder to further reduce odor. Washing your hair does not have to be done daily. Depending on your hair type and the exposure it gets, you need to shampoo at least once a week, and more frequently based on personal preference and need.

Lastly, keeping our nails clean and short and away from our mouth will reduce the number of germs and bacteria that can be transmitted both to others and to ourselves. You can pay attention to the accumulation of particles under the nails or add a nail brush to your hand washing routine to further reduce buildup.

Oh, and regarding the Q-tip question: it is actually not recommended to use Q-tips for your ears. They are fun to paint with, though.

Health Maintenance

A woman aged 21 and older should schedule an annual wellness exam with a provider specializing in reproductive health. During this exam, all your general health concerns will be addressed as well as general screenings for issues like depression or safety at home. Your exam will typically start with a comprehensive list of questions. This helps your provider know what to focus on and thus provide better care. This is your story, and it's perhaps the most important part of the visit. Based on these questions the provider will also decide what physical exam to perform. They will then ask about your family history. This will help determine your risk factor for health concerns including breast and other types of cancer. You will have the opportunity to talk about how to maintain a healthy lifestyle and prevent disease. It's also a chance for you to get referrals you may need to see other healthcare professionals.

Typically, a routine wellness exam will include taking and charting your vitals and weight, listening to your heart and lungs, checking your thyroid and your skin, and a breast, pelvic, and abdominal exam. Unless you have a specific concern, a young woman (under age 21 and possibly, even older than that) who has no prior history of physical intimacy does not need a pelvic exam. It is well within your rights as a patient to share that you do not wish to have a pelvic exam. If the provider continues to push the issue without a specific medical need or concern, you do not have to remain in that practice or in that exam room. It is also important to note that whether or not the provider understands where you are coming from, they should respect your personal needs and desires and work with them.

Routine examinations give your provider the opportunity to provide preventative care and treatment for common health concerns. At the time of this publication, the recommendations are for women between the ages of 21 and 65 to have a PAP smear done once every three years. If you have a specific concern or health history these guidelines may not apply to you; you should discuss this with your provider.

Your provider will also have some questions about your physical intimacy to ascertain that there are no problems or concerns in that area. Issues like vaginal dryness, spotting, and a change in libido can all be connected to overall health concerns. Naturally, a discussion about your menstrual cycle as well as your reproductive history is to be expected. It is important to share whether you are actively trying to get pregnant or are having trouble getting pregnant. In general, a good rule of thumb is that if you're unsure about what to share, err on the side of sharing too much rather than too little.

Speak to your Provider about Taharat Hamishpachah

Own it. Providers see a lot of variation in how cultures and religions approach health in general and birth and intimacy in specific. Some cultures seem to foster a

Appreciating Our Bodies: Inside and Out

sense of pride in their distinctions while others veer towards the apologetic. Either way, a good provider will respect your needs and accommodate them. There is no reason to apologize for your beliefs. This is true in general and even more so when our belief is Torah. Please come into this discussion with confidence and avoid phrases like "this will sound silly but…." or "I know this is weird…". Use statements like "According to Jewish law which I practice…" This states the facts and grants credibility to what you are asking for. Your provider will respond to the confidence with which you share information.

Choose well. Make sure you are using a provider who honors your wishes and beliefs. Pay attention to how they respond to the conversation you are having; are they receptive or dismissive? If they ask follow-up questions or make sure to take note of your needs in the chart, you can rest assured they will respect your religious needs. In medicine, our job is to figure out how to make medicine work for our patients. If your provider is not willing to entertain options that work within your belief system, this is a good indication they are not a good fit for you.

Use accurate language. The words "getting clean" is confusing to anyone who isn't *nidah* literate. You are not "dirty" or "clean", you are *nidah* or *tehora*/not *nidah*. Unless they are an observant Jew or *nidah* literate provider, be sure to offer a working definition for the term *nidah*. If you're asking questions regarding whether an exam or procedure will make you *nidah* or not, explain the reasoning for your question. Below this essay, you will find a handout you can use or paraphrase from.

Tone. Be aware of the tone you are using while communicating with your providers. They will be less receptive if you are defensive, demanding, or dismissive. You want an open and respectful dialogue on both ends.

Prepare. Prior to a procedure such as a colposcopy, uterine biopsy, IUD insertion, PAP smear, or even when the provider is prescribing medication, you may want to ask some of the following questions, always in an open and respectful manner are:

1. Can you explain how the procedure works?
2. Will this medication or procedure cause vaginal bleeding or spotting?
3. Will the procedure affect the cervix or beyond?
4. Is there a way to schedule the procedure while I am already a *nidah*? Explain why that's helpful for you.
5. If the procedure or medication causes me to bleed or spot, how long should I expect the bleeding to last?
6. At what point can I insert a *bedika* cloth vaginally?

Vulva/Vaginal Health and Hygiene

We are often fed the narrative that our nether regions should have either no smell or a distinctly pleasant odor. The reality is that every woman's vagina and vulva region have a smell unique to them. If the odor is not foul or repulsive there is no cause for concern. The vagina is a self-cleaning organ. The natural discharge that your body produces will wash away anything of concern and balance out the pH to prevent infection and maintain vaginal health. We try our best to not interrupt the body's natural pH; there is no need for any internal cleaning, including douching, at all. In fact, using commercial cleaning agents will likely disrupt your vaginal pH and increase the likelihood of infection. The only thing you need when you are cleaning the outer vulva region is warm water and possibly a mild, non-fragranced soap.

It is important to choose underwear that is made from breathable and naturally moisture-wicking material such as cotton so that our vulva area is cool and dry. Although some women are more comfortable using pantyliners on a regular basis, it does trap moisture, and moisture in a warm area can lead to bacterial growth. This is the same reason we want to change out of our wet swimsuits and workout clothes as soon as we can.

When we clean ourselves after using the bathroom, we always want to wipe from front to back. We want to keep any bacteria away from traveling forward into our vagina. It is also important not to reuse towels. Always wash and replace your towels or washcloth after you use them. Bacteria can cling to the surface of the towels and grow; reusing them can bring that infection to you.

The foods we eat also influence our vaginal health. Foods high in simple carbs and sugar provide food for yeast to grow. Fermented foods like yogurt, promote the growth of the good bacteria in your vagina and help prevent infections.

Our body is made up of interconnecting organs; the lifestyle choices we make will affect our reproductive health, our hormones, and inner organs. Getting enough sleep, reducing stress, drinking enough water, and eating nutrient-dense foods will all affect our cycles and reproductive health.

Vaginal infections

The top three vaginal disruptions that women encounter are Bacterial Vaginosis, Vulvovaginal Candidiasis, and a UTI. Not only will they cause a woman to be uncomfortable, but they can lead to *tahara* issues and related spotting and staining

Appreciating Our Bodies: Inside and Out

that may look like *nidah* blood but is not. These infections are easily treated. By familiarizing yourself with the signs of these disruptions you can address them in a quicker and more effective manner.

Bacterial Vaginosis (BV)

Overgrowth of vaginal bacteria (a certain amount is normal) can lead to inflammation and an infection called bacterial vaginosis or BV for short. This is the most common infection for women aged 15-44. Some of the symptoms you may notice when you have BV are:

- A fishy vaginal odor
- Pain, itching, or burning in your vagina or while urinating
- Watery white or gray discharge

Bacterial Vaginosis is treated with oral or vaginal antibiotics. It is especially important to treat BV during pregnancy because it can lead to preterm labor. Abstain from intercourse until you have completed the course of antibiotics. Probiotics (with *Lactobacillus*) in pill form or in the form of fermented foods like yogurt will help recolonize the healthy vaginal bacteria.

Vulvovaginal Candidiasis (Yeast Infection)

The second most common infection in women of reproductive age is vulvovaginal candidiasis or a yeast infection. Pregnant women in the second and third trimesters are more prone to getting yeast infections as well as those who are on certain medications or have uncontrolled blood sugar levels. Yeast infections are more common with increased estrogen levels in the body like during pregnancy. Maintaining good habits to promote vaginal health will also help prevent yeast infections. If you have a yeast infection you might notice:

- Vaginal or vulvar itching
- Vaginal discharge with a consistency of cottage cheese
- Vulvar itching or pain

These symptoms may worsen the week before your period.

Up to 20% of women may have an asymptomatic yeast infection that does not need to be treated. Many women treat what they think is a yeast infection– but is actually not– with over-the-counter antifungals. It is important to see your provider for an accurate diagnosis. If you are diagnosed with a yeast infection, your provider will either prescribe a topical cream or a pill to take. They are both equally effective; it depends on your preference. You can also self-treat with 600mg of boric acid capsules placed vaginally. **It is important to note that this can be FATAL if swallowed.** Increase your intake of fermented foods like yogurt, sauerkraut, and kombucha, or add a daily probiotic pill to your daily routine.

If you have four or more yeast infections in a year or are pregnant your provider will take your infection very seriously.

Urinary Tract Infections (UTI)

About 50% of women will have a UTI sometime during their lifetime. Some women are more prone to contracting a UTI due to their physiology; pregnancy can also make you more susceptible. Diabetes, incontinence, contraceptives (i.e. spermicides), and a new spouse can all lead to increased UTIs as well for other reasons.

Often when you have a UTI you will notice:

- A change in urination (a burning sensation, incontinence, or increased frequency are common)
- Pain at the sides of your lower back
- Fever and chills (which you may or may not suffer)
- Sometimes you may even notice blood in your urine

A UTI may be treated with an antimicrobial medication, and you should feel better within 28-72 hours. Keep in mind the general vulvar health tips given earlier with a specific focus on how you wipe, and drink an adequate amount of water. If you are still feeling the same symptoms go back and get retested so that the medication can be more targeted. If your symptoms are severe, prolonged, or reoccurring you may have to do some imaging and treat it more aggressively. This is also one of the things tested during a first prenatal visit to make sure you don't have too much bacteria in your urine as it can adversely affect your pregnancy.

Herbal sitz bath for vaginal yeast infection:

    1 TBSP tea tree oil

    2 TBSP cider vinegar

    2 cups warm water

Herbal therapy for UTI:

Work with an experienced alternative medicine provider or herbal literate provider who can guide you on the exact combination and dosage for your particular situation and circumstance.

1. Uva-Ursi (not for pregnancy)
2. Thyme
3. Marshmallow root
4. Echinacea
5. Vitamin C

Self Breast Examinations

While recommendations regarding self examination and preventative screening have become less stringent over the years (due to a high false positive rate and a high rate of unnecessary intervention), breast cancer remains the most commonly diagnosed cancer in women in the US. Both pregnancy and breastfeeding reduce the risks. If you had an early period or late onset of menopause, as well as known genetic or family history of breast cancer you can be at higher risk. Taking hormone replacement therapy for menopause is also associated with a higher risk for breast cancer.

Taking all the above into consideration, a woman of average risk (lacking any of the above-mentioned risk factors) should not do regular breast exams. You should however know how to do one in case you notice something concerning.

The standard age to begin screening through mammography is between forty and fifty years old, with testing done either every year or every other year. By fifty years old every woman, regardless of medical history should at minimum be getting a mammogram every two years. If there is cause for concern, you will have more frequent testing. Mammograms are no longer recommended at 75 years and above.

The HPV (Human Papillomavirus) Vaccine

The HPV vaccine prevents precancerous cells from developing by prophylactically preventing the infection that causes these cancers. There has been a 40% decrease in cervical, vaginal and vulvar cancer in women as well as anal and oropharyngeal cancer in both genders amongst the population who have been vaccinated since this vaccine was rolled out in 2006. Contrary to popular belief, this vaccine is relevant for all people, including the *frum* population that does not engage in intimate relations before marriage, or with multiple partners.

HPV vaccine can be given from age 11-26. If given up until age 15 you only need 2 doses, given 6-12 months apart. If administered after 15 years of age you will need a third dose. There is less benefit to having the vaccine after age 26 due to probable exposure; however, if you think you are a candidate, speak to your provider about whether the vaccine is right for you.

Pap smears

Every year roughly 50-60 million Pap smears are done in the US with 3.5 million coming back abnormal. The goal of a Pap smear is to prevent cervical cancer through checking for HPV and CIN3, as well as CIN2 if post-childbearing. The hope is that if we can track precancerous cells, we can prevent cancer from developing. It is possible that the more frequently and more widespread the HPV vaccine is, the less frequently we will have to do Pap smears.

A Pap smear is an internal exam in which after a speculum is inserted to visualize the cervix, a "spatula" and a "brush" or a "broom" (it looks very much like an elongated q-tip (usually pink) but is made of plastic and has abrasive edges that increase efficiency in harvesting the cells) is inserted to remove cervical cells for testing in the lab. This test can be scheduled at any point in your cycle. However, according to the American Society of Clinical Oncology, it is best to schedule it 5 days after your period.

The current guidelines state that from the age of 21-29 women should have a Pap smear done every 3 years. From ages 30-65 women can continue with this same protocol every 3 years or every 5 years if done with specific HPV testing. Stand-alone HPV testing can also be done every 5 years. After age 65 if a woman has had no abnormal Pap results, there is no need for further testing.

If you have had a hysterectomy but still have a cervix, testing is advised. One similarly continues to do the testing if vaccinated against HPV.

Personal Lubricants

Not all *kallot* — or women of any age or stage, for that matter — will need a personal lubricant. It is, however, a bedroom staple. For women who are not naturally well lubricated, a personal lubricant gel can help make intimacy more comfortable and

Appreciating Our Bodies: Inside and Out

enjoyable. Lubricants can be purchased online if one is uncomfortable buying them in person.

Whether you are trying to conceive or not, it is prudent to look at the lubricant you are using. Lubricants can enhance your pleasure but they can also cause pain, breed infection, or cause other harm. Some lubricants hinder sperm movement and life span due to their chemical makeup; you most certainly do not want to use those when trying to get pregnant. Be aware that this is not due to their containing spermicides. In other words, these gels will not actively prevent pregnancy but they can hinder your chances. Even if you're not trying to conceive, check if your lubricant has parabens or fragrance or promise a certain sensation; those lubricants contain ingredients that can irritate your sensitive vulvovaginal region and cause pH disruption. We want to maintain the vaginal pH (less than 4.5) level to avoid infection. It is important to note that anything that disrupts the natural state of your vagina can also inhibit pregnancy. Examples of this are douching or using vaginal creams.

The following lubricants can be used safely throughout life– including menopause– and come recommended for vaginal use (take care not to spread in the vulva, as it can lead to possible UTI infection).

- Uber lube
- Slippery stuff
- Good clean love
- Emu oil

If you don't have access to the lubricants on the list, search for a lubricant that is hydroxyethylcellulose-based. These lubricants don't decrease sperm motility and are the most like natural vaginal mucus.

Recommended lubricants that do not inhibit conception and are recommended when actively trying to conceive are:

- Pre-Seed
- Baby Dance fertility lubricant
- Conceive Plus
- Yes Baby
- Sage culture oil

More natural alternatives are:

- Coconut oil
- Olive oil
- Aloe Vera (most sperm-friendly)

Baby oil doesn't affect motility but can cause vaginal irritation and is not recommended.

Keep in mind that some of the recommendations above may not work for all women, so if you see that you or your spouse have a specific sensitivity, move on to a different recommendation. In addition, keep in mind that if you are dehydrated your vaginal secretions will also decrease.

Self-Care and Preventive Medicine

Our relationship with our body is usually shaped by the messages we get from a young age about how our body should look and what is considered "pretty" or "healthy." We internalize those messages, work, and sometimes even struggle to reach that ideal. When and if we do, we get external feedback on how impressive and noteworthy, inspirational even that journey is.

Our bodies are meant to come in different shapes and sizes. We have a mitzvah to take care of our bodies and that includes all aspects of it; It does not mean we need thin bodies but rather that we need healthy bodies. Our bodies are our vessels through which we can accomplish much positivity and goodness in this world. Our bodies are deserving of proper care.

It is important to shift the focus to healthy habits and lifestyle changes rather than a number on the scale. If you are getting joyful, consistent movement in your day and eating nutrient-dense foods you are more likely to have long-term healthy habits. On the other hand, if you are punishing yourself for a piece of cake by exercising and not eating you will create unhealthy long-term habits. Below are some sustainable, long-term, healthy habits we can all incorporate into our lives:

Nutrients- Eating a variety of nutrient dense food nourishes us. Therefore it is important to pay attention to the foods we are bringing into our homes and onto our plates. Using fruits and vegetables of all different colors is bound to give us a solid base in nutrient density. Adding high quality fats like avocado and olive oil will help with energy and satiety. Fermented foods help with gut flora which promotes overall health. High quality protein like wild caught salmon and pasture raised poultry rounds out the meal. Limit processed foods, refined sugar, and low nutrient foods. Make your plate pretty and your food tasty. Enjoying the foods you're consuming will help you keep consuming healthy foods. What you are choosing to eat has a lasting effect on both your physical and spiritual health, so make it intentional.

Hydration- We tend to think we are drinking more than we are. Being intentional about our hydration is important. Our body weight is up to 60% water. Water is an essential part of who we are. Hydration affects our brain function and our energy levels, so the more we drink the better our brain function and energy levels are. It is also our body's natural detox resource, it will help remove bodily waste and help clear your body of things it doesn't need. This results in clearer skin and fewer infections. Drinking water may even help you lose weight and maintain blood pressure levels at an optimum level. The amount we need to drink is person specific but drinking at least 12 cups is recommended for most of us. Even mild dehydration can have deleterious effects both physically and mentally.

Movement- Find movement you enjoy, even if it's dancing in your kitchen. There are so many health benefits to exercising and moving more. Your muscles get stronger which improves your stability and balance as well as your overall ability to physically get things done. Weight bearing exercises improve bone health, which is important for women as we age. The increase in heart rate improves oxygenation and brain, lung, and heart function. There are also reduced symptoms of anxiety and depression in those who exercise. There isn't one size fits all, but find the thing that you enjoy doing or it won't be sustainable. Remember it's all about joyful movement.

Sleep- None of us feel we get enough sleep. The truth is we probably don't. Sleep is important for all our bodily functions, as well as our hormones and emotional state. Most of us need six to eight hours of sleep (more at certain times of our lives). Some of the things you can do to improve your sleep include: creating a sleep schedule, turning off electronic devices, having a cool dark room to sleep in, and creating a bedtime routine. With more sleep, we feel better, accomplish more, stay healthier, and even become smarter.

Stress Management- In a society that is both fast-paced and values more and more of everything, stress is not only inevitable but high. Long-term, chronic stress can impact our health both physically and emotionally. In addition to managing the stress and limiting obligations, it is important to take time to reground and recenter yourself. You can accomplish this by meditation, prayer, going out with friends, gardening, reading a good book, going for a walk, having time alone or with people (depending if you are an introvert or extrovert), exercise, or deep breathing. What will work for one person will not work for others; find the time and what works specifically to nourish yourself. When the cup is empty there is nothing to pour out of it for another. If you don't fill yourself up you cannot give to those around you. Taking care of yourself is not a selfish thing.

Joy- How can we talk about living our lives in a healthy manner without talking about living it joyfully? There's a reason we are supposed to serve Hashem with *simchah*. When we do things joyfully we do it holistically; with every aspect of ourselves. Laughter and joy release endorphins which reduce stress and make us feel good. Joyful activities are immune boosting and lower our blood pressure. Infusing joy throughout our day also makes our *avoda* in this world beautiful and personally meaningful. So look out for moments of pleasure, gratitude, and joy and intentionally include them in your day. They are not extras. They are essential.

Structure- Having a sense of *seder*, structure, to our day supports growth in a spiritual sense and growth within our relationships, with those around us and with Hashem. Making sure there is a time and place when things occur, a place for things to go, and a clean organized space around us is crucial. Lack of structure creates chaotic, dysfunctional relationships and does not allow us the *menuchah,* rest, to pursue our spiritual or physical endeavors.

Spirituality- Connecting to Hashem is empowering. Hashem is our life source and sustains us; connecting to Hashem is connecting to our essence. Everyone connects to *ruchniuyut,* spirituality, differently. For some it's music; listening to a soulful *niggun* or heartfelt song. For others, it's action; doing something for someone else to get out of the space of ego and heaviness. For yet others it's learning; the mind connection and ability to process lofty ideas create paradigm shifts and changes in perception. Whatever it is for you– and this list is not comprehensive– make sure you include G-dliness and spirituality in your day to day existence.

Mentor- Look for role models and connect with them. The Lubavitcher Rebbe spoke very strongly about having a *mashpia*, spiritual mentor, in your life. A mentor can encourage and even empower your personal growth. A mentor should have more life experience and knowledge than you have and can see things from a different perspective than you do.

Community- We are not meant to travel through life alone. Being part of a community sustains us spiritually and emotionally. We get support and perspective through the connections we make with those around us. It is important to get out and work on making those connections. If it means volunteering, going out to a *shiur* or community event; reaching out and connecting to neighbors or old friends is crucial. Sometimes it is hard to make these connections in communities where everyone seems to have someone, but keep putting yourself out there and you will find your micro-community and they will become your people.

At some points in our lives, we can incorporate all of the above aspects and more, and at other times only a few might be feasible. It is understood that our growth and self-care don't always follow a linear pattern and that is okay. If we are cognizant of what we would ideally want to achieve it is that much more probable that we will incorporate additional self-care items within our day-to-day lives.

Mental Health Awareness

The first step is knowing if your mental health is suboptimal; this can happen to anyone at some point in life. When regular behavior patterns shift, it is always a good idea to explore why. If someone starts eating or sleeping too much or too little, has little to no energy, or is suddenly angry, these are signs that a deeper conversation is in order. Mood changes, lots of unexplained aches and pains, the absence of joy in activities previously enjoyed, or struggle with daily responsibilities are all signs of something being off kilter.

Because there is still so much stigma surrounding mental health issues, it is important to clearly state: if you are experiencing mental health challenges, it is not your fault. Our mental health is affected by a lot of complex factors, many of which we don't control. Some of them are genetics or epigenetics, infections, brain injuries, prenatal damage, exposure to toxins, and trauma. Simple things like unbalanced hormones can cause big shifts in how we feel inside and manifest externally. If you feel (or someone who loves you notices) that something is awry, contact a licensed mental health professional and schedule an assessment.

Below are listed some of the most common mental health challenges that face women:

Depression- Women are twice as likely as men to suffer depression. Depression is when you are overwhelmed with sadness and feelings of worry. It can last for a short time and reoccur or it can be constant. Depression can manifest in retreating from previously enjoyed activities, crying more than usual, having a hard time getting through the day or even getting out of bed, or feeling sick. There are screening tools your provider will use during wellness visits to best care for women who are suffering from depression. Sometimes depression can manifest during pregnancy and it can feel like something is doubly wrong with you as you should be happy and glowing and you feel awful. Remember it is not your fault, there is nothing you did wrong that causes depression to occur. Reach out to your provider and set up an appointment to get the support you need.

Depression can be treated with a combination of medications, therapy to learn coping mechanisms and tools, as well as overall health and wellness regimens. Some of the complementary therapies in addition to standard treatments available include, taking an Omega 3 fatty acid supplement daily, using bright light therapy, moderate exercise for 30 minutes a day, massage, and acupuncture.

Anxiety- Anxiety is feelings of worry, fear, or nervousness about situations or events; most people experience this. Anxiety as a disorder is when this affects your daily living or when non-threatening events feel threatening. Women are more likely to have panic disorder, generalized anxiety, and specific phobias. A panic attack is an intense overwhelming feeling of anxiety and can be followed by more generalized feelings of worry or stress. Because panic attacks are unexpected and thus unnerving, many women will experience anxiety in between attacks. Specific phobias manifest as fear of a specific situation or event, such as fear of heights, water, or animals. This can also manifest as social phobia; extreme anxiety and self consciousness in social situations. You can experience feeling watched, judged, or embarrassed in disproportionate amounts.

Women are more prone to anxiety disorders due to the shifts in hormones that occur during the menstrual cycle. Other factors that play into anxiety are past trauma or genetics.

Anxiety can be treated by a combination of medications and therapy. The therapy will help deal with past trauma as well as help you develop coping mechanisms and tools to better manage the day-to-day symptoms. Medications will help manage the symptoms and increase the levels of serotonin in your brain which will make you feel better.

Some helpful complementary therapies in addition to standard treatment include yoga, meditation, mindfulness, connecting your spirituality, vitamin B12 supplements, chamomile tea, Inositol, and passionflower supplements.

Perinatal Mood and Anxiety Disorder (PMAD)- It is estimated that 10-20% of women will develop perinatal mood or anxiety disorder. This refers to when women see symptoms such as depression, anxiety, sleep disturbances, obsessive thoughts, lack of joy, panic attacks, strong feelings of overwhelm, or hopelessness. According to the WHO, perinatal depression affects 13% of women and is the most common of PMADs. Perinatal depression is depression that occurs during or after pregnancy. It presents similarly to regular depression or anxiety but isn't necessarily a lifelong challenge. It is important to make a distinction between perinatal depression and the "baby blues." The first two weeks post birth are a roller coaster of hormonal shifts, physical exhaustion and lack of sleep and it is normal to feel weepy and overwhelmed as you transition to motherhood. The baby blues pass within two weeks of birth. If your symptoms persist beyond two weeks it is important for your health and your baby's long term health to reach out for help. All the above recommendations regarding regular depression apply for perinatal depression as well. Regardless of which mood disorder one may develop in the perinatal period it is important to not be ashamed and to reach out for support. If one previously suffered from PMAD, this is important information to disclose in subsequent pregnancies so that a support plan can be put in place and help mitigate future challenges.

Eating Disorders- Women account for 65% of all those with eating disorders, and 85% of those affected by anorexia and bulimia are women. It is a common misconception that having an eating disorder is a choice. Eating disorders are caused by a complex combination of genetics, trauma, and underlying health issues. Many women experiencing eating disorders are also experiencing depression and anxiety. It is important to find the right combination of nutritional counseling, medical care, and medications that work best for the individual. Therefore, treating eating disorders usually require a team based approach consisting at minimum of a mental health clinician, dietitian, and a general medical clinician. In many cases, it is important to also have the family members come in for therapy. It is important to note that if a patient with an eating disorder is not stable, care is likely to be taken care in an inpatient setting.

Anorexia describes severe restriction of caloric intake. There are many factors that can cause one to develop anorexia; these factors can be environmental, psychological, or social. People with anorexia can see themselves as fat and be obsessed with weighing themselves, restricting their food intake, and exercising too much. These are not healthy behaviors and cause tremendous emotional and physical suffering. Over time anorexia can cause infertility, brain damage, and organ failure amongst other lifelong issues.

Bulimia nervosa describes a cycle of binge eating followed by purging through forced vomiting, use of laxatives or diuretics, or an inordinate amount of exercising. People with this condition may be underweight, average-weight, or overweight. Some of the symptoms family and friends may notice include a chronic sore throat, compromised tooth enamel, acid reflux, or stomach upset. Bulimia Nervosa can also lead to strokes and heart attacks from the electrolyte imbalance.

Binge eating disorder manifests as a lack of control over food intake. It is the first part of bulimia without the purging aspect. Unsurprisingly, those who suffer from binge eating disorders are usually overweight or obese. Symptoms include eating when you're full to the point of being uncomfortable, eating very quickly, secretive eating, and intense feelings of shame and guilt associated with your eating. The treatment for binge eating disorder focuses on the psychological aspects over the physical aspects.

PTSD- Women are twice as likely to have PTSD after a traumatic event. This can happen after a natural disaster, personal trauma, accident, or injury. People with PTSD have intense memories and emotions related to their experience long after it is over. They may also experience strong emotions of anger, sadness, or fear. This can cause them to feel isolated from others around them who have not experienced the same event as they have. There are three categories of symptoms that can occur. Intrusive thoughts, flashbacks and memories, and disturbing dreams can make the person feel like they are reliving the event. The person may choose to avoid all events and people, even items, that remind them of the traumatic event. Conversely, sometimes the person suffering PTSD won't be able to remember the event at all or may rewrite the events to blame themselves. They may even have the inability to feel joy and happiness or create negative thoughts and beliefs about themselves. Lastly, they may have changes in their reactivity. This means they may have extreme anger episodes, reckless or self destructive behavior, become easily startled, or have trouble sleeping or concentrating.

Treatment includes cognitive therapy, EMDR, exposure therapy, and medications. TMS (Transcranial Magnetic Stimulation) is a non-invasive and painless technique that stimulates the brain and is used for the treatment of PTSD. It is important to deal with PTSD using multiple modalities as it is a more complex mental health challenge and you want to make sure your subconscious and conscious parts are both being supported.

Some of the complementary therapies available for PTSD are acupuncture, moxibustion, meditation, and deep breathing exercises. Art therapy for PTSD is something that some people may find helpful as well and has been used since the 1970s.

OCD- OCD stands for Obsessive Compulsive Disorder. OCD causes someone to have the same thoughts (obsessions) again and again as well as repeat the same behaviors (compulsions) over and over again. There is no pleasure in the rituals and it causes them significant problems in their daily life. Sometimes OCD is accompanied by tic disorders which can be either small repetitive movements or vocal tics like throat clearing or grunting. Some people have specific triggers that will set off their

OCD; some triggers can be avoided while others cannot. There is a definite genetic component involved in OCD and tic disorders, as well as a link to past trauma. In rare cases children may develop OCD (and other personality and behavior changes) after a strep infection; this is called PANDAS.

For *Taharat Hamishpachah* observant women, OCD can manifest within the *mikvah* process. Due to there being different ways this disorder manifests itself, the disorder in relation to *mikvah* may be different in different women. It is important to work with both a *rav* and a therapist if you are being affected by this. If you are unsure how to start the process, reach out to your *kallah* teacher who can further direct you.

Psychotherapy is used in conjunction with medications to help give coping mechanisms and tools to the individual. A specific subset of CBT, cognitive behavioral therapy, is used effectively to treat OCD. Exposure and Response Prevention (ERP) is administered by placing the client suffering from OCD in a controlled and supported environment whilst being exposed to their triggers. They receive specific tools to avoid or mitigate the compulsions that usually occur after exposure to these triggers. TMS is also used effectively for OCD (this modality is explored in PTSD). Sometimes it is also beneficial to enroll in comprehensive outpatient and residential treatment programs when daily functioning is affected.

PMS VS PMDD- Most of us are familiar with PMS (premenstrual syndrome). PMS is a series of symptoms that occur in conjunction with fluctuating hormonal shifts that happen around our period. Some of the common symptoms are bloating, moodiness, acne, less energy, and breast tenderness. About 75% of women experience PMS around their period, but less than 10% (some say as little as 3%) experience PMDD (premenstrual dysphoric disorder).

Essentially PMDD is a more acute form of PMS. It can interrupt daily life and have an effect on intrapersonal relationships and overall mental health. It is a chronic condition that needs to be addressed in a prompt manner. PMDD can be addressed through prescription medication. Some of the complementary therapies available for PMDD are a combination of dietary changes (decrease salt, caffeine, alcohol, and sugar), exercise, stress management and Vitamin supplementation (B6, calcium, and magnesium- see below). There is also some research indicating that Chasteberry can reduce the symptoms.

It is important to note that when using medications or therapy for any of the above mentioned conditions it may take a while to find the right medication or the right dosage of a particular medication, the therapist with whom you click, or the right complementary treatment. It is important to keep working at it and not give up on yourself. When you feel the issue is under control and you are feeling better do not stop the regiment that has brought you to this place. Keep maintaining the positive changes. If you want to taper or stop taking medication or going for therapy, do it with the support and guidance of a licensed professional.

Whether you have a temporary mental health challenge or a more permanent one it is important to reach out for support and connect with people who have successfully navigated the same syndrome. Support groups can give you access to new research and tools as well as success stories to encourage and support personal growth. Remember that struggling with things internally or externally is simply part of being human. Some of us have more common struggles and some of us have one with a name attached to it. Either way, it is important to have a growth mindset and to be open to treatment and support so that you can be the best version of yourself. Don't let a diagnosis hold you back from achievement and growth. Take care of your body inside and out so that you are able to serve Hashem from a place of health and well-being *b'guf u'benefesh*, in body and in soul.

If someone you love or care for is struggling with mental health challenges it is important to be there to support them. Check if you have an unconscious bias towards mental health challenges and understand that these syndromes are not a choice but a medical condition. No one chooses to have these struggles. Sometimes a spouse, friend, or family member is the first one to notice signs or symptoms of any of the challenges stated above, in that case, be sensitive in how you broach the topic. Encourage your loved one to speak to a mental health provider who will support them, offer emotional support, and help with daily tasks as needed. There are resources available if you need guidance and support such as support groups, online forums, and books. When you are the caregiver it is equally important to remember to take the time to make your own emotional and physical health a priority.

Lifestyle Changes that support Good Mental Health:

- Daily exercise
- Adequate sleep
- A nutrient dense diet
- Good hydration
- Taking on a hobby that helps you destress
- Connecting with others
- Reaching out for help if needed

Nutrition for Hormonal Health

An overall, non processed, nutrient dense diet:

- B6 reduces bloating, such as brown rice.
- Manganese reduces cramps, and can be found in walnuts, almonds, and pumpkin seeds.
- Boron reduces cramps, and can be found in avocados, prunes, bananas, peanut butter, and chickpeas.
- Calcium reduces cramps (1,000 mg/day). It can be found in dairy, sesame, almonds, and leafy greens.
- Vitamin E is an anti-inflammatory, and can be found in olive oil and broccoli.
- Iron treats anemia, and can be found in meat, fish, leafy greens. Consume iron alongside Vitamin C.
- Omega-3 reduces inflammation, and can be found in flaxseed and salmon.
- Water reduces bloating.

When you take care of yourself– body and mind– you are able to reach your full potential, as well as take your rightful place within your family unit and broader community. Keep in mind that recommendations in medicine do change and make sure you keep updated. Let's keep learning and growing and taking care of your health.

Handout for your provider regarding *Nidah*

What causes nidah status:

Within Jewish law, *nidah* status is conferred on a woman any time she experiences the flow of uterine based blood. Cervical dilation (even without issue of blood) may cause *nidah* status as well.

What are the practical applications for a woman while in the state of nidah:

Whilst in a state of *nidah*– for the duration of her menses (or for a minimum of five days from dilation of cervix or staining or spotting) and for one week after the minimum five days – a woman and her husband may not enjoy intercourse, physical expressions of affection, or even touch. The minimum duration of separation due to *nidah* is twelve days. Her state of *nidah* ceases with immersion in a *mikvah*, ritual pool, after the requisite twelve (or more) days. Understandably, this discipline can be difficult for the couple; certainly, any additional time apart is taxing. Therefore, whenever possible it is helpful to schedule procedures while a patient is already in *nidah* status.

Labor and Delivery:

At some point during the laboring process, a woman will enter *nidah* status. For this reason, it is common for a doula or female family member to be present. During cervical examinations and during the actual birth the husband will likely leave the room or position himself in such a way that he cannot see his wife's private parts. Especially during the actual birth he might step outside of her room or retreat to a corner where he may recite psalms or other prayers. This is the strongest support he can provide his wife within the framework of their faith and practices. The Jewish laws of modesty are also important at this time; if the provider can be cognizant of that and give the laboring woman a helping hand to ensure that she can maintain her modesty (within reason, of course, such as with her head covering or her upper body), it will be greatly appreciated.

Birth Control:

Because having children is considered a religious commandment rather than simply a lifestyle choice, observant women will consult with their Rabbi concerning the use of contraceptives, and if and when they choose to do so, about which is the best option from the perspective of Jewish law. Certain forms of birth control are unacceptable to religious couples; providers can expect the observant patient or couple to express a specific preference for one form over another.

••••

Rivky Boyarsky, APRN, CNM, is a certified Chabad Kallah teacher and lecturer on *Taharat Hamishpachah* and topics of women in medicine, Torah, Hashkafa, and Halacha. She is currently in training to become a Bodeket. Rivky has spearheaded "Conversations with our Children" through mikvah.org as well as many other lectures available on podcasts. You can follow her podcast 'bodies & souls' on all streaming platforms, or on her website www.bodiessouls.com. Find her contact information on mikvah.org and on Instagram, where she shares her knowledge of Torah and women's health.

Helpful Resources

For Mental Health referrals that are specifically geared to the Frum community call Relief at 718-431-9501 or email info@reliefhelp.org or visit their website www.reliefhelp.org.

For addiction, sexual abuse, and associated mental health issues contact Amudim at 646-517-0222.

For Postpartum Support call Sparks helpline at 718-277-2757, they can provide therapy, support groups, and resources from past classes on relevant topics. Their website is www.sparkscenter.org.

For general information on mental health and to locate treatment services in your area you can call SAMHSA Treatment Referral Helpline, 1-877-726-4727. Speak to a live person, Monday through Friday from 8 a.m. to 8 p.m. EST.

If you or someone you know needs emotional support or is suicidal reach out 24/7, even on Shabbat or Yom Tov to the National Suicide Prevention Hotline 800-273-8825.

Channie Gurkov Akerman, RN

The Bodeket

A *Bodeket* is Hebrew for a woman who examines. She is sometimes referred to as a *Bodeket Taharah*, since a *Bodeket* examines a woman for *taharat hamishpachah* matters. Spotting and staining do not automatically cause one to be *nidah*; the source may be *dam makkah*, blood from a wound. When a woman finds a blood stain that she suspects is not menstrual blood, she will ask a *rav* about her *nidah* status: *nidah* or not *nidah*? Often, the *rav* will be able to establish her *nidah* status simply by looking at the stain. Many times, however, when looking is not enough and more information is necessary, the *rav* will send her to a *Bodeket* to be examined and to determine the source of the bleeding. A *Bodeket* will perform an exam and will be able to see if the blood is coming from the uterus or from elsewhere. Uterine bleeding will usually cause a woman to be *nidah*. However, other bleeding which is not from the uterus (for example, from the outer cervix, vaginal walls, or labia), whether in a minute or large amount, will rarely cause a woman to be *nidah*. After the exam, the *Bodeket* will provide a report to the *rav*. The *rav* will then give a *halachic* determination of her *nidah* status.

This exam can prevent a woman from being *nidah* unnecessarily. It can actually save her a month! It can prevent husband and wife from being separated at a time when *halacha* does not require separation. Instead of being *nidah*, she will be in a state of *tahara*, ritual purity. All this, from a simple exam!

How to determine if you should see a Bodeket:

Menstruation, or the period as it is commonly known, is bleeding that a woman expects to see on a monthly basis. However, there are times throughout a woman's life when she may find unexpected bleeding. This may appear on her underwear or she may find it on toilet paper after using the restroom. The bleeding may be small dots of blood or it may be large stains or any size in between. It may be red, pink, orange, brown, or various shades of these colors. This bleeding is commonly referred to as "spotting" or "staining."

As mentioned above, bleeding from a wound is non-*nidah* bleeding and is referred to in *halacha* as *dam makkah*. Bleeding from the uterus almost always causes the *nidah* status. Can a woman determine the origin of the bleeding on her own? If you are having your period, then the origin is certainly the uterus and causes one to be in the category of *nidah*. However, if spotting or staining is found and you know that it is not due to your period, can you guess its source on your own?

Here are some guidelines to help you decide.

Spotting or staining from a wound:

- Is commonly bright red
- Does not usually flow out onto toilet paper and underwear
- Commonly bleeds only when the wound is touched
- Commonly not accompanied by pain

Spotting or staining from the uterus commonly:

- Drips or flows
- May occur spontaneously, without the area being touched
- May be various deep shades of red or brown

These guidelines can help you determine for yourself the origin of the bleeding. This will be helpful information to provide to your *rav*. He will then *pasken* your *nidah* status, or he may send you to a *Bodeket* for further clarification.

Remember, spotting and staining are common during the childbearing years and are rarely a cause for alarm. However, if you have any medical concerns, visit your healthcare professional. Likewise, if you find any spotting or staining during the post-menopausal stage, visit your healthcare professional.

Your *rav*, healthcare provider, and *Bodeket* are there to help you. Reach out to them.

Understanding Dam Makkah

Dam makkah is blood that comes from a wound (from the outer cervix, vaginal walls, or labia), trauma, or naturally occurring injury to delicate tissue and therefore does not cause a woman to be *nidah*. Blood that originates from the uterus is the kind of bleeding that causes one to be *nidah*. (A wound in the uterus is a complex situation that will not be addressed here.) At times, *dam makkah* may interfere with a successful *hefsek taharah* and achieving clean *Bedikot*. It may even be noticed on underwear or toilet paper used in the bathroom. (Please note that there is no *halachic* obligation to look at used toilet paper and so a woman should avoid doing so unless it is medically advised.)

These non-uterine wounds may not necessarily be considered a "medical wound" or pathological finding or be of any health concern at all. In fact, many wounds are only considered wounds *halachically* and would not be considered a wound medically. Most of these wounds do not cause any pain at all.

Some common sources of wounds are a cervical ectropion, most commonly referred to as cervical erosion, polyps, the stitch site after delivery of a baby, and a prolapsed uterus.[1] Urinary tract infections are sometimes accompanied by bleeding from the bladder; a *rav* should be consulted for this situation. Other causes of a *makkah* are excessive *Bedikot*, *Bedikot* done in a rough manner, rough washing of the vaginal canal, and waxing in the area.

During different stages of a woman's reproductive cycle, she may be more prone to wounds. Nursing mothers as well as post-menopausal women tend to have a drier than usual vaginal canal which can lead to bleeding when touched. During pregnancy, the vaginal canal and surrounding area may be engorged with blood, making these areas more prone to bleeding on contact. During the postpartum stage, the labia, vaginal canal, and cervix may also bleed when touched until complete healing takes place. Usually, the bleeding caused by these situations would be *halachically* determined as *dam makkah* by the *rav*.

Various birth control methods (consult a *rav* for permissibility) can have an effect on the integrity of the vaginal canal and cervix, causing these areas to bleed when

---

[1] Cervical ectropion (also called cervical eversion or cervical erosion) is a normal, common condition in which the cells from the inside of the cervical canal, known as columnar epithelium, protrude out through the external os (opening) of the cervix onto the outside surface of the cervix. These cells are redder and are more sensitive than the cells typically on the outside of the cervix, which is why they may cause symptoms, like bleeding and discharge, for some women.

touched. This too would be considered *dam makkah* by the *rav*. Certain medications, whether prescribed or purchased over the counter, can have the same effect.

Some gynecological procedures and tests can cause bleeding of the cervix or vaginal canal due to slight trauma caused by medical instruments. This bleeding would usually be classified as *dam makkah* and would not cause a *nidah* status. A *rav* should be consulted.

Any sighting of blood that one suspects is not uterine bleeding must be presented, along with all relevant information, to a *rav* for halachic determination. The *rav* will use the concept of *teliyah* to "attribute" the bleeding to a wound and not from the uterus if such is the case. Many times, the *rav* will require additional information provided by a physical exam. A trained and certified *Bodeket* can perform this exam to verify the source of any bleeding. She will then provide a report to the *rav* who will *pasken, halachically* determine, whether or not the blood is *dam makkah*.

One may prevent or at least minimize the question of *dam makkah* altogether by not looking for stains. Other than during the *Shivah Nekiyim*, the seven clean days, it is advisable to wear dark (if your *rav* allows) or colored underwear, not to look at toilet paper or at the toilet water, and not to perform *bedikot* which are not *halachically* required at the time. In this way, one will save a lot of aggravation and not become *nidah* unnecessarily. If, for medical reasons, it is necessary to be aware if you have any bleeding, please consult with your *rav* about how to do so while minimizing *shailos*.

If a woman is not able to obtain a clean *bedika* on her own due to a *makkah*, she can visit her *Bodeket*. A *Bodeket* can usually perform the *bedika* for her in a way that the blood of the *makkah* will not spread onto the *bedika* cloth. The *Bodeket* can sometimes suggest a treatment for the *makkah*. A *Bodeket* can also perform a *bedika* for a woman who has a physical impairment such as an injured back or broken arm.

Dam Nidah

Dam nidah is blood that originates from the uterus. When a woman finds blood, whether a flow or a drop that came from the uterus, she will enter the status of *nidah*. The most common cause of *nidah* is menstruation. However, there are other causes of uterine bleeding that would also cause one to be *nidah*.

More invasive gynecological testing that necessitates dilation of the cervix and beyond, treatment procedures, and surgery can cause uterine bleeding that may be *nidah* bleeding. A *rav* should be consulted to determine the *nidah* status as not all bleeding from medical intervention is actually *nidah*.

Some women may experience occasional breakthrough bleeding (spotting and staining) while using hormonal contraceptives. IUD insertion and removal can cause some bleeding from the uterus. An IUD, whether hormonal or non-hormonal, may also cause spotting or staining until the body adjusts to this foreign object. Consult with your *rav* if you experience staining or spotting due to any form of contraception.

Pregnancy may cause uterine bleeding due to reasons that are inconsequential or due to reasons that require medical attention. Although a woman is not menstruating during pregnancy, uterine bleeding at this time would cause her to enter the *nidah* status. Any significant bleeding during pregnancy should be checked by a healthcare provider.

Fertility testing and treatment may cause bleeding from the uterus which may be considered *dam nidah*. Fertility treatment using hormonal agents may cause uterine bleeding that would be considered *dam nidah*.

"Unexplained Uterine Bleeding" is bleeding from the uterus that has no medical known factor. This bleeding is not menstruation but it does cause the *nidah* status. This bleeding may occur sporadically or cyclically. It is important to verify with your healthcare provider what the source of the blood is and, only if it is medically advisable, to ignore it. This is especially important for a woman at the perimenopausal stage.

When finding unexpected spotting or staining there is no reason to panic. Spotting and staining during the reproductive years is rarely a sign of dire disease. You have time to call your doctor and schedule an appointment to determine the cause of the bleeding. However, If you have significant heavy bleeding which is not your period, call your healthcare provider or Hatzalah right away.

The next person to call is your *rav*. Not all uterine bleeding causes one to enter the status of *nidah*. A *rav* can verify your status based on your individual circumstances. Sometimes the *rav* will direct you to a certified *Bodeket* to determine if the blood was actually uterine in origin.

Staining and spotting are common during the reproductive years. Your healthcare provider, *rav*, and *Bodeket* are there to help you.

Preventing Halachic Questions

When a woman finds a blood stain or spot, she must consult a *rav* about her *halachic* status. However, the only time one is obligated to look or notice if there is any blood or bleeding is during the *Shivah Nekiyim* the seven clean days and certain specified days on your personal *mikvah* calendar. At all other times, one *should not* look to see if there is bleeding. Looking for bleeding when not obligated to do so is looking for trouble. It can cause one to become *nidah* unnecessarily. If your healthcare professional has instructed you to look out for bleeding, consult your *rav* for guidelines in this situation.

Not looking for bleeding is not cheating the system. It is obeying the system. *Halacha* advises one not to look for bleeding and to prevent oneself from noticing blood during times when it is not *halachically* mandated to look or check.

The following is a list of practical suggestions for women who tend to notice or look for bleeding. These suggestions will help you avoid having a question for the *rav* in the first place. Remember, these suggestions do not apply during *Shivah Nekiyim*.

1. Wear colored underwear – stains found on colored garments are ruled less strictly *halachically* than stains found on white underwear. Please note, one must wear white during *Shivah Nekiyim* unless advised otherwise by a *rav*.

2. Do not look at toilet paper before flushing it. Throw the toilet paper in the bowl before standing. Looking at toilet paper is also not *halachically* required during *Shivah Nekiyim* and *onot* of separation.

3. Use colored toilet paper in case you have a difficult time not looking at the toilet paper. Stains found on colored items are less strict for *halachic* purposes. Since various opinions on this matter exist, ask your *rav* regarding your particular situation.

4. If you have a private bathroom, consider hanging a "Do Not Look" reminder sign on the wall of your restroom.

5. Do not look at the toilet water after using the bathroom. If you have a very difficult time not looking at the toilet water, add blue toilet cleaner to your toilet (example: Tidy Bowl TM). Flush the toilet before standing.

6. Use colored sheets on your bed. (White sheets should be used during *Shivah Nekiyim*.)

7. During intimacy, spread a thick, dark-colored towel across your bed. Do not leave white undergarments on your bed. Clean up after intimacy with dark

washcloths; do not use fresh wipes. Do not look down at the sink or shower drain afterward.

8. If you like wearing panty-liners, ask your *rav* if you may use black panty-liners.

9. If using a vaginal applicator (for example: for medication) *do not* look at the applicator upon removal. Have a black or colored garbage bag ready for the direct disposal of the applicator. Close the bag and dispose of it.

10. Only perform *bedikot* when *halachically* required. *Do not* do a *bedika* at any other time just to see "what's going on" unless specifically told to do so by the *rav*. Blood found on items inserted vaginally are ruled very strictly *halachically*. If you are not sure if a *bedika* is required, ask a *rav* before doing one.

If You Don't Live Near a Certified Bodeket

Here is a guide for what to do if you find unexpected spotting or staining and you don't have the luxury of living near a certified *Bodeket*.

If you find spotting or staining that you suspect may be of non-uterine origin, you will need to rely on your healthcare provider, whether it is your physician, midwife, or similar provider, to determine the origin of the bleeding. Once you have gathered the pertinent information from your provider, consult with a *rav* as to your status.

Often, *halachic* wounds which may be significant in determining your *nidah* status may be overlooked by your healthcare provider since these types of *halachic* wounds are usually totally insignificant from a medical and/or health point of view. By asking a number of key questions you can guide your healthcare provider to obtain the findings necessary to relate to your *rav* so that he may *pasken*.

Questions to ask your healthcare provider *before* the exam so that s/he knows what to look out for:

1. Is there any bleeding from the uterus?

2. Very important question: Is there an ectropion? Is the ectropion bleeding? If the ectropion is not bleeding, touch it with a swab; does that cause it to bleed? If it does not bleed when touched with a swab, does it bleed when touched with a *bedika* cloth? (Please provide your healthcare provider with a *bedika* cloth so that he/she can touch the ectropion with the cloth.) Ectropion is the most common cause of non-uterine bleeding.

3. While doing the exam do you see any lesion, cyst, erosion, polyp, or any other irregularities on the cervix? Is it bleeding? If it is not bleeding, touch it with a

swab; does it then bleed? If it does not bleed when touched with a swab, does it bleed when touched with a *bedika* cloth? (Please provide your healthcare provider with a *bedika* cloth.)

4. While doing the exam, do you see any lesions or irregularities on the vaginal walls? Is there any bleeding from the vaginal walls? If it does not bleed, touch it with a swab; does it bleed then? If it does not bleed when touched with a swab, does it bleed when touched with a *bedika* cloth? (Please provide your healthcare provider with a *bedika* cloth.) The vaginal walls are not a common source of bleeding.

5. Examine the labia. Is there any lesion, cyst, or other irregularity? Is it bleeding? If there is no bleeding, touch it with a swab; does it bleed then? If it does not bleed when touched with a swab, touch it with a *bedika* cloth; does it bleed then? Is there an episiotomy site that is not completely healed? Does it bleed? If not, does it bleed when touched with a swab? With a *bedika* cloth? (Please provide your healthcare provider with a *bedika* cloth.)

6. Could the exam itself lead to any spotting or bleeding? If so, what is the source of this bleeding?

7. Would you expect any bleeding found during the exam to be constant, intermittent, or only to occur when the area is touched?

8. How much bleeding would you expect to see?

9. How long would you expect the bleeding to last?

These questions are a guide for you to inquire in the case of unexpected spotting or staining that you suspect is non-uterine bleeding. It is *not* a guide for a routine exam or for an exam that includes a procedure. The questions asked in those situations would be somewhat different and should be asked to your *rav* or *kallah* teacher.

The above guide will hopefully help get you to the *mikvah* on time.

Brides and Newlyweds

Many *kallahs* are unsure if they are making their *bedikot* properly. Some are unsure of their anatomy, and a verbal explanation from the *kallah* teacher is not sufficient for them: they need hands-on instruction. Some *kallahs* are anxious about making *bedikot* because of their lack of experience.

Newlyweds, too, may have concerns due to lack of experience. They may still be unsure if they are making their *bedikot* properly. They may not be sure if they have consummated their marriage, or they may be afraid of intimacy.

A *Bodeket* with experience in *kallah* and newlywed instruction can be an invaluable source of guidance and reassurance. During an appointment, the *Bodeket* will be able to provide answers to the following questions:

1. How do I make a *bedika*?
2. Did I do my *bedika* properly?
3. How to have intimate relations?
4. How long does it take to figure out and be comfortable having intimate relations?
5. Is my anatomy normal?
6. Is my hymen completely open yet?
7. How does pleasure in intimacy happen?
8. Is pain normal during the first occurrence of intimacy? The second? The third? How much pain is normal?
9. Positions for intimacy in special circumstances?

The *Bodeket* is qualified to answer many more questions as well.

Many young women have questions about the hymen. There are three openings in the female genital area. The urethra is the tube through which the urine exits and is generally too small for the insertion of a finger. Another opening, the rectum, is for a bowel movement and allows stool to exit. The vaginal opening is the middle opening and allows the menstrual blood to exit. The baby emerges through this opening during birth, as well.

The hymen is a round, flexible band of skin or tissue with a hole in the middle, configured at the opening of the vagina. The hymen is somewhat stretchy and there is always a hole in the hymen. This allows for the insertion of an average size lubricated finger or a tampon without causing damage or tearing of the hymen. Every hymen is different, just as every ear or nose differs from one person to the next. The hymen looks similar to a hair scrunchie in the sense that the hymen tissue may appear ruffled and the hole may not be apparent until you hold it open a little. During the first occasion of intimacy, the hymen may stretch/tear open to become a larger opening. This may cause some discomfort or pain and bleeding; this is part of a very normal process. This may even happen several times until the hymen is stretched open completely, and it is no reason for concern. Some women are especially relaxed and the hymen will stretch easily with barely any discomfort at all. Every woman is different.

When doing a *bedika* as a *kallah*, it may be difficult to insert your finger through the opening in the hymen while it is wrapped with a *bedika* cloth. Therefore, insert your finger only as deeply as instructed by your Kallah teacher. Once your hymen is completely opened through marital relations, you will be able to insert your *bedika* cloth-wrapped finger deep into the vaginal canal.

If you experience any difficulty making a *bedika* before or after marriage or if you have difficulty consummating your marriage, ask your *kallah* teacher for a referral to a certified *Bodeket*, one who has the extra bride/newlywed training to assist you. A *Bodeket* will be able to screen for any problems and issues that may be present. She will then refer the young woman to a *rav*, medical provider, pelvic floor physical therapist, or mental health therapist as needed.

There is no need for a *kallah* or newlywed to spend several months with anxiety or uncertainty. A visit to a competent, caring certified *Bodeket* can quickly put her at ease and clarify the situation.

Understanding the Role of a Bodeket

To practice as a *Bodeket* a woman must be a certified women's healthcare professional such as a physician, midwife, registered nurse, physician assistant, nurse practitioner, or an EMT. Most *Bodkot* are registered nurses. She must also be trained in the laws of *taharat hamishpachah*. Only after that is she ready to do an apprenticeship training with a certified *Bodeket*, which usually lasts from 3 to 6 months depending on the number of clients she examines during this time period. All three components of training are necessary.

Some *Bodkot* have extra training in other areas such as bride and newlywed instruction, intimacy, and vaginismus training. However, a *Bodeket* is not a therapist and should not be relied on for therapy. Nor is she a *rav* and therefore will not provide a *psak*, *halachic* determination.

A lay person is not a *Bodeket*. This would not be safe for the woman she is examining and is a grave insurance liability for the alleged "practitioner."

A *Bodeket* must maintain confidentiality, be gentle, and be discreet. It goes without saying that a *Bodeket* must be a G-d fearing, Orthodox Jewish person.

It is advisable to ascertain the training, experience, and reliability of the *Bodeket* before choosing a *Bodeket*. You can do this by asking your *rav*, *kallah* teacher, or *mikvah* lady, or by asking the *Bodeket* directly.

A professional certified *Bodeket* can be a valuable provider of care for your *halachic* needs as well as your feminine needs. A *Bodeket* can be of service from the time that you are a *kallah* until you reach menopause. She will give you the time, patience, and instruction that you deserve.

Channie Gurkov Akerman, RN and certified *Bodeket* for more than 25 years, was trained in Israel and the United States. She has been endorsed by prominent Rabbonim and numerous authors of *sefarim* on *taharat hamishpachah*.

Helpful Resource:

Tahareinu

www.tahareinu.com

For assistance with issues related to *taharat hamishpachah*, women's health, fertility, and sexual dysfunction.

Shayna Eliav, CNM

A Jewish Mother and Midwife's Guide to Pregnancy and Childbirth

Congratulations, you're expecting a baby! Or maybe you aren't yet but are thinking ahead, which is wonderful. I want to share some pearls of wisdom I have collected over the years I have worked in this field, both philosophical and practical in nature. I am confident they will stand you in good stead during your own labor and birth, *b'ezrat Hashem*. May it be in a good and auspicious time.

First of all, it's important to keep in mind that being pregnant and giving birth are natural functions of the human body. A woman's body was designed to nourish, birth, and feed a child. This is truly an example of *niflaot haborei*, the wonders of our Creator. For proof, we need to look no further than *Sefer Bereishit*, the Biblical book of Genesis. The name "Chava" means the mother of all the living. Giving life to and nurturing children as they grow was the primary mission with which Hashem entrusted Chava, and by extension, womankind at large. We may have many roles, some of which are deeply rewarding, but there is none more personal or essential than that of mother. Indeed, it is the closest that human beings can come to creating *yesh me-ayin*, something from nothing. As such, I believe that mothering also provides an incredible opportunity for a woman to grow as a human being. The day you give birth to a child is certainly not just another day in your life. It can be a life-altering experience – one you emerge from feeling awestruck, accomplished, humbled, at once exhausted and energized, and overall more alive and connected to Hashem. A positive experience gives you the confidence to take on the challenge of motherhood and can be a strong bonding experience for the new or growing family. On the flip side, a negative childbirth experience can be emotionally devastating. So I encourage you not to look at birth as only a means to an end, but to make a conscious shift towards actively embracing this transformative journey.

Allow me to share a story that illustrates this point. I heard it from Penny Simkin, author and mother of the professional doula movement. Early in her career, she was teaching childbirth education classes which were being held in the cafeteria of a nursing home. One evening, an elderly woman walked into the class, quietly took a seat in the back, remained there for the duration of the class, and then left. The next week, the same woman returned and again sat quietly in the back. The third time she came, she stood up and asked if she could share something. Penny gave her the stage, having no idea what she was going to say. The elderly woman then stood up and recounted each of her birth stories. Penny concluded by saying that she wasn't sure, based on this woman's age and frail appearance, if she remembered what she ate for breakfast that morning, yet she remembered her birth experiences in vivid detail. Not only did she remember them, but they were so precious to her that she waited week after week for the opportunity to share those memories with people she believed wanted, perhaps needed, to hear her message. They were etched deep in her heart. I believe that this is true for all women. I also believe that if we are going to carry an experience with us until we reach the age of 120, it makes sense to invest in it and do what we can to make it the most positive experience possible.

And now for my travel tips... fasten your seat belt. It may be tempting to skip over some sections, but this guide is organized in a step-by-step fashion. Even if you are more advanced in your pregnancy, I encourage you to read through all the points below to make sure you haven't overlooked anything.

Pre-Pregnancy

Start preparing now, even if you're not pregnant. To start with, make an appointment with either a midwife or an OBGYN. (We will discuss how to make that choice later.) It is valuable to develop a relationship beforehand so that once you are pregnant, you have someone you can call with any concerns. I have had many women with whom I had no prior relationship call me in early pregnancy worried that they may be miscarrying. They weren't my patients but they had no one else to call. Establishing care beforehand for what is termed "preconception care" can help prevent that. A preconception visit involves reviewing your health history, having a physical exam, and perhaps doing some bloodwork, to make sure that you are in overall good health. I am not trying to imply that you need to avoid becoming pregnant until every single item below is checked off the list. Rather, the point is that it's never too early to prepare for a healthy pregnancy. It's also never too late to make positive changes. Below is a list of things to consider:

- Take 400 mcg of folate or folic acid daily. Methylfolate is thought to be the most bioavailable form. Ideally, you would start as early as three months before you may become pregnant. The reason is that adequate folate stores are needed to help the baby's spinal cord develop normally and reduce the possibility of the baby having a serious birth defect called spina bifida. The most critical time to take a folate supplement is in the first month of pregnancy when you often don't know you are pregnant. In fact, you may decide to take that folic acid pill for the duration of your childbearing years. However, more isn't necessarily better. Avoid products that have a significantly higher dose (as some prenatal vitamins do) unless you have extra risk factors and your provider has prescribed the higher dose.

- Take a Vitamin D supplement. I recommend 1000-2000 IUs of Vitamin D. (All vitamins and supplements must be certified as kosher.) Ideally, your provider will test your Vitamin D level and prescribe an appropriate dose to optimize your level. It seems as if not a month goes by when science isn't discovering some amazing new benefit of Vitamin D. But because Vitamin D is normally made by the skin's surface is exposed to natural sunlight, those who stay indoors much of the day and have most skin surfaces covered when outdoors generally don't build up adequate Vitamin D levels.

- Visit a dentist. Periodontal (tooth and gum) infections are a known cause of preterm birth, so it's important to have your dental health in check. Also, catching any cavities early will help you avoid the need for mercury fillings, which are toxic, in favor of nicer-looking, safer white compound fillings. X-rays, if needed, are safe. Just make sure to have the lead apron covering your belly.

- If you have any pre-existing health issues, such as hypothyroidism or diabetes, definitely pay a visit to the appropriate specialist. Even if your family doctor managed these concerns until now, pregnancy, with its innate hormone changes, can complicate things. The appropriate specialist will be an important member of your team throughout pregnancy. Hopefully, everything will proceed smoothly and you will never need the specialist, but it's always best to be prepared.

- Check your vaccination record. You should know whether you either recovered from or were immunized against Rubella, Varicella (chicken pox), and Measles. The reason is that those viruses can pose a danger to the baby if contracted during pregnancy. Please note that these particular vaccines cannot be given during pregnancy, or for four weeks prior to conception. If you are already pregnant and are not immune, take precautions by avoiding anyone with those illnesses. You can receive these vaccines after giving birth if you choose.

- Consider taking probiotics, especially if you have a history of frequent urinary tract infections, vaginal yeast infections or bacterial vaginosis. Some research also shows that taking probiotics might reduce your chance of having a positive Beta strep culture. Beta strep (also termed "B strep" or "GBS") is a commonly found bacteria (about 25% of women test positive) which is harmless to adults but potentially harmful – even deadly – to babies who contract it during birth. Women usually get checked for Beta Strep at around 36 weeks of pregnancy. Those who test positive need antibiotics while they are in labor. While this treatment has definitely shown benefits for babies, there are some downsides involved. First, a woman with Beta Strep needs to have an IV inserted and receive at least one dose of antibiotics four hours before birth. Trying to time arrival at the hospital can be tricky since you have no way of knowing when you will actually give birth. You don't want to come too late, but you don't want to come too early either as this can lead to more intervention. Plus the longer a woman is in the hospital the more doses of antibiotics she will receive, which isn't ideal for mom or baby's gut flora. Clearly, it's preferable to not have Beta Strep at all, so if a product as simple as probiotics can possibly ward off the infection, it's worthwhile to take it. Make sure to get a good quality product, which incorporates multiple strains. They are usually available in the refrigerated section of a health food store. Some contain dairy, so speak to your rabbi about kashrus aspects of probiotic supplements.

- Don't leave out mental health. As you are probably aware, pregnancy can have a very real impact on your emotions. If you are struggling now, have relationship issues, or have a history of mental health issues, the support of a good therapist can be critical in helping you smooth out the bumps you may experience during pregnancy or after giving birth. Anyone who takes psychiatric medications should see their prescribing provider well in advance of conception as medications may need to be adjusted or changed altogether. Many psychiatric medications can be continued, so don't make assumptions. Self-weaning is not recommended.

- Avoid alcohol. A sip of *kiddush* wine is fine. The issue of drinking four cups on Pesach warrants a consultation with your *rav* and provider. That's because alcohol in pregnancy can lead to birth defects, and no amount has been determined with certainty to be safe. The most sensitive period for the fetus regarding alcohol consumption is from 4-12 weeks after conception, when the major organs are developing. Later in this guide I mention drinking a little bit of wine while in labor to help you rest. This is Okay because your baby is fully formed at that point.

- Read up on the *minhagim* surrounding pregnancy. Chabad.org has a comprehensive listing that will be very helpful to you and your husband.

- Lastly, consider your living environment. You are probably aware that cigarette smoking and alcohol use are bad for both pregnant women and unborn babies, but did you know that fathers' cigarette and alcohol use has also been linked to birth defects? Plus, second and even third-hand smoke (such as if a household member smokes outside and their clothing, skin, and hair absorb the smoke) carries risks for the entire household. If your husband is struggling with bad habits, maybe this information will motivate him to make a positive change. I also encourage you to do what you can to reduce chemicals in your home overall. Get a carbon monoxide alarm and use healthy alternatives to conventional cleaning products. (Check out the Environmental Working Group's (EWG) Guide to Healthy Cleaning available online to compare commercial products.) Open your windows daily, air out your freshly dry cleaned items before you put them in the closet, make sure you don't have lead paint on the walls, don't use foreign-made ceramic utensils or foreign spices (they may contain lead), get a water filter… The list continues, but I don't want to overwhelm you. If you want more information about this, go to ewg.org, a database with a wealth of information based on scientific facts. Toxins are everywhere in our environment, and to a certain extent our systems can handle them. But we can reduce the load on our bodies (and our children's immature bodies) by guarding what comes into our homes.

Nutrition Before and Through Pregnancy

Stay healthy with good nutrition, both before and after conception. This is a broad topic, so I will try to keep it simple. Many women rely on their prenatal vitamins as "nutritional insurance." While prenatal vitamins are important and recommended (and are easy to find with kosher certification), they contain only micronutrients, not macronutrients. Macronutrients are protein, carbohydrates, and fats, and all of these are absolutely essential for the health of a woman and her developing baby. Your individual needs will vary slightly based on your pre-pregnancy weight and whether you have one or more babies in the womb. As a general rule you need about 80 grams of protein, 250-350 grams of carbohydrates, and 50-75 grams of healthy fat every day. A balanced daily diet would look something like this:

- Three servings of protein (about 20 grams per serving) plus smaller protein-containing snacks (think nuts, hard-boiled eggs, veggies and hummus, yogurt, granola)
- Five or more servings of vegetables, including at least two servings of leafy green or yellow vegetables (the deeper the color, the greater the nutritional content)
- Four to five servings of whole grains
- At least two servings of fruit (emphasize low sugar fruits like berries and apples)
- Five servings of healthy fats, like avocados and olive oil
- Omega 3 fatty acids, including at least 300 mg of DHA which is essential for brain health. The most readily available kosher source for this is salmon. Six ounces of salmon once a week meets the requirement. Good vegetarian sources of EPA (which the body uses to convert into DHA) include chia, flaxseeds, and walnuts. Tuna should be eaten rarely in pregnancy since it is high in mercury.
- Calcium-rich foods or a calcium supplement (1200 mg daily). Supplements should include magnesium and are best taken at night for the added benefit of helping promote restful sleep and reducing leg cramps. The pills are large, so if you have a hard time swallowing large pills, consider a powdered or chewable form. Calcium and iron (present in most prenatal vitamins) don't absorb well together, so make sure to separate them by at least two hours. There are many calcium supplements on the market with kosher certification.
- Iron-rich foods/ Iron as needed. Your provider will draw your blood to check if you are anemic. If you are low in iron, it will take at least three to four weeks of daily supplementation to boost your iron levels, so start right away.

Adequate iron levels help maintain your energy level, are critical for the baby's growth, enable your uterus to contract effectively during labor and after birth, help protect you from losing too much blood after birth, and help you feel more energetic sooner postpartum. Healthy iron levels may also play a role in decreasing postpartum depression. Depending on your levels, you may need to increase iron-rich foods or take a supplement, or both. If you are feeling tired all the time, this is a tell-tale sign of iron deficiency, so mak e sure to mention it to your provider. The iron typically prescribed is a bit harsh on the stomach, but there are many forms of iron available for purchase. Some popular iron supplements have kashrus issues, but there are others that do not, like "MyKind Organics" and "Blood Builder."

- 12 cups of water per day. Hydration is essential for many body functions. If staying hydrated is hard for you, get a one liter water bottle and make a goal to fill it three times a day. Drink the first liter by lunch, the next one by 4 pm, and the third one by about two hours before bedtime (so you aren't in the bathroom too many times at night). If you are looking for a more interesting flavor, try drinking caffeine-free teas, infusing lemon or other fruits in your water, or diluting 20% juice with 80% water.

A healthy diet will help you feel strong, reduce complications, help you gain an appropriate amount of weight, and help ensure that you grow an appropriate-sized baby for your body to birth. For more detailed guidance, look at the work of Lily Nichols, RDN at lilynicholsrdn.com.

Early Pregnancy

Morning sickness: If you are feeling very nauseous, no matter what time of day it is, this is often referred to as morning sickness. While it is entirely normal – even a positive sign of a healthy pregnancy – morning sickness can be very difficult. If you are suffering morning sickness, or its more severe manifestation, known as hyperemesis gravidarum (HG), please be aware that there is help for this too. Milder cases of morning sickness respond well to lifestyle changes like switching to small, frequent meals, high-protein snacks before bed and even in the middle of the night, moving slowly in the morning, using ginger (such as in the form of hard candy or "Preggie Pops") and avoiding "trigger" foods or odors. This might mean someone else has to cook for you for a bit. That's Okay! Vitamin B6 (25 mg two to three times a day) can also help. However, if you do all of the above and are still vomiting every day (or multiple times a day), you may need medication, so reach out to your provider for advice. Nausea medications are quite safe; the malnutrition and misery that can come with severe nausea is not! If you are losing weight and have signs of dehydration, get help immediately.

Get prenatal care – early. At face value, it doesn't seem like much happens at most prenatal visits. Weight check, blood pressure, measuring the belly, listening to the heartbeat, the provider asking a few questions, maybe a blood draw – these may not seem significant to you. And in some offices, you might wait an hour or more for a visit that lasts 5-10 measly minutes. This makes some women hesitant to go to all the scheduled visits, which is understandable. But please go anyway. Here are a few reasons why:

Starting with the first appointment, early care is important to establish an accurate due date. Some women don't have regular cycles because of breastfeeding, chronically irregular cycles, or recent birth control pill use (including those that may be taken prior to a wedding). This can make dating a pregnancy challenging; however, the earlier you are seen for care, the greater the possibility of determining an accurate due date. Establishing an accurate due date is very important. First, if your due date is inaccurate, your provider might be led to believe that the baby is either too small or too big, which could result in extra testing (sonograms) as well as considerable anxiety. Or you might pass your due date by a week or more, tempting your provider to induce your labor, which can be necessary in some situations but in this scenario could occur for no real reason. You can achieve accurate dating by charting your cycles, the fertility awareness method (check out tcoyf.com), or frequent pregnancy tests (you can get large quantities very cheaply online). An early sonogram is also a way to arrive at an accurate due date, although no more accurate than what a well-kept cycle calendar will provide in most cases.

A word about ultrasound/sonograms: The American College of Obstetricians and Gynecologists (ACOG) recommends at least one sonogram during pregnancy. They do not recommend routine ultrasounds at every visit. It should be noted that the Rebbe considered ultrasound technology to carry risk of harm to the baby, and thus for use only when necessary. Of interest, ACOG guidelines note "ultrasonographic energy delivered to the fetus cannot be assumed to be completely innocuous, and the possibility exists that such biological effects may be identified in the future." Therefore, it is advisable to have an ultrasound when information is needed that can only be acquired through use of this technology, and when that information has the potential to change the medical plan of care. You can simply ask your provider, "Will the results of this test change my care? Is there any other way to get this information?"

Coming to regular prenatal visits helps establish what is normal for you, and therefore it makes any deviations easier to appreciate and interpret. In clinical terms we call this a baseline. For example, if at seven months your belly is measuring a little small, this would be worrisome if you had not been seen in a while, but if you had been coming regularly and it was noted that while you were always a bit on the small side, but growth was steady and consistent, the overall picture would be much more reassuring. Skipping visits gives the provider less information to work with. This is one of the main reasons that many providers won't accept patients after a certain point in pregnancy.

At the end of pregnancy it is critical that you be seen more frequently (usually every two weeks in your eighth month and weekly in your ninth month) because this is when complications of pregnancy, most notably preeclampsia, which can be life-threatening, are more likely to surface. Those simple checks that are done during prenatal visits can pick up on smaller problems and keep you and your baby out of harm's way.

Lastly, regular prenatal visits offer an opportunity for you to create a relationship with the person, or people, who will be at your birth. However, if you find yourself coming out of your prenatal visits feeling that something is missing, that the care you are receiving is impersonal, that you feel so rushed that you forget your questions – don't ignore your feelings. You are not alone in feeling this way. This is exactly the same sentiment that caused me to seek out other options with my first baby. Pregnancy isn't a mechanical process and prenatal care shouldn't make you feel like you're on a conveyor belt. This is a sensitive time, and birth is a very intimate, sacred experience. You need to feel comfortable with and fully trust the person that is going to be attending your birth. But even if you haven't found your dream provider yet, please get care somewhere while you are figuring it out.

How To Choose a Medical Care Provider

- Choose a care provider thoughtfully. How do you find the right care provider? Finding a care provider is a lot like finding a *shidduch,* match. It's a big decision and the candidates are on their best behavior when you meet them, which makes you wonder if you are actually seeing their true colors. You may try to get references, which helps if they give you specific details. But it doesn't help much if the reference merely uses general adjectives like, "wonderful" and "amazing." You need to know what it is that's amazing. It is important to have your own priorities straight, because you might meet someone great, but the real question is, "Is s/he great for you?"

First of all, you really need to make two choices: setting and provider. "Setting" means where you will give birth – hospital, birth center, or home birth – and "provider" generally refers to an obstetrician or midwife, although in some areas family practice physicians provide obstetric care as well. I advise deciding on the setting before the provider, because most providers only practice in a specific setting. It does you no good, for example, to find a home birth midwife that you connect well with if your preference is a hospital birth. By way of analogy, don't shop in the Apple store if you are looking for a phone with an open app store which you can only get with an Android device.

- **Setting**: While hospital birth is by far the most common setting choice in the U.S., it should not be inferred that it is the only safe choice. In England and Canada about 5% of births are planned out of hospital, and in the Netherlands that number is around 30%. Many high quality studies have been done comparing outcomes of women with low-risk pregnancies planning home births or birth center births to similarly low-risk women planning hospital births, and most have come to the conclusion that home birth is equally safe for women with low-risk pregnancies. There is, however, an important difference: hospitals use much more intervention and surgery to get the job done. Interventions and surgery carry real risks. It is also important to note that while non-drug forms of pain relief (such as freedom of movement and access to showers and tubs) are far more available to a woman having an out-of-hospital birth, anesthesia – including epidural anesthesia – is only available in the hospital setting. Furthermore, any complications that arise during a home birth will require hospital transport. It is essential that this be available in a timely manner, generally considered to be under 30 minutes. Remember, just because the outcomes are similar doesn't mean that all outcomes are good. Even in a low-risk pregnancy, unexpected complications can arise, some of which would have been better handled in a hospital with the additional staff and technology. There is no "no-risk" option. Every woman has to choose the risks (and benefits) that are acceptable to her. Many women are thrilled to find out that there is an option that gives them the comforts of home, the opportunity to develop a one-on-one relationship with the midwife who will be with them during birth, and an opportunity to labor free of unnecessary interventions like fetal monitor belts and IV lines. It is absolutely essential for a couple considering a home birth to be aware of the safety data. Deciding on a home birth is work. This is because it's not a default choice in our culture. Anyone who makes this choice will find themselves defending that choice to family and friends, and having researched the scientific facts enables them to do that. But more importantly, this kind of research will help prevent regret and guilt in the event that things do not work out as planned. Good resources on home birth safety include ontariomidwives.ca/home-birth-safety, and hencigoer.com/articles. At the end of the day, a woman must process the information, search her heart, and give birth where she truly feels most comfortable. A patient's state of mind is critical to the success of treatment, and that this is especially so in obstetrics. I have known women who had "accidental" car births on the way to the hospital because they didn't really want to have their baby in the hospital. And there are the women whose labors did not progress at home because deep down they were not totally comfortable with a home birth. In labor one cannot escape the "moment of truth," so it's best to face it early on.

- **Provider**: Currently in the United States, about 90% of births are attended by physicians and about 10% by midwives, mostly Certified Nurse Midwives (CNMs). This is very different from the system in most European countries or Israel where midwives take care of the majority of low-risk birthing women. In those countries, OBGYNs are reserved for higher risk patients. Interestingly, these countries all report better outcomes in terms of healthy mothers and healthy babies, using fewer interventions, and lower cesarean rates than in the U.S. Midwives take pride in helping a woman achieve a vaginal birth. I have worked with OBGYNs who truly believe there is no advantage to vaginal birth over cesarean. Midwives are generally more patient with long labors, provide more positive encouragement, and have tips and tricks to help laboring women. They are also usually more open to birth in alternate positions and support a gentle birth less likely to result in tearing. This doesn't mean that you should not use an OBGYN. Some OBGYNs are well aware of the risks of using too many interventions and do their best to avoid them, while having the expertise needed in more complex situations. And if you have risk factors, you may need to use an OBGYN (although in some cases you can have midwifery care in collaboration with an OBGYN). When interviewing a potential provider, ask a lot of questions, focusing on the issues which are most important to you. One very important question is "What is your c-section rate?" If they say, "Not very many," or "I really try not to do c-sections," push for a concrete number. I know providers with a 5% rate and some whose rate approaches 50%, so this question has real potential to make a big difference in your care. Again, I focus a lot on cesarean rates, because they can come with heavy consequences, especially for women who are planning large families. This doesn't mean that cesareans are never warranted – quite the contrary! Sometimes they are the only safe option. However, experts estimate that a nation's cesarean rate should be about 15%, whereas the U.S. rate in 2018 was 32%. That means well over a million women in the United States every year may be getting unnecessary surgery.

Whatever the letters behind their name, the right care provider should meet these criteria:

- Skilled, experienced, having good judgment, but not self-important or egotistical. Each labor and birth are unique and demand not only expertise, but humility and flexibility. When a provider toots their own horn or talks down to you, that should be a major red flag.

- Good bedside manner: patient, compassionate, confidence-boosting, and respectful. You should feel heard. You should be given options and included in decision-making, not have things done to you or be bossed around. I have seen serious trauma inflicted by providers who used their position of power to intimidate the women they were supposed to be caring for to get them to accept their plan of care. It's inexcusable.

- Uses interventions appropriately: Abundant research is available in many areas of obstetrics, and a good provider should be keeping up with the research and not just repeating outdated practices they learned when they were training. This is referred to as evidence-based practice. Reading good childbirth education books and going to a solid childbirth education class should give you some insight into which routine obstetric practices are evidence-based and which are not. For example, denying a woman in labor food and water and attaching her to an IV instead is not an evidence-based practice in this day and age, although it still takes place widely. Another outdated practice is the use of continuous electronic fetal monitoring in low-risk labors. It doesn't improve outcomes and has been shown to increase cesarean rates – not to mention being uncomfortable for the mother. I highly recommend checking out evidencebasedbirth.com, which explains research on many topics in childbirth to help you make informed decisions. I also recommend Lamaze.org's Six Healthy Birth Practices.

- The provider's labor induction policy: According to the Gemara "there are three keys which Hashem does not entrust to an intermediary (an angel): the key of rain, the key of birthing and the key of *techiyat hameitim*, resurrection of the dead."[1] The time of birth is also connected to one's *mazal*. As such, from a spiritual standpoint the time of birth should not be tinkered with without good cause. Certainly any condition that could be a risk to the mother's or baby's life is a valid reason. This would certainly include preeclampsia, pre-existing diabetes, or cholestasis, for example. But often the reasons given fall in the gray area, in which case one should consult their *rav*. Until not long ago the standard of care was to wait up to two weeks past the due date to induce labor unless complications arose (while doing fetal monitoring and limited sonograms to ensure safety). However, more recently the trend has been to push for earlier "deadlines"– 41, 40 even 39 weeks. But the statistical average for a first-time mom to go into labor is about 41 weeks so aggressive induction policies inevitably lead to large numbers of women being induced. Moreover, some providers like to "sweep the membranes" during weekly prenatal visits in order to encourage labor to start naturally. This involves inserting a finger through the cervix and into the uterus, and according to some *halachic* authorities renders a woman *nidah*, even if no blood is seen.

- Female: The Rebbe felt that if a female provider is available who is equally competent to a male provider, that a woman should preferably use the services of the female provider.[2] This is both because of modesty issues and because a woman is more likely to be sensitive to another woman's feelings and needs. From my experience watching male and female OBGYN residents in training, this is absolutely true. If a woman is going to use the services of a male provider, she needs to remember that the laws of *yichud* are still in effect.

---

1   *Taanis* 2a.

2   From a letter dated 23 Tevet 5748, and printed in *Healthy in Body, Mind and Spirit* vol 2 page 180.

- Practice philosophy: Someone can be a wonderful, kind, knowledgeable provider but have a very different philosophy about childbirth than you. Identify what your style is and look for someone who understands and will support that, not merely tolerate it. Just as you wouldn't hire a portrait photographer to shoot an action event, or a classical pianist to create a lively vibe at your wedding, don't hire a doctor (even with a great reputation) whose patients all get epidurals if you are dreaming of a water birth (to use an extreme example). If not, you are almost guaranteed to be disappointed. Once you identify your style, you can narrow your search and find the right fit.

- Hire a doula. Labor support is a basic human right. Research has repeatedly shown that women who have continuous labor support have better outcomes in ways that are readily measured: increased satisfaction, higher Apgar scores for newborns, lower cesarean rates, less use of pain medication, less postpartum depression, and the list goes on…. In fact, one of the lead researchers was apt to say, "If a doula were a drug, it would be unethical to withhold it." But who should that person be? Can it be your husband? Your mother or your sister, your nurse? And if you have a midwife, do you need a doula? Isn't she like a two-in-one? Let's examine this more closely.

  A doula should be knowledgeable and experienced in supporting women in childbirth, and not responsible for any medical decisions. This person's only job is to provide you with continuous labor support, meaning that they need to be there for you from the time that you call them until after you have given birth.

  Midwives and nurses may certainly pitch in the labor support effort, offering suggestions and direction, some wise words, or a hand to hold, but they have to be focused on the clinical aspects of your care first and foremost, so they really cannot be your doula. They may also be caring for other patients at the same time, making true continuous labor support impossible.

  Mothers and other female relatives have been the classic doulas of generations of women. Certainly there is nothing greater than a mother's love and dedication to her child in times of distress or vulnerability. But there can be a few pitfalls in relying on one's mother for primary labor support. First of all, some mothers really want to do this for their daughters but have a hard time seeing them in pain. Their emotions can cloud their judgment. I once had a mom suggest a c-section when it was completely not indicated, because it was so hard for her to see her daughter in pain. Secondly, nowadays most mothers haven't been to many births besides their own, so they may have a very set idea of what birth is like based on their own experiences. This can make it difficult for them to understand when labor unfolds differently than it did for them. For example, if the mother's labors were all six to eight hours, she may become distraught if her daughter has a 36 hour labor because she may see this is horribly abnormal when actually it is not. She might also be tempted to impose her values. For example, if she had all natural births she might try to dissuade her daughter from having an epidural even though her daughter has thoroughly considered the facts and decided on this option. It's also important to remember that labor support can be physically strenuous, often involving long hours, need for massage, and helping the laboring mom with position changes. This is a serious commitment. Sometimes mothers are able to provide this kind of continuous, non judgmental support. At other times it may make more sense to have a doula and allow the mother, sister or friend to play a secondary support role.

- Become a partner in your care. An educated consumer is more likely to be a happy consumer. Research shows that women who felt that they were involved in decision-making during their childbirth experience reported higher levels of satisfaction. This doesn't mean that your care provider will neglect his or her medical duties and leave things totally up to you. It means that they will present the relevant information about risks and benefits to guide you in making a decision. This is very important in situations where there isn't a single clear right or wrong choice. This kind of informed choice conversation takes into account that each person will make different decisions based on their individual circumstances and personal values. To be more concrete, here is a common scenario:

- A woman who has had a previous cesarean is pregnant a second time and contemplating the options of a vaginal birth after cesarean (known as VBAC) or a repeat cesarean. She learns that there is a 0.5% statistical chance (1 in 200) of having a serious complication called a uterine rupture if she attempts a vaginal birth, whereas the possibility of this happening is minimal if she has a repeat cesarean. On the flip side she learns that each additional cesarean increases her risk of having issues with the placenta, such as placenta previa (where the placenta covers the cervix) or placenta accreta (where the placenta adheres to the wall of the uterus and may not be able to be removed, requiring a hysterectomy). All of these situations can be life-threatening for both mother and baby. While there isn't a hard-and-fast rule about how many cesareans one can have, the risks rise with every additional surgery. Furthermore, while not all providers will offer the option of a VBAC after one cesarean, far fewer will offer that option after two previous cesareans, and fewer still will offer it after three or more. Clearly the decision is not black-and-white. One person would say, "One in 200 is too high in my mind – I will have another cesarean." Another would say, "I really don't want another cesarean. The recovery is difficult. A cesarean carries its own risks and may also limit the number of children I will be able to safely have. I would rather try for a vaginal birth and rely on my medical team to act quickly in the rare event that there is a complication."

Neither choice is right or wrong. Unfortunately, however, women don't always get to make true informed choices in childbirth. I remember talking to one woman who had had multiple cesareans. She asked, "What are the chances of a uterine rupture happening during an attempted VBAC?" When I told her that it's one in 200, she was shocked. "That's it?!" she said. "No one ever told me the number. My doctor made it sound so scary, and my impression was that the likelihood was very high." That doctor did not give her patient an informed choice. The facts I have cited above are well-established by research and should have been shared with her. But in our healthcare culture, patients too often don't get involved in their care, and they simply wait for the provider to make the decisions. Many providers are accustomed to this and stop trying to involve the patient. Some get so accustomed to it that they believe they are entitled to live on that pedestal regarding every patient. When a patient starts asking too many questions, such providers feel challenged or even annoyed. Other providers honestly wish their patients were more involved because they recognize the benefit of being a provider-patient team. I encourage you to seek the second type of relationship. I know this may require that you put in a lot of work to find this type of care provider, but I believe that it is absolutely worth the effort.

Before Birth

Become educated about pregnancy and childbirth. This will help you decide what kind of birth you want, and it will also help you be an active partner in your care. After all, it's hard to have a conversation on a topic if you're missing essential vocabulary.

- Start with some light reading, such as "Giving Birth with Confidence" by Judith Lothian or "Labor of Love" by Rachel Broncher to gain a general picture. Then watch some well-prepared videos to get a feel for what it's like to be in labor, especially in different settings. Continue to read more if you like, based on the questions you have or the options you want to explore further.

- Try to avoid listening to women recount their horror stories and be very careful on social media. You need positive messages. As the Rebbe said many times, *"tracht gut, vet zain gut,"* "Think good [positively] and it will [ensure] be good [a good outcome]." This doesn't mean that you avoid relevant facts, but do avoid negative discussion which only serves to increase your anxiety with no benefit.

- Next, locate a comprehensive childbirth education class with an experienced instructor that covers several major areas: the natural process of labor and birth, stages of labor, explanation of interventions and why they may be needed, how to advocate for yourself, and coping skills. Try not to get overwhelmed by the different methods that exist – and there are quite a few. Some of them, notably those using some form of self-hypnosis, hold out the promise of a pain-free birth. This can be possible to some degree, but it's not the reality for most women. If you feel drawn to these methods and ideas, I suggest that you take a general childbirth class series that offers a broader range of coping techniques, and then take a supplemental course in the specific technique that interests you. The reason is this: if you develop only one tool and that tool doesn't work for you at some point during your labor, you will need some others to choose from. In a nutshell, don't put all your eggs in one basket. Also note that self-hypnosis is different from classical hypnosis. Classical hypnosis is guided by someone else, and it is controversial in Jewish law.

- All of the above may be a process that takes months. Don't worry about figuring everything out right away. Just begin and see where the process takes you. As questions come up, start initiating conversations with your provider during prenatal visits to hear their take on some of these topics. It will be informative, and it will also help you decide if the two of you are truly a good fit. For example, if you express interest in giving birth in a squatting position after seeing images of women doing so in videos, and your provider laughs and says, "that's impossible," then you have a picture of what you can expect from that provider.

- Optimize your mind, body and soul. Here are suggestions for simplifying what sounds like a tall order:

- Body: Research has shown that physical exercise is not only good for you, but can help you have a shorter labor. Don't take up new sports or intense exercise in pregnancy, as you are more prone to injury during this time. But, with your provider's approval, you can likely continue any pre-existing exercise routines, possibly with modification. If you haven't been exercising regularly recently, then try brisk walking or swimming. Prenatal yoga is also excellent, but be aware that yoga is a spiritual practice rooted in *avodah zarah*, idol worship, so I suggest finding a "kosher" yoga class or video taught by a Torah-observant instructor, which avoids certain problematic poses and all chanting. Also avoid Bikram yoga, or "hot" yoga, as it raises core body temperature. This is not safe in pregnancy, nor are saunas or hot tubs. I also highly recommend the "Daily Activities" featured on the Spinning Babies(™) website, which help to support balance in the pelvis which allows labor to progress more smoothly.

- Mind: We already discussed self-hypnosis (*halachically* compatible). If you are taking a course in one of these methods, I encourage you to use these techniques on a daily basis for general relaxation. If not, then consider looking into some guided meditations. Make sure to avoid meditations which use any spiritual imagery. In my classes I taught "directed breathing." In this technique, you touch a spot on your body and then imagine that you are sending your breath to that spot. You can easily practice this at night before bed, putting your hand on your lower belly, and imagining that you are directing your breath into the area that your hand is touching. But I warn you: your baby will likely start kicking in response to the attention. This technique works nicely to cope with the contractions in early labor. Also, look around for some good positive affirmations that resonate with you. Get some mini poster boards and write the affirmations in pretty colors. Hang them up around your house so that you see them during the last several weeks of pregnancy, as well as in labor. You can take a few to the hospital or birth center, which will also send a powerful message to the staff about what kind of environment you are trying to create.

- Soul: Our Sages tell us that childbirth is a time of potential danger.[3] As always, Torah, *tefillah*, and *tzedakah* help! You might give extra *tzedakah*, *daven* for a good outcome when you light Shabbat and Yom Tov candles, make a meal for another woman who recently gave birth, or take on a *hachlata tovah,* good resolution. Being scrupulous in the details of *taharat hamishpachah* is critical. Review the *halachot* with your husband – it's an opportunity to spend quality time together doing a mitzvah. You will likely both be rusty on these laws (especially *harchakot*) after so many months of (hopefully) not needing to keep them, but they will come into effect at some point in labor, so a refresher is in order. The Rebbe spoke many times about the importance of enveloping

---

[3] *Shabbat* 31b.

the newborn in a holy environment and the singular importance of placing a *shir lamaalot* card or placard which contains chapter 121 of *tehillim* and additional *pesukim*, in the birthing room.[4] The Rebbe explained that the verses themselves act as a protection and encouraged the wide promulgation of this custom. The Rebbe explained that most generally, healthcare practitioners understand that the success of their efforts hinges in no small part on the patient's positive state of mind. They therefore strive to alleviate concerns and anxieties. This is especially true when it comes to birthing. He therefore felt that hospital administrations will show little resistance to this idea. In fact, many hospitals approached regarding this matter readily agreed to hang pieces of art that actually have the *tehillim* and the accompanying *pesukim* worked into the artistic motif in their labor and delivery rooms.

- Bring one for yourself and one for the baby (both copies should be *kis b'toch kis*, double wrapped). Chapter 121 of *Tehillim* focuses on having faith in Hashem. Connecting to one's faith increases tranquility, and helps a woman surrender to the experience. I was once assisting another midwife at a Jewish woman's birth who while fully dilated, was unable to push effectively. The birth team was trying many techniques for close to two hours, when I got an idea. I asked the laboring woman, "Can I put a prayer under your pillow?" She agreed and remarkably the baby was in her arms five minutes later!

- Note the Chabad custom; After the baby's birth, the *shir lamaalot* card should be placed in his or her bassinet which becomes the child's "*Beit Chabad.*" As is true for every *Beit Chabad*, it is fitting that a *Sefer Chitat* and *pushka*, charity box, be placed in the bassinet as well.[5]

Labor

What about labor? I want to leave the technical details of the birth process and learning coping skills to your childbirth education class, because it deserves more attention. But I will share some important points that deserve to be emphasized.

---

[4] From a talk from the Rebbe on 19 Kislev 5747 regarding things one should be careful about for the safety of the woman giving birth, including at the hospital (edited version printed in *Hitvaaduyot 5747*. Vol. 2. p. 37. *Teshuvot U'Biurim BeShulchan Aruch*. p. 446). Rivkah Slonim shared: My husband and I are *shluchim* in Binghamton. NY. We happened to be expecting the birth of a child when the Rebbe spoke this *sichah*. We therefore wrote to the Rebbe asking if in light of his most recent teachings, we should make alternative plans as my doctor was affiliated with— and I was therefore set to deliver our baby in (Our Lady of Lourdes) a Christian Hospital which has crucifixes hung in every room etc. The Rebbe advised us not to transfer out of that practice for this reason. He further wrote: what is the connection between what you described (concerning the hospital) and your putting a *shir lamaalot* and other holy things near the bed of the infant? We understood from this rhetorical question that the main emphasis was on making sure that both mother and baby (after delivery) were protected by the *shir lamaalot* etc.

[5] *Sefer Hasichot* 5747 *chelek aleph* p. 327; *Likutei Sichot* volume 26 p. 420.

- Early labor is the time for rest. And unless there is some medical reason to come to the hospital early, it's best to stay home. You may have heard that you need to walk to "get things going." You may be tempted to sit nervously wondering when things will pick up. Slow down. You have to take this step by step. The uterus needs to have this time to coordinate its muscle fibers, kind of like a warm-up. A walk can be fine, but don't wear yourself out. And if you are already worn out because contractions started at the end of the day before you had a chance to get sleep, then you absolutely must rest, and may need some help to do so. You can take a bath, have a glass of wine, and put yourself to bed with a heating pad or hot water bottle (filled with very warm, not boiling hot water). If you want it on your back, find a stretchy skirt or exercise pants with an elastic waistband that you can tuck it into so you don't have to hold it. Many midwives recommend 50mg of Benadryl for tired moms who are experiencing a long early labor. Even if you can't sleep, hopefully you will be relaxed enough to breathe through the contractions and really rest in between. You may wonder if there is any point if you're not able to actually sleep. There is. Even resting five or six minutes at a time helps. Every bit of energy that you can save up will be useful later. Think of it like putting money in the bank: everyone wishes they could make big deposits, but small deposits add up too. Also make sure to drink eight ounces of liquids hourly and eat now since you probably won't want to eat later. In my experience, a woman who is highly motivated to have an unmedicated birth, can usually be successful as long as she has two things: adequate energy and a good team. Once a woman is physically exhausted, the chances of giving birth without pain medication drop significantly. Saving your energy starts before labor too. If you are pushing yourself too much at the end of your pregnancy, this will take a toll. Be sensitive to your need for rest every day, especially as your due date draws closer.

- In active labor you need to alternate between rest and activity. Generally you need to move during the contractions and rest in between. Changes of position help labor progress more smoothly once it has reached this stage. Try positions that shift the pelvis such as lunges with one foot on a chair, alternating sides, leaning forward and doing "figure 8"s with your hips, and walking up and down stairs. I recommend buying your own birth ball. They cost about $20 on Amazon. Just make sure to buy one that includes an air pump for inflation and is appropriate for your height. (If you are between 5'1" and 5'8", the 65 cm size is usually a good fit.) These simple balls are amazing because they help facilitate many positions that wouldn't be possible otherwise. If you are in a hospital bed attached to wires and monitors, you can still change positions near the bed. You can also move in the bed, rotating from one side to hands and knees and then to the other side.

- Use water. Showers and baths often reduce pain levels dramatically. Many hospitals do not offer baths. Most have showers, although getting to use them is a little tricky if your provider wants you attached to the fetal monitor all the time. Hopefully, either your provider will agree to monitor intermittently (usually 20 minutes on the monitor and 40 minutes off), or your hospital will have wireless, waterproof monitoring available so that you can use the shower. Try spraying the shower wand directly on your lower abdomen or lower back during contractions. This one tool helped me more than anything else in my own labors.

- At some point in active labor you will need to either get to the birth center or hospital, or make sure your home birth midwife gets to you. Always call ahead and make a plan with them before coming in. If you have a doula, one of the major advantages is that she can help you determine when is a good time to go so that you get there neither too early nor too late.

- Pushing – wow! You're almost there! It takes a lot of energy to push a baby into the world. If you feel a very strong (i.e. uncontrollable) urge to push, then do! Usually your provider will examine you first to make sure that the cervix is completely dilated, meaning out of the way. But if you are just feeling a little pressure – even if you are fully dilated – it's usually best to save your energy and breathe through it. Your uterus will push the baby down – this is called "passive descent" or "laboring down." It cuts down on the amount of time you actually have to spend doing intense pushing. That's not only helpful to save your strength: it might also help you avoid a cesarean since most hospitals have a certain time limit on how long a woman can push before they decide that it isn't working. Since the clock only starts with active pushing, laboring down helps you get ahead without "losing time." I was once at a birth where the woman was overwhelmed by the intensity of the pushing phase. She asked the doctor, "How long will this last?" The doctor replied, "No more than three hours." Poor woman! She wanted to know how long she would need to push (which of course was impossible to know, but completely natural to ask), but the doctor instead answered with how long she would be allowed to push before a cesarean would be done.

- Avoiding tissue damage. It used to be routine to cut an episiotomy. Then doctors realized that a woman's tissues were created to stretch, and that natural tears generally heal better than cuts. According to current recommendations, episiotomies are reserved for situations where the baby is almost delivered but needs to be born a bit faster. In normal situations, though, a baby can often be born over a totally intact perineum. This is not the result of any magical oil or potion, but primarily four things:
- Good nutrition – healthy tissue stretches better than unhealthy tissue.
- Position for birth – studies show that some positions lead to less tearing than others. Being flat on the back and deep squatting increase tears, whereas side-lying and all fours positions decrease tears.
- Slow, controlled birth – as the baby is about to crown, your provider may give you some feedback, perhaps asking you to stop pushing at some point, or to give little pushes while he or she supports the perineum. The goal is to keep the baby's head from emerging too fast which can cause tears. Communication is key.
- Perineal massage might help first-time moms, but the research isn't spectacular, so it's certainly not a "must." Here is a helpful handout with instructions: https://www.ouh.nhs.uk/patient-guide/leaflets/files/10938Pmassage.pdf
- But what about epidurals – good, bad, neither or both? Let me sidestep that trap at the beginning. Getting an epidural is not a moral issue. It's a personal choice. From my perspective, that choice boils down to three points: 1) concerns about the risk of side effects, for which there is factual information to inform your decision; 2) one's overall outlook on childbirth; and 3) attitudes toward pain (which may be able to be reframed but may also have deep roots that have to be honored). Let me unpack those three points:
- Risk of side effects – Without going into the nitty gritty (which is best left to your reading and your childbirth education instructor), let's just summarize and say that epidurals work very well for pain relief and can be especially beneficial for tired moms experiencing very long labors. But there is a fair amount of research that indicates that they may increase the rate of cesareans (especially if given early) and instrumental (forceps or vacuum) births. There is also a small but real set of side effects associated with epidurals, which include risk of spinal headache, infection and long term back pain. For your information, the chance of becoming paralyzed by an epidural is less than your chance of being struck by lightning G-d forbid, unless you have certain, rare medical issues. That

being said, I have seen women who saw the epidural as an enemy or who had intense fear that something would go wrong. I think that such thinking creates unnecessary stress. I prefer to think of it as a tool – not the first one I reach for, but one that I'm grateful exists. The epidural is less likely to slow labor if done after five centimeters when strong contractions are present. So even if you decide to have an epidural, consider waiting it out a bit.

- Outlook on childbirth – Some women see this as an adventure, a challenge – sort of like running a marathon or climbing Mt. Everest. It doesn't feel good when you're doing it, but the "high" and the sense of accomplishment afterwards is an unbeatable feeling. In fact, just as runners get "runner's high" – which is a burst of the feel-good hormones called endorphins – women in labor get a burst of endorphins too. In fact, the longer the labor, the more endorphins a woman's body produces. Women in labor also produce high levels of oxytocin, the hormone that causes contractions, which has a secondary effect of promoting bonding and loving relationships. This is no accident, but also an exquisite example of *niflaot haborei*. Hashem wants mothers to "fall in love" with their babies at first sight, so He created a cocktail of hormones to be released during the childbirth process that promotes those feelings. This is why many consider childbirth to be a "peak" experience. Women who have given birth without pain medication often report a feeling of empowerment, a feeling that they can do anything. I know for myself, at age 22, the unmedicated birth of my first son was one of the proudest, most accomplished moments in my young life. Seeing the triumphant "I did it!" expression on women's faces is one of the greatest highlights of my work as a midwife.

- Attitudes about pain – Normally in life when you have pain it means that something is wrong. But in birth it is quite the opposite. Leaving theories of painless childbirth aside, when the contractions get stronger it means that progress is taking place and you are getting closer to birth. It's a good sign. Looking at it this way can help decrease psychological distress, which is important because psychological distress has the effect of magnifying the physical distress. But let's be honest: it doesn't make the pain go away. So the question remains: "How do you feel about pain?" When I used to teach childbirth classes, I would explain the risks of epidurals, and then say: "Some people will look at this and say, 'Why should I accept any risk? It's only pain! Other people will hear it and say, 'Hey! Pain is a big deal to me, and the chance that anything negative will happen is really small.'" So they will opt to take the epidural. Either choice is Okay! The point is for everyone to have real, informed choices they can make. Because when an anesthesiologist comes into a labor room holding the meds and rattles off a list of potential side effects when you are in pain, it's not realistic to think that you will make a rational decision at that point. A little tool I find helpful is to ask yourself before labor, "on a scale of 1 to 10 where 1 = "I want the epidural as soon as possible," 10 = "I don't want an epidural no matter what" and 5 = "I don't really care either way," where do you fall on the scale? This helps those around you to better understand your goals, because their job is to support you in reaching your goals. They shouldn't have an agenda of their own.

- Now if you read all this and aren't inspired about having some peak experience, I understand. I had six unmedicated births because I figured if I had to give birth anyway, I might as well aim for the ultimate birth experience if possible, but honestly I'm the last person to engage in an extreme sport or try to climb a mountain. It just depends on how you feel about it. This isn't a competition, and you are no less a mother because of the kind of birth you did or didn't have. Your job is not to keep up with anyone's expectations, but to make the best, healthiest choices possible, which includes taking your peace of mind seriously. You deserve to be an *em habanim s'mecha*,[6] "a mother of children is happy", period.

- One last note about epidurals: It isn't guaranteed that you will be able to get one. Your labor might go too fast, the anesthesiologist might be needed for an emergency, you could have a medical condition (like low platelet count) which makes the procedure too risky, or you might get the epidural and find that it doesn't work so well for you (yes, it happens). I will never forget a birth I attended early in my career as a doula. I had just been hired the previous day. Someone had encouraged the mother to hire a doula to improve her chances for a VBAC and she was scheduled for an induction the following morning. She was 100% set on having an epidural, but when the anesthesiologist arrived, he informed her that her low platelet count significantly increased her risk of complications from an epidural. She wasn't comfortable taking the risk. It was very difficult for her to change her mindset and cope with the pain that she had had no intention of experiencing, but I coached her through it, and she ultimately gave birth vaginally. Afterwards she told me that if I had not been there to help her she would have requested a cesarean because there would have been no way she could have coped by herself. I don't think she was exaggerating

---

6   *Tehillim* 113;9.

to make me feel good – it was a rough labor for her. I also have no doubt that she went on to have many more children. I'm proud that I had a role in enabling that to happen. I have also seen women get an epidural that does not fully relieve their pain. I don't want to cause you added anxiety – 95% of the time the epidural is successful. I would, however, encourage you to have coping skills and labor support in place in the event that you encounter an obstacle with an epidural.

Giving Birth on Shabbat

Regarding Shabbat there is a question as to how many people may accompany a woman. Most *poskim* agree that at a minimum a husband and doula are permitted; however, additional people may or may not be permitted. One should ask one's *rav* in advance.

A husband's emotional support is critical for his wife throughout pregnancy, labor, and childbirth. However, in my opinion there are different types of support that women typically need in labor. In early labor, which can last several hours or easily an entire day, the contractions are lighter and usually irregular. It's best to try to rest and not focus on the labor too much, so at this point a woman generally appreciates her husband's company. Taking a stroll together, laughing, eating a meal, napping, foot massage – these are the kinds of activities that are helpful in early labor. And since most women aren't *nidah* at this point, the husband is usually the best candidate for the job. Anyone else may make her feel like the proverbial "watched pot." However, once labor intensifies, women usually need the wisdom and touch of an experienced woman, someone who has helped many women and can reassure her with words like, "I know it's hard... you have come so far... let's just focus on this contraction..." etc. To a woman in labor, it feels more authentic and believable to hear certain messages from another woman. An experienced doula also knows how to use her hands to relieve the pain with massage, counterpressure, and knowledge of different positions. Research has also shown that husbands report a more positive experience when there is a doula, because she takes pressure off of him. A husband can offer words of affirmation – "I'm so proud of you... you're amazing... I can't wait to meet our baby... I am so excited... I know that you will be a wonderful mother" and so on which gives his wife tremendous *chizuk*. But more uniquely, the husband is his wife's protector. He will stand up for her and advocate for his family with medical staff if need be. He will help her process information about any decisions that might need to be made. He will *daven* and say *Tehillim* for her, as is our custom.[7] With one of my children, I was having a difficult labor and my husband arranged for a group of people to *daven* for me – all at 3 am! A baby girl was born a short time later, and I was extremely grateful for his help. My experience is that if there is a full team present – a carefully chosen care provider and doula – the husband should not feel marginalized; on the contrary, it can be a very warm bonding experience for the couple and newborn if he is nearby. But barring an emergency which might necessitate his physical help (like a baby suddenly being born at home with no one else present), he shouldn't need to do anything that Jewish law doesn't permit.

Halachot in childbirth are not complicated, but there are some differences of opinion amongst *poskim*. Please don't wait until you are in labor to ask, as you may not be able to reach the *rav* at that time. Certain things are clear: a woman who has experienced vaginal bleeding or who is in the pushing stage is definitely *nidah*, and therefore all *harchakot* must be observed. Beyond this, there are some differences of opinion as to what other circumstances might render a woman *nidah*. Some *poskim* consider loss of the mucus plug (a brownish jelly-like discharge which sometimes happens in early labor or in the days preceding labor), having reached a certain dilation point, or breaking of the bag of waters to also render a woman *nidah*. When the laboring woman is being examined or at any other time that she is uncovered, her husband must be sure to walk out or look away. The Rebbe felt very strongly that the husband should not be in the labor/delivery room during the actual delivery even if he were to look away and not touch his wife.[8] Please consult your *rav* well in advance to determine how that applies in your situation. We have to remember that holding fast to Torah is the conduit for blessings. We also need to remember what's happening: A soul is making its way into this world. Just as a couple is careful to conceive that child in *kedusha*, it's critically important to usher that life into the world in *kedusha*. There is a great deal a husband can do within the realm permissible by *halacha* and this should be his focus.

Once you cover your bases, relax. There is a saying, "If you fail to plan, then you plan to fail." *Hishtadlut*, effort, is critical. We have to do our part. But birth is not like saving money for a house or studying for a test, in which if you perform certain behaviors you will have fairly predictable results. That's because there is no one set pattern to labor or pregnancy. This is why you should never compare your birth to

---

[7] *Sefer HaChassidim* p. 487; *Sefer Hatoldot Maharash* p. 20. According to the instructions issued by the *Tzemach Tzedek* to his sons during the birth of the Rebbe Maharash, the following chapters of *Tehillim* are recited: 1, 2, 3, 4, 20, 21, 22, 23, 24, 33, 47, 72, 86, 90, 91, 92, 93, 104, 112, and 113 to the end.

[8] *Teshuvot U'Biurim BeShulchan Aruch*, p. 445.

anyone else's – because it was different to begin with. One woman can have a smooth, manageable six hour labor and another person can have an exhausting three day labor. One woman has serious complications and the next sails through pregnancy with only minor aches and pains. We are all different and our experiences are different. Maybe it's this natural variation that often makes people think, "why bother to plan?" in the first place. They figure "what will be will be." It's all up to Hashem, right? Of course it is, but in life we always have to balance between *hashgacha pratit* and *hishtadlut*.

It is my hope that this article will serve as a guide to help you take smart, logical steps towards achieving a healthy pregnancy and birth experience. But don't take it too far. Some people are overly focused on trying to do everything "right" and can't relax, losing the precious gift of *menuchat hanefesh*. While it's important to put in effort, try to remember that you can't control the outcome. You have to make good choices, then "let go, and let G-d." *Bitachon* is a powerful thing. If you find yourself being overly attached to your birth plan, or generally anxious, consider the following meditation: place your carefully crafted, dearly held vision of the birth you desire into an imaginary balloon. Send this balloon up to the Heavens with a prayer: "Master of the World, this is what my heart desires. I have done what I can do to make it happen, and now I'm giving it over to You. I trust that everything You do is for the good, and that You will take care of me." Take a few deep breaths and notice what you are feeling in your body. Acknowledge it, write down a few words about it, and repeat the meditation until you are able to let go more freely.

In conclusion, I want to bless you, dear reader, with strength and clarity, with beautiful births, and with healthy children born *b'sha'a tova*. May you have endless *yiddishe nachat* from all of them, and may you find meaning and joy in every part of the journey. *Hatzlacha rabba!*

Your Baby Has Arrived!

Mazal tov! The baby's here! What now?

Do the natural thing – hold your baby in your arms. This is the prize you have worked for! As long as the baby is stable, he or she should be placed directly on your body after birth and ideally remain there for at least the first hour. This is often termed "the golden hour" as it is during this time that babies are generally wide-eyed and primed for bonding. Routine procedures can either be done while the baby is on you, or delayed. There are many benefits to the baby derived from skin-to-skin contact, including:

- Better body temperature maintenance
- Improved ability to absorb nutrients
- Crying less often
- Improved weight gain
- Higher blood oxygen levels
- More stable heart rate and breathing
- Improved brain development
- Higher breastfeeding success rates

If you are feeling weak after birth, your doula or female friend or family member can hold the baby on your abdomen or chest so that you don't actually have to do anything. If any stitches are needed, looking at the baby can serve as a good distraction.

- Wait to cut the umbilical cord. Waiting at least one full minute ensures that the baby gets the majority of the blood from the placenta, resulting in less anemia in both the short and long term. This leads to better oxygenation, fewer infections, and maybe even some neurological benefits. This blood is rich in stem cells, which are often harvested for treatments for people suffering from many ailments, including cancer. Delaying the clamping and cutting of the cord means that your baby is getting a full dose of stem cells right at birth. You also have the opportunity to do a mitzvah with these stem cells by donating whatever is left after the cord is clamped to "Gift of Life," which matches this blood to others in need. Go to Jcord.org for more information.

Breastfeeding

When you are ready, initiate breastfeeding. The benefits of breastfeeding for the baby are almost too many to enumerate, including:

- Stronger immune systems
- Fewer gastrointestinal problems
- Fewer colds and ear infections
- Lower rates of Sudden Infant Death Syndrome (SIDS)
- Fewer hospitalizations
- Fewer childhood cancers, especially leukemia
- Lower risk of developing diabetes
- Fewer cavities

- Less likelihood of becoming obese
- Less likelihood of developing heart disease

Mothers who breastfeed have a lower risk of:

- Breast cancer
- Ovarian cancer
- Diabetes
- Cardiovascular disease
- Osteoporosis with aging

May we all merit to conceive and bear healthy children and raise them to Torah, *chuppah* and *maasim tovim,* good deeds, in good health and with great joy.

Shayna Eliav, CNM is a proud mother and grandmother. She currently works as a midwife in New York City, fulfilling her long-nurtured dream of helping women and babies on this miraculous journey.

Sarah Eichler, IBCLC

Mother's Milk
A LACTATION PRIMER

Your body's readiness to provide nutrition to your baby is automatic and one of the greatest wonders of the universe. Your ability to breastfeed and your baby's ability to suckle, while natural, do not present seamlessly and in the same manner for each woman. Be proactive, not reactive, when it comes to breastfeeding. The more you know before having the baby, the easier the transition you will have to a breastfeeding mother.

Among the many body changes, women notice when they become pregnant, is a change in their breasts' appearance. The areola, which is the dark area around the nipple, gets larger and darker. The nipple may become larger and protrude slightly. You might notice some little bumps on the areola. These are called Montgomery glands and they secrete a fluid that hydrates the areola while also releasing a scent that is said to smell like amniotic fluid to a baby. Another big adjustment for newly pregnant women is the growth in breast size. This transformation is the first step your body takes in getting ready for lactation. Once the baby is born and the placenta is delivered, your body recognizes that you need to provide milk and begins transitioning from producing colostrum (your baby's first milk) to making mature milk. Colostrum is high in protein and dense in antibodies and immunological properties that help protect your baby from disease they may be exposed to in their new environment.

Colostrum is the first form of protection for your baby. As your baby's first food, it will help colonize their gut with healthy microbiome. It also contains a laxative-like substance. Frequent and effective breastfeeding in the early days will help ensure a timely *brit* as it helps the baby's body eliminate bilirubin. Colostrum stimulates early passage of meconium stools that are rich in bilirubin and reduces the possibility that bilirubin will be reabsorbed into the bloodstream and cause jaundice.

Hashem created our bodies with the amazing ability to produce custom milk for each of our children. How does our milk change and increase? As our babies latch and start to suckle for the first time, they stimulate increased levels of prolactin and oxytocin. These hormones cause the milk to be expelled from the breast, also known as the milk ejection reflex (MER) or letdown.

When you are having your letdown, you may feel a tingling sensation. Some people experience it as a feeling of fullness, or a rush inside their breast. You may notice this feeling when you hear a baby cry or if you start to think about your baby. For first-time moms, this feeling generally starts a few weeks after birth. Sometimes the mom doesn't feel it at all, and that's totally normal too.

Immediately after birth, place your baby on your chest, skin on skin. Taking that moment to just hold the baby, enjoy their scent and warmth and their soft skin. It is an incredible time that has important benefits for both mother and baby. Babies will bond, be more calm, have their temperature regulated by the mom, and breathe comfortably when they are skin to skin with you. They can also smell you, and this will start the wonderful process of your baby finding your breast to get her/his first meal. For some babies this can take 20 minutes; for others, an hour. But throw away the clock, turn off your "I must help my baby latch" thoughts, and just watch what the baby will do. If the baby was taken away for whatever reason and brought back to you wrapped like a burrito, unwrap that baby down to their diaper and start skin to skin contact with your baby at that moment.

Believe it or not, if we just hold the baby, they will start to touch, lick and move towards the breast, ending in a big, deep latch. They will start to suckle at the breast, initiating a huge increase in your oxytocin which not only helps your milk be pressed out into the baby's mouth, but helps you to bond with the baby, as well as helping expel the placenta, essentially ending the birth process. For some moms who had an intense birth, this quiet and peaceful time with the baby can help them center themselves while bonding with their baby. Remember, this can be done at any time. I also encourage my clients to have skin to skin contact with their babies from time to time during the first few weeks of life. It's so easy, especially if we stop and think how most of the time we have to undress the baby to change their diaper anyway. And this extra touch adds a whole new level of bonding physically, hormonally, and emotionally.

Generally a few hours after birth, once that baby has had some great bonding and breastfeeding time with you, the baby goes down for a nice deep sleep.

How do we know when the baby is ready to eat again? Let's talk about all-important feeding cues. New moms need to recognize them so they won't end up with a screaming and frustrated baby who now has no patience to latch. After all, babies want their food immediately. Having the baby near you helps as babies show earlier signs when their mom is close and the mom can see the signs and respond to them faster.

Your Baby's Feeding Cues

- Fluttering of the eyes – This may look as if the baby is sleeping, and very possibly they are in a light sleep just before waking up. This is a great time to start setting up your breastfeeding location.
- Movement of the mouth – This looks like small movements of the mouth. The baby might also stick out their tongue, licking their lips.
- Rooting - Have you ever seen someone touch a baby's cheek and how the baby moves towards that side? This is called rooting and is a reflex so that the baby will feel the mom's breast/nipple to then latch.
- Movement of the body – Now the baby is awake and they are starting to move to try and find the breast. At this stage, you want to unwrap the baby as soon as possible and latch.
- Last, and a late sign, is crying. Once the baby is crying, some people take advantage of the open mouth and latch. This may work sometimes. However, if you notice that the baby is so frustrated that they are not latching, take a different approach. Hold the baby and let them suck on your finger or a pacifier. Calm the baby down and then try to latch. You will find that a calm baby will find it easier to latch on.

Being attentive to your baby's cues is a wonderful method, not only for feeding but for early parenting. It will help you understand when they are hungry vs. wanting a diaper change or maybe just wanting to chill with their parents. Watching for cues will also allow you to find your rhythm in breastfeeding. In addition, I find new moms tend to be more relaxed once they let go of the idea that babies should be on a schedule at such a young age.

How often should the baby be eating? The colostrum is a powerful thick liquid which allows the baby to slowly practice their suck-swallow-breathe pattern. Frequent nursing sessions are normal, and the average baby will nurse around 8-14 times in the first 24 hours. What about after the first day?

What goes in must come out. Count your baby's diapers to see that it is getting milk. An easy way to remember this is:

- Day 1 - Minimum 1 pee, 1 poo
- Day 2 - Minimum 2 pees, 2 poos
- Day 3 - Minimum 3 pees, 3 poos
- Day 4 - Minimum 4 pees, 4 poos
- Day 5 and on - The American Academy of Pediatrics (AAP) suggests a minimum of 4-6 pees and 3-5 poos each day.

Next we check the color. The pee should be clear or a light yellow. The baby's stool will start off being black and thick. This first poop is made up of meconium. As the baby starts to take in more milk the poop will change color and consistency: from black to brown, then green, and finally an orange or yellow cottage cheese-like poop. If your baby is getting formula then the poop will be more brown/green in color with a paste- or cream-like consistency. If you see the pee is getting darker or not as frequent as suggested above, and/or the stools are not frequent and are not changing color, then reach out to your pediatrician or lactation consultant to figure out why.

Babies' appetites increase over time. They are not born to take in 2.5 oz at once, but rather very small amounts of milk. So don't worry if you are not producing a large amount of milk immediately. It takes about 6 weeks for your milk to become fully established and for you to develop your full capacity for milk storage. If you are concerned, firstly, the more you breastfeed, the more milk your body will produce. If that is not working, seek professional help from an IBCLC (International Board Certified Lactation Consultant) who will be able to assess and advise you. They will be able to guide you on how to increase your milk supply and give you options on how to feed your baby in the meantime.

Latching and Nursing Positions

There are a variety of ways to hold the baby while s/he latches on for nursing.

To latch – Line the baby up with you, either nose to nipple or philtrum (the midline groove in the upper lip) to the nipple. You can gently tap or swipe your nipple to induce a sucking reflex. As the baby starts to open its mouth to latch, bring them towards you. As s/he feels the nipple in its mouth, s/he will close to seal and then suck the breast in.

Cradle Hold – This is probably the best-known position and is great when the baby is older as there isn't much control or support offered. The baby will lay tummy to tummy with you, their head in the cradle of your arm or crook of your elbow. The mom then gently brings the baby to the breast.

Cross Cradle Hold – Many women find this to be the easiest position when they are just beginning; it provides the mom with control and the ability to see clearly if the baby is latching. If you are latching to your right breast, your left hand will be placed on the baby's back with your hand supporting the back of the baby's neck and shoulders. Your right hand holds and shapes the breast. As the baby is opening its mouth, you bring the baby to the breast.

Football or Clutch Hold – Hold the baby on your side, supporting the back of shoulders and neck. Use pillows to support the baby's weight. The baby should be aligned on your side, ribcage to ribcage.

Side Lying – Lay on your side and place the baby on its side. Use your upper hand to bring the baby towards you. Be careful that the surface you are lying on is not too soft and that the baby can't roll or have its face inadvertently covered by a blanket or pillow.

Laid Back Nursing – Have baby tummy to tummy with you. Lie back in a reclining position with your hand wrapped around the baby to give him/her support. Move your hand to bring the baby closer to your body if needed.

Common Breastfeeding Challenges

*Painful nipples: This can happen in the first few weeks of breastfeeding, and most of the time it's due to improper latch. If the baby isn't latching on correctly, the nipple is not reaching deeply enough into the baby's mouth. Then the baby ends up pinching the nipple over and over which causes blisters, cracks and sometimes bleeding nipples. The first thing to do is check the latch. Make sure the baby's mouth is nice and deep on the breast, not just on the nipple. Also, remember you're not a pacifier. If the latch doesn't feel good, it likely isn't. Nipple creams can help with the healing but if the latch isn't corrected, pain may just get worse.

*Engorgement: When the milk comes in, the breasts can become very full and hard. Frequent nursing and massage help not only prevent engorgement but also help stop it. Using a cold compress can help reduce the swelling. A warm compress or shower can be helpful *only* if you massage or express your milk. I find alternating between the two works best. Some women will place cabbage leaves in the bra; this helps to reduce the swelling. Change the cabbage leaf when it wilts (about 10-20 minutes). Repeat if necessary, but not too often, as cabbage can dry up your milk. Once you are feeling relief, it's time to start using massage.

*Flat or inverted nipples: If you notice before having your baby that your nipples don't protrude, you might want to see a lactation consultant who can give you tips for the first few days in the hospital in case the baby doesn't latch on easily. One tool which often helps is called a nipple shield. It's a thin silicone nipple-shaped tool that you place over your nipple. This allows the baby to latch directly onto your breast. I call it "training wheels" for breastfeeding. Eventually a baby should be weaned from it, usually before the baby is 6 weeks old.

*Sore back for moms: Most moms will laugh, wondering, "What does my back have to do with breastfeeding?" Trust me, I've seen some of the most inflexible women become professional contortionists during breastfeeding, which can result in real back pain. Please make sure to arrange for yourself a comfortable spot for breastfeeding. Have different sized pillows, or even a commercial breastfeeding pillow, available to help you support your baby's weight and save your back. Remember to center yourself in your space and then bring the baby to you. Even if you lean in to latch the baby, make sure to sit up once it is latched. If you don't feel comfortable, readjust yourself. Your back will thank me for this advice.

This special time with your baby will pass quickly. Hashem has created an easy way to bond and give love to our children through breastfeeding. Our breasts are positioned near the heart, which brings our babies close to us, allowing us to interact with our children while they nurse to bond and connect. Our breasts also heat and cool our babies. If we look at a thermal image, when a woman breastfeeds her child, the breast looks like an upside-down heart. New babies can see 25 centimeters in front of themselves. Amazingly, that is the approximate distance between a baby and their mother's breast. In Straight from the Heart, a beautiful book about the Torah perspective on mothering and nursing by Tehilla Abramov, she notes that the placement of our breasts is near our face and heart, unlike other mammals in whom the breasts/udder are near the bottom/back of the animal, far away from the face.[1] This illustrates that breastfeeding is not only about nutrition as it is in the case of animals, but for connection and bonding.

---

1   *Brachot* 10a.

Mother's Milk: A Lactation Primer

In fact, Rabbi Yehudah Hachassid wrote in his famous *Tzavaah* (Will), that when nursing her newborn child for the very first time, a mother should begin on the left side because the baby should have his first meal from the place that's closest to the seat of understanding – the heart.[2]

Sometimes it can be hard to focus on nursing. We may feel we are missing out on other things or being held back by this choice. It's so important to understand and remember that no one else but you can do this for your child. Throughout history, women could have chosen a wet nurse, yet many did not.

וחנה לא עלתה, כי אמרה לאישה: עד יגמל הנער והבאתיו ונראה את פני ה׳, וישב שם עד עולם. ויאמר לה אלקנה אישה: עשי הטוב בעיניך, שבי עד גמלך אותו, אך יקם ה׳ את דברו. ותשב האשה ותינק את בנה עד גמלה אותו.

But Chana did not go up [to Shiloh], for she said to her husband: "[Let us wait] until the child is weaned. I will then bring him and we will appear before Hashem, and he will reside there forever." Elkanah her husband said to her: "Do what seems good to you; stay until you have weaned him. However, may Hashem fulfill His word." The woman remained and nursed her son until she weaned him.[3]

Chana, who *davened* for a child for many years and finally merited to be a mother, chose to stay home in order to nurse her child even when her husband went to the *Mishkan* to give thanks to Hashem. She did this, the Rebbe pointed out, although she was a *neviah,* a prophetess, and could have merited great revelations. Our priority is our children.[4]

The Top Three Questions About Breastfeeding

1. *What are the benefits of breastfeeding?*

Breastfeeding offers significant benefits for both mom and baby. Research continues to indicate the incredible way in which Hashem's "formula" supports our children right from the start. Breastfeeding protects babies from infections and illnesses that include diarrhea, ear infections, lower respiratory infections, and pneumonia. Breastfed babies

---

[2] *Knesset Chachmei Yisrael,* siman 214.

[3] *I Shmuel* 1:22-23.

[4] *Sichot Kodesh* 5734, vol. 1, pp. 24-29.

are less likely to develop asthma and Type 2 Diabetes. Children who are breastfed for six months or longer are less likely to become obese. Breastfeeding also reduces the risk of sudden infant death syndrome. Incredibly, when you or your baby is sick, your milk composition will change, providing your baby with more antibodies and immune system-boosting properties.

Dr. Lawrence Noble, a neonatologist, who presented at a conference I attended, spoke about the effect breast milk can have on a child's health. If only we knew, he said, how any amount, even a few small drops, can make an impact on the child's life. The more breast milk, and the longer the child receives the breast milk for, the more positive the benefits will be. "Each drop is gold. We know so little about breast milk, but what I know is that it's miraculous," said Dr. Noble.

Necrotizing enterocolitis (NEC), is a disease that affects the gastrointestinal tract in premature babies, or babies born before 37 weeks of pregnancy. Those babies that were given breast milk exclusively were 6-10 times less likely to develop NEC.

Breastfeeding also helps with mood. Oxytocin is in your milk, which makes your baby feel good and connected with you. It also helps you connect with your baby. Have you ever noticed how babies look sleepy after breastfeeding, or how moms are tired after nursing? Yes, that's right: the prolactin hormone your body produces during breastfeeding aids with sleep[5].

There are significant health benefits for women who breastfeed too: studies have revealed a lower statistical chance of certain cancers, less chance of postpartum mood disorder, and that nursing can help you burn the extra calories you gained while pregnant.

Another great benefit is that the milk is always there, waiting, available for your child at the perfect temperature and flavor. This helps by giving you a break from washing bottles, or if you're running out of the house, there is one less item to pack and prepare.

---

[5] Dysphoric Milk Ejection Reflex (D-MER) is an abrupt emotional "drop" that occurs in some women during the "letdown" (before milk release) and continues for not more than a few minutes. The brief negative feelings range in severity from wistfulness to self-loathing, and appear to have a physiological cause. Some women can have physical symptoms as well, such as nausea, a pit in the stomach, or another "warning" sensation. Some women feel an eversion to breastfeeding as well. There are several effective treatment options starting with meditation, music, and other distraction techniques until these feelings pass. For more severe symptoms, medication can be helpful as well.

2. What if I can't breastfeed due to prescription medication I must take, a lifestyle issue, or a physical or mental health issue? What can/should I do if I have a child with special needs who can't breastfeed the way I dreamed?

Remember, breastfeeding is not one-dimensional. What might work for one mom and baby might not work for you. Breastfeeding takes time and is a learned skill. It also involves two people (or more if you have multiples). There are so many aspects required in order to make breastfeeding work. And for some moms it just doesn't work out the way they expect it to. It's okay to let go of the idea of perfection, of being "the best mom." I learned that the best mom is a happy mom, a mom who is balanced and can enjoy her baby.

Sometimes I meet a mom with a pre-existing health condition that she feels may impact her ability to breastfeed. If you fit that description, speaking to a lactation consultant before birth can help you decide if breastfeeding will work for you. Some moms with mental health challenges like anxiety or depression may just need extra support, which may come in the form of physical support like extra help around the home and/or emotional support through seeing a therapist, sleeping more, or medication. Planning ahead and understanding how all the new changes may impact you will make the transition easier. Many new moms think that because they are on medication they will be unable to breastfeed. In reality, many medications are safe, and those that are not can sometimes be replaced to create a safe breastfeeding experience. If any of this applies to you, definitely speak to your doctor and do your research in advance. https://www.infantrisk.com/ is the most up-to-date website (as of the publication time of this book) regarding medications for pregnant and nursing mothers.

If you are not breastfeeding your baby – such as if, for example, you have been discharged from the hospital and the baby is in the NICU or the baby has a cleft palate and can't nurse until after they have their surgery – you may choose to pump. This can be a wonderful way to connect with your child by giving them your milk. Speak to a competent *rav* who understands the unique benefits of breast milk and the pertinent *halachot* for help with navigating pumping on Shabbat and Yom Tov. Don't rely on hearsay about *halacha*.

If the baby is unable to breastfeed, there are important techniques you can use to foster a great connection with your newborn. Lots of skin to skin contact during the first few days and weeks is wonderful, as I have described above. If you want to give your baby your milk in a bottle, start expressing your milk as soon as possible. Hand expression during the first few days of life is more stimulating than pumping, but if you're too overwhelmed and pumping will work for you, do that to start your milk production. This might seem simple, but it's a good idea: be the one to give the bottle to the baby whenever possible. Switch sides while giving the bottle so the baby can develop their peripheral vision. Communicate and talk to the baby while giving the bottle.

3. How can I best prepare to be successful?

Even though breastfeeding is normal and natural, it's a learned skill. The key is setting yourself up for success. We know that the ultimate breastfeeding duration is directly related to the confidence a mom has during the first few days. That is why taking a class before having the baby is one of the best ways to prepare. A live class with a lactation consultant can help you learn basic latching techniques and understand what's going to happen during the first few days. It will also provide you with a person you know and feel comfortable with to contact after the birth if you have any trouble. If you don't have someone to turn to locally, a virtual class that can be interactive would be another great option. Books, articles or websites can be extremely helpful; make sure you are gleaning information from sources that are research rather than opinion based. Gain knowledge in advance, but also get help when you need it. There is no reason to be shy or to wait until the situation is out of hand.

When I had my first baby, I was convinced that I knew exactly what to do. I had read multiple books, watched a variety of youtube videos, and read articles on the web. But when I had my daughter, it turned out that all the information I learned was helpful only to a certain extent. My daughter ended up losing too much weight and her jaundice level almost landed her in the hospital to be put under lights. Thank G-d I had an amazing pediatrician who told me my baby needed more food and suggested I give her formula. I said I wanted to breastfeed and was referred to an IBCLC who gave me personalized guidance. It's possible that I could have found the information online, but I wouldn't have known how to implement it. She gave me a plan so I was able to build up my milk supply. My daughter gained weight and she didn't have to go to the hospital. Sometimes all the planning we do helps us know when to seek professional help, which is all-important.

Persistence and Commitment: For some new moms, mastering breastfeeding can take days and sometimes weeks. I had one client who only reached the point of feeding her baby 90% breastmilk after three months. This was an older mom in her late thirties who had some markers for IGT (Insufficient glandular tissue, which means she might not be able to have a full milk supply). When I first saw her, the baby was unable to latch on to her breast and she was feeding her adorable baby formula only. We set two goals: to get the baby to the breast and to build up her milk supply. During the first week she reached the point of feeding her baby 10% breastmilk. She was so excited, and I joined her in her joy. A few weeks later the baby was latching and I showed her how to use a supplemental nursing system. This way the baby could get the supplement while at the breast. She was thrilled with the idea. It was a challenge but she persisted. I told her I was there for her and that she was doing an amazing job. We adjusted her plan as the pumping was becoming too much of an effort for her, so I told her to focus on the baby, bonding and breastfeeding. I suggested that she stop pumping only if she felt like it. (Sometimes I use pumping as a way to increase milk supply if the baby is struggling to drain the breast.) I didn't hear from her for a while, but when I finally got the call I was full of joy that she was feeding her baby 90% breastmilk. This mom taught me important lessons: sometimes it takes longer to reach our goals than we think it will. Persistence and commitment are the key to success. Take each day and each nursing session as they come. Just because you give your baby one bottle, it will not make or break your breastfeeding journey: it depends on what you do at the next session. And sometimes that bottle gives you the break you need.

For many working women today, going back to work only after the first six weeks after childbirth may not be an option. Pumping and having someone give your breastmilk to your child while you are away is an amazing option. When you get home you can nurse. There is no reason your baby shouldn't be able to switch from breast to bottle.

Support: Getting support from friends and family is important. If you don't have anyone in your family who breastfeeds, that's okay. Listen to them, but also understand that if they have not breastfed a baby they may not be able to give you the information or advice you need. Speak to your husband before the baby comes. Tell them the amount of time it takes for a baby to nurse and to learn the skill. Let him know that it will be challenging and that you will need him to support you and be your cheerleader during the first few weeks. Find a support circle outside the family if necessary – this could be friends or a local breastfeeding support group. Now with the easy availability of virtual classes and support groups, you don't even have to leave your home to join. Many are moderated by professionals. Or find your local La Leche League, a mother-to-mother breastfeeding support organization which has branches worldwide. Find professional help that you are comfortable with. Every lactation consultant has something to offer. Sometimes it requires talking to a few people until you find the right person to help you. Or sometimes it takes talking to a few people to get the information you need. Keep searching and find the support that works for you. Speaking to friends and family members who have used a lactation consultant can help you find someone with a good reputation.

Trust yourself: Everyone is unique. I once helped a mom whose 5-month-old baby had not gained any weight in the past month, and the pediatrician was concerned. The mom mentioned her milk supply had dipped and that she didn't feel as full as she used to. I asked her what had changed in the past month. She responded that she had started to sleep train her baby, who was now sleeping about 6-7 hours straight at night. I asked how it was the first week. She said, "I was waking up so full that it was painful, but after a few nights things became regulated." She reported that nothing changed during the day. Then the lightbulb went off in my mind. I explained to her that breastmilk works by supply and demand. Her waking up every morning so full was telling her body she didn't need so much milk anymore. The other issue was that nothing changed during the day: she wasn't making up those lost nursing sessions in the daytime. Essentially, *she was weaning*. "But," she said, "this didn't happen to my sister or sister-in-law who did the same thing." Of course it's possible that that technique did not impact her relatives' milk supplies as quickly as hers. But it only matters what happens to your body, not to others. We made a plan so she would replace the missed nursing sessions during the day, as the extra sleep at night was extremely important to her. The lesson: what works for one might not work for another. It's vital to listen to your intuition and body. If you think something is wrong, trust yourself.

End Note: Why I Chose to Become a Lactation Consultant and Personal Challenges

My journey to becoming a lactation consultant started even before I had my children. I've always loved to learn about a variety of subjects. One day an acquaintance spoke about a lactation consultant they saw and questioned her training. I became curious and decided to find out what was involved. To become an International Board Certified Lactation Consultant (IBCLC) takes years, not days or weeks as I thought. It requires multiple college courses, 90 hours of human lactation education, and a minimum of 500 clinical hours (not just observation). Most IBCLCs take an average of four years to complete the requirements. When I had my own baby and met with my lactation consultant Freda Rosenfeld, she mentioned off-handedly, "You'd be really good at this." I responded quickly, "I just had a baby and am not changing my career."

Four months later, after doing further research, I knew this is what I wanted to do. I loved the idea of helping other women and the blending of science with the art of breastfeeding. I enjoy solving mysteries when a client can't communicate her needs or even questions. It has been my honor to help women through their journey of breastfeeding. My goal with each client is to meet them where they are. Many times my own personal journey and struggles allow me to relate to them on a deeper level.

Sometimes I see new moms who have been inundated with information, much of it conflicting. I'm there to be their guide or "personal Google." I keep my information up to date and evidence- based by attending conferences and online webinars. I also share what I see works experientially. Transparency is vital; sometimes information passed from mother to mother beats all science. It's important especially for first-time moms to know that *you know best*. It's your baby; you are with them 24/7. Sometimes we have to say thank you and move on after receiving unhelpful information from well-meaning family members. Remember, a lot of advice is based on personal experience; what works for one woman and her baby may not work for you.

My own journey includes only one exclusively breastfeed baby. My other three were supplemented with both breastmilk and formula in a bottle. I can tell you it was hard. Have you ever heard the saying, "The shoemaker's kids don't have shoes?" I guess I'm the lactation consultant who does not have milk. I can joke about it now, but it was a painful journey to get to this point. I will share some lessons I learned along the way.

Giving your baby a bottle of your breastmilk is also amazing. You can still bond with your baby even if you don't breastfeed. For example, my first child was exclusively formula-fed from about 4.5 months old. I was very conscientious about being the one to give her the bottle and about holding her close to me while she drank her formula. I'd switch sides, as I once heard that breastfeeding helps babies develop their peripheral vision. Even once she was able to hold the bottle herself, I'd still try to hold her in order to achieve the best possible bonding experience I would have gotten if I was breastfeeding. Paying attention to all these details was a choice I made and I don't regret it for a moment. Each time I found it hard I'd remind myself, "This is just a short time in her life. Grab it and hold onto it because the time will pass quickly and before you know it she will be an independent toddler." Oh, and if I couldn't give the bottle, my husband or the person giving her care would be the one to give it.

Sarah Eichler is an International Board Certified Lactation Consultant (IBCLC) and a Certified Doula through DONA International. She is also a Lamaze Certified Childbirth Educator and Hypnobabies Childbirth Hypnosis Instructor. Never one to stop learning, Sarah is currently studying to be a Body Ready Method (BRM) certified practitioner to help pregnant women prepare their body for birth.

Sarah, herself a mother of four, was inspired to become a lactation consultant after experiencing her own breastfeeding challenges. Sarah maintains a private practice in Brooklyn, New York where she sees clients in person and via virtual consults and classes. Find Sarah on her website saraheichler.com and Instagram @thesaraheichler where she posts daily on matters related to birth, breastfeeding and the postpartum period.

Eliana Fine, MD
Bat-Sheva Lerner Maslow, MD, MSCTR, FACOG

Pru U'rvu:

UNDERSTANDING FERTILITY AND INFERTILITY

Introduction

Conception is a very precise and careful balance of steps that do not always fall into place. That is why even young potentially fertile couples do not always conceive right away. The natural pregnancy rate per menstrual cycle is about 25% for young couples (under 30 years old) and drops to less than 10% for couples when the woman is over forty. That means that even for couples in the height of their fertility, only about 1 out of every 4 who are trying to conceive will succeed during any given month! That being said, about 60% of young couples will conceive within 6 months, and 80% within 12 months. The definition of infertility is having tried to conceive for a year without success. Infertility is common. It is estimated that 1 out of every 6-8 couples will experience infertility in their lifetime. Infertility can be caused by dysfunction in any of the below outlined steps needed to achieve a pregnancy. Thankfully, there are many therapies available to treat the various causes of infertility.

The Menstrual Cycle and Fertilization

The menstrual cycle can be divided into three phases: the follicular phase, ovulation, and the luteal phase. An interplay of several different hormones drives the menstrual cycle. While the bleeding phase of the cycle is the most noticeable, the critical action is taking place behind the scenes. To begin a menstrual cycle, the brain must signal the ovary to select an egg, also called an oocyte. The oocyte grows in a fluid filled cyst on the ovary called a follicle. This phase of the cycle is called the "follicular phase" and usually spans the first 10-14 days of the cycle. During this time, the follicle produces estrogen, which helps build up the lining of the uterus in preparation for a potential pregnancy. When the egg is ready, the follicle and the brain then coordinate "ovulation," releasing the egg into the pelvis. The follicle now becomes a "corpus luteum" (a more solid appearing cyst on the ovary) and switches to producing progesterone, which will support the lining of the uterus should a pregnancy occur. This part of the menstrual cycle is called the "luteal phase" and typically lasts about 14 days. If the egg is fertilized by sperm and successfully implants in the uterus, it will start to produce HCG (human chorionic gonadotropin). HCG signals to the corpus luteum to keep producing progesterone to support the pregnancy. Without HCG, the corpus luteum stops producing progesterone after approximately 14 days. As the progesterone levels fall, the uterine lining sheds, and menses begins.

The above coordination between the brain and the ovary needs to be precisely timed so that the egg and sperm can meet under just the right conditions. After ovulation, the egg is picked up by the fallopian tube and carried toward the uterus. When a couple has intercourse, millions of sperm swim from the vagina through the cervix into the uterus and towards the tubes in search of the egg. Both the egg and the sperm that finds it need to be healthy in order for fertilization to occur. Once fertilized, it will take the embryo 5-7 days to divide from one cell into hundreds of cells and be ready for implantation. Over the course of this week, the embryo will journey through the tube into the uterus, where a lining will have been growing under the influence of estrogen in the follicular phase and now will be precisely coordinated by the influence of progesterone after ovulation. If the embryo has all the right components, and it finds a perfect spot in the uterus, it will implant itself in the lining and start secreting HCG. The HCG will signal to the ovary to continue progesterone production, which will prevent the shedding of the lining that would have occurred with the next period. HCG also starts a cascade of changes in the body even before a woman will ever recognize she is pregnant.

Causes of Infertility

Sometimes, infertility is caused by disorders of ovulation, where the quality or supply of eggs is healthy but the communication between the brain and the ovary is disrupted, so the menstrual cycle becomes irregular. Menstrual irregularities, not getting a cycle every month, are common in young women who are within 7-10 years of their first period. However, irregularities can be a sign of other issues, like polycystic ovarian syndrome (PCOS) which is a common hormonal disturbance in young women, issues with thyroid or prolactin, or very rarely a premature loss of the egg supply. Women with PCOS or other forms of ovulation dysfunction, do not release an egg in a predictable way, which can make it difficult to know when is the optimal time for conception.

Women can also have mechanical issues with their reproductive tracts that make conception or pregnancy more challenging. Obstruction or dysfunction of the fallopian tubes, uterus, or cervix could lead to infertility or miscarriage in some women.

There are other causes of infertility as well. Male-factor infertility, caused by issues with the male reproductive tract or sperm supply, is just as common as female-related causes. Up to a third of infertility cases will be exclusively caused by male-related issues (and another third are a combination of male and female related issues or unexplained infertility). Unlike the woman's limited egg supply, men produce new sperm every single day. As a result, the sperm supply is very susceptible to environmental factors. Smoking, alcohol intake, weight gain, weight loss, and illnesses have all been shown to decrease sperm counts or impact sperm motility (the sperm's ability to swim towards the egg). Thankfully, most of these effects can be temporary. However, it does take about 90 days for the body to develop new sperm cells, and any positive lifestyle modifications might take 3-6 months to significantly improve sperm.

Infertility evaluation and Treatment

Thankfully, there are many very successful treatments for couples experiencing infertility and it is important to seek out medical care sooner rather than later. An infertility evaluation is recommended for couples who have been trying for at least 12 months if the female is under 35 years old, 6 months if the female is older than 35 years old, or at any time if she is experiencing irregular cycles or if either spouse has a medical condition that could predispose them to fertility issues.

An infertility evaluation will typically involve a doctor asking questions about the menstrual cycle and timing of intercourse, hormonal bloodwork and ultrasound of the ovaries to assess the egg supply, and an ultrasound of the uterus to look for any structural abnormalities in the uterus. It may also include a special X-Ray study of the fallopian tubes called a hysterosalpingogram (HSG). The doctor may want to know about any medical conditions or lifestyle issues that could affect male infertility and at some point may want to look at the semen under the microscope to assess whether there is an issue with the sperm count, shape, or motility. This can be done in several *halachically* appropriate ways, so one must consult a *rav* who specializes in the field of infertility.

At times, couples keeping the laws of *taharat hamishpachah* may find that ovulation occurs prior to going to the *mikvah*. This is sometimes referred to as *halachic* infertility. Short cycles, leading to early ovulation, should be evaluated by a physician who could work together with the couple and their *rav* to help address the issue.

Treatment for infertility might include medications like clomid or letrozole that strengthen the communication between the brain and the ovary to help assist with ovulation, or a "trigger shot" that induces ovulation to occur in a very precise window of time. An intrauterine insemination (IUI) may be used to help carry the sperm as close as possible to the ovulating egg. Sometimes surgery might be recommended to correct an issue with the male or female reproductive tract.

While IVF may be the most aggressive option of all the treatments, it affords the highest success rates. IVF involves stimulating the ovaries to grow multiple eggs at a time and then removing those eggs from the body with a very minor procedure called an egg retrieval. The eggs are fertilized in the lab (that's where the term "in-vitro fertilization" comes from) and the fertilized embryos are cultured until they are developed enough to implant in the uterus. IVF allows for testing of the embryo for chromosomal abnormalities which might prevent pregnancy or lead to a miscarriage. This is done with a technique called pre-implantation genetic testing for aneuploidy (PGT-a). If both partners are known carriers for a genetic mutation that could affect their children, IVF embryos can be tested for their particular mutation using preimplantation genetic testing for mutation or PGT-m. Once an embryo and the uterine lining are prepared for implantation, a doctor places the embryo very gently into the uterus in a procedure called an embryo transfer. If there are additional embryos, they can be frozen for a future attempt at pregnancy. It is a long process but one that is thankfully highly successful for most couples. There have been over 7 million babies born worldwide since IVF was first introduced in 1979. It is one of the most incredible miracles of the modern era.

Female Age and Fertility

The risk of infertility significantly increases as a woman ages. This is because both the quantity and quality of her eggs declines. Women are born with all the eggs they will ever have. Over time, the egg supply dwindles and when a woman runs out of eggs, her menstrual cycles will stop and she will go into menopause. However, the ability to conceive ends many years before a woman reaches menopause, due to the quality, or chromosomes, in the eggs themselves.

A healthy human egg should have 23 chromosomes. A human sperm also has 23 chromosomes. Healthy humans generally have 46 chromosomes, 23 from their mother, and 23 from their father. The woman's eggs are extraordinarily protected from environmental factors that damage other cells in the body. For example, skin cells and blood cells can only survive for a few months. The egg can survive for decades! However, over time, errors accumulate in the chromosomes of eggs, leaving some with too many chromosomes and others with too few. The scientific term for an abnormal number of chromosomes is aneuploid. Aneuploid eggs tend to either not fertilize or not implant; if and when they do, the pregnancy will typically end as an early miscarriage. As women get older, more of the eggs they carry will have chromosomal abnormalities. Therefore, there are likely to be more months during which they won't conceive. Thus naturally, the time required to conceive and the rates of infertility increase as women age. The most common cause of miscarriage (more than 90% of cases) is an aneuploid embryo, and as a result miscarriage rates increase as women get older. Extra chromosomes can also lead to syndromes like Down Syndrome, which occurs when there is an embryo with an extra copy of chromosome 21. While such conditions are thankfully still rare, chromosomal abnormalities like those that produce Down Syndrome increase as women get older as well.

More and more single women, or those with medical conditions, are exploring egg freezing (only with *halachic* consultation) as a way to preserve younger, healthier eggs for the future. Given that infertility rates increase as women age, mostly as a result of more of the eggs being aneuploid, preserving "young" eggs can increase the chances that a woman will attain her desire to have a family should she experience infertility in the future. The success rates with infertility treatments, like in-vitro fertilization (IVF), are directly related to the "age" of the eggs being used. Egg quality peaks in the woman's late 20s and early 30s. If a woman froze her eggs at 30 and then required IVF at 40, by using her 30 year old eggs rather than her 40 year old eggs she will nearly triple her chances of having a baby from the treatment!

Infertility, primary or secondary, is painful. For many the pain is compounded by the surprise, almost shock, at just how complicated conception can be. When conception happens naturally, not many stop to think about the magnitude of the miracle. When conception does not happen quickly and easily, a new world of information must be confronted and navigated in an effort to find a solution. Today we are privileged to have many reproductive technologies available and many infertile couples, with the help of Hashem, experience their own miracles. This essay is presented as a primer on the topic to help young women understand the complexity of conception and what next steps would be recommended in the case that they do not get pregnant as quickly as they had hoped.

Eliana Fine MD is an OBGYN resident at Stony Brook University Hospital. She received her Medical Degree from the Renaissance School of Medicine 3-Year MD Program in 2021. Previously, she received her Bachelor's degree in Biology from Stern College for Women-Yeshiva University in 2018. In her first year of medical school she co-founded the Jewish Orthodox Women's Medical Association, JOWMA, a 501(c)3 non-profit organization dedicated to providing support, mentorship, and networking opportunities to Jewish female physicians, trainees, and pre-medical students, as well as providing preventative health and women's health education to the Orthodox Jewish community. To date, JOWMA has over 350 members. In addition to her responsibilities as an OBGYN resident and past-CEO of JOWMA, Eliana is the mother of a 4 year old boy and 1 year old girl. She is an aspiring Reproductive Endocrinology and Infertility specialist.

Dr. Bat-Sheva Lerner Maslow is double board certified in Obstetrics & Gynecology and Reproductive Endocrinology. She is a reproductive endocrinologist and the Director of Research at Extend Fertility, where she specializes in counseling women about their fertility and options for fertility preservation. In addition, Dr. Maslow provides the full spectrum of infertility care at Extend Fertility and Premium Health Center, both in New York City. Dr. Maslow frequently lectures and writes on the intersection of *halacha* and reproduction, and is often called upon as an adviser for questions related to *hilchot nidah*. She serves as the Director of Medical Education for the North American Yoatzot Halacha Program and sits on the founding board of directors of the Jewish Orthodox Women's Medical Association (JOWMA).

Helpful Resources:

www.Boneiolam.com

www.Atime.org

www.puahfertility.org

Aimee Baron, MD

The Dream That Was:
UNDERSTANDING PREGNANCY LOSS

You're twenty and the first in your family to get married. It all happened so quickly – a family friend suggested a *shidduch* and five months later, you were playing house. And then before you knew it, you were craving strange foods at crazy hours, and vomiting the rest of the time. On your due date, the baby was still comfortably nestled inside and taking his sweet time. Four days later, you realized that it had been a while since you felt him kicking. Your baby, perfectly formed, with your lips and your husband's ears, was stillborn.

You're 28 and you just got married. Your friends have been paired off for years, and each has one or two kids with more on the way. *Baruch Hashem*, you become pregnant within a few months and are finally feeling like you can breathe. Your dream of having a full, bustling home is on its way to becoming reality. And then on a routine visit to your OB at eight weeks, your baby has no heartbeat. And in an instant, all your hopes and dreams come crashing down around you.

You're 36 and excited about your latest pregnancy. Your six kids are thrilled at the idea of having another baby in the family, and you actually feel pretty good this time around. At the 20-week ultrasound, the doctors share that your baby has multiple anomalies that are not compatible with life outside the womb. Further testing reveals a horrific genetic disorder. The doctors recommend terminating the pregnancy. After you speak to a *Rav* who specializes in this field, that's exactly what is done. But you can't seem to move on from the intense grief and guilt.

•••••

Pregnancy loss is horrible.

It's a mismatch between expectations and reality. It's the life you're supposed to be living, but somehow you're stuck in an alternate version, where everything has turned upside down since your baby died.

Your family and your community expect that you will have a child by your first wedding anniversary. You expect to have children when you want to have them and to stop only when *you're* ready to do so.

You're supposed to be pregnant for nine months. You're supposed to give birth on or around your due date. You're supposed to hear your baby's first cry. You're supposed to watch your baby grow, smile, and laugh.

And yet, you don't.

And everyone else around you is seemingly going on with their perfect lives, not knowing how your world has just been shattered. You don't wear a sign to announce how much you are suffering inside. You wake up, go to work, go to the supermarket, go to *simchot* and mask the pain. This dichotomy between what's expected and reality, between putting on your best face and your inner pain, is what makes pregnancy loss so hard.

First, some definitions:

Miscarriage is the loss of a baby that is less than 20 weeks gestation. Somewhere between 10-20% of known pregnancies end in loss, but many scientists suggest that the number is higher than that, and is closer to 25%, as many losses happen so early, when a woman does not know that she is pregnant.

Stillbirth is a fetal demise at greater than 20 weeks gestation. It occurs in 1 in 160 pregnancies yearly in the United States, leading to about 24,000 stillborn babies.

Ectopic pregnancy is when an embryo implants itself somewhere other than the uterus, usually in the fallopian tubes. This pregnancy is not compatible with life, and can also endanger the mother.

Termination for medical reasons is termination of the pregnancy (only with *halachic* consultation) because of a genetic or other medical condition that would significantly impact the baby's quality of life, lead to an early death, or is not compatible

The Dream That Was: Understanding Pregnancy Loss

with life. Sometimes, the pregnancy causes a life-threatening risk to the mother and may need to be terminated as well.

Once a woman finds out that her baby has died, there is a whirlwind of choices that she must make in conjunction with her husband, her *rav*, her family, and so forth.

Delivery:

If your baby is less than 20 weeks gestation, there are a few options.

Some parents opt to let the body deal with the pregnancy naturally (in consultation with their doctor) and will wait, sometimes for weeks, for the pregnancy to pass. Others choose to take medicines to induce labor, so the process is initiated by them, but still managed by a doctor.

Many opt for a surgical procedure most often referred to as D&C or D&E, Dilation and Curettage or Dilation and Evacuation, which removes the pregnancy. These are usually not done by your OB; They are done by another physician trained in this area. Your doctor will give you the name of some specialists in your area, and usually will also help you set up the appointment. It can take a while to get an appointment, and you may have to wait a number of days to get the procedure done.

If your baby is older than 20 weeks gestation, often the decision is made to have the mother labor and deliver the baby. If the baby is breech, a cesarean section is a possibility.

What happens when the baby is born? Do I need to bury him/her?

If the baby is removed by a surgical procedure and is between 12 and 20 weeks, some *poskim* hold that the baby does not need to be buried. Others hold differently. Ask a *shaila*.

If the baby is over 20 weeks, the baby is usually buried. (Speak to your hospital and/or *rav* to confirm this.) Standard practice is to call your *rav* and follow his suggestions regarding:

- which *chevra kadisha* to call
- naming the baby/*brit*
- touching the baby
- holding the baby
- taking pictures
- making hand/foot molds (done by many hospitals)
- where the baby is buried

- attending the funeral
- sitting *shiva*
- putting up a tombstone
- lighting a Shabbat candle/*Yahrzeit* candle
- *Yizkor*, etc.

There are a few *halachot* in this area that one should be familiar with when experiencing this type of loss; don't hold back from talking to your *rav* and asking your questions.

In years past, the *rav* and the grandparents of the baby made all the decisions for the parents, including the naming and location of the baby's burial, and wouldn't tell the parents. The prevailing wisdom at the time was, "If you don't know anything about it, you'll forget about this baby and move on with your life." The theory was that it was best not to dwell on negative things. Presumably, this was done because the infant mortality rate was extremely high until the advent of antibiotics and modern medical technology, so it was common for nearly all families to have experienced loss.

Here is my suggestion: If the family decides that they do not want to name the baby, hold the baby, take pictures of the baby, or know where the baby is buried, please have someone from the family be in charge of staying in contact with the hospital, funeral home, and *chevra kadisha* to archive these details. In this way, if or when the family does want more information years later, it will be possible to obtain it.

In our day and age, the evolving views on the psychological health of the mother and the parents of a baby who dies, point to the clear benefits of a different mindset. Perinatal loss is a huge stressor on both parents, accompanied by many intense feelings for everyone involved. The more those emotions are squelched, the more the body holds onto those memories and events in ways that can impact one's health and immune system. Working to repress those experiences can overly tax the mind and the body. The more one represses them, the more they can interfere with one's life.

Current recommendations urge parents to talk about the loss and to share their thoughts with anyone who will listen. This is because the more anyone talks about the difficult issues in their lives, the less alone they feel as they deal with the pain and suffering.[1] Classic studies suggest that putting your feelings into words, a process called

---

[1] Research from U.C.L.A. (Psychol Sci 2007 May;18(5):421-8. doi: 10.1111/j.1467-9280.2007.01916.x *Putting feelings into words: affect labeling disrupts amygdala activity in response to affective stimuli*, Matthew D. Lieberman, Naomi I. Eisenberger, Molly J. Crockett, Sabrina M. Tom, Jennifer H. Pfeifer, Baldwin M. Way.

"affect labeling," can diminish the stress response when one encounters –and be less affected by–issues that are upsetting.[2]

Researchers also discuss traumatic experiences and how undergoing talk therapy has a positive impact on a patient's health and immune system. Another study on trauma argues that holding back thoughts and emotions is stressful. A person has negative feelings either way, but they have to work to repress them.[3]

What is it about miscarriage, stillbirth, ectopic pregnancy, or termination for medical reasons that elicits such a strong reaction; that makes this experience so difficult?

Generally speaking, the intensity of the grief is correlated with two factors: the gestational age of the baby and how long it took a couple to become pregnant. The longer one is pregnant, the more opportunities one has to form an attachment to the child. The positive pregnancy test, seeing sonogram pictures, feeling fetal movement, preparing for the baby's arrival – all of these things help cement the relationship between parents and the baby. Most families have deeper levels of pain and grief, and suffer longer, after a stillbirth as opposed to an early loss. (Although anecdotally I can tell you about numerous couples who fell into a deep depression after an early loss, and the families who seemed to plow forward after a later loss.) For families who have struggled to become pregnant due to infertility, a physical or mental illness, or a multitude of other reasons, the loss is even more devastating.

Within the framework of loss, the pain and suffering associated with pregnancy loss are unique because:

- The loss is sudden and unexpected
- Wrenching decisions have to be made about naming, spending time with the baby, the burial, and so forth
- There are often no physical reminders or mementos as there would be with an older child or an adult

In addition, no one is comfortable discussing loss, let alone the end of a pregnancy. It is a unique kind of pain that is difficult for the immediate family, and how much more so for those surrounding them in the community and workplace. Families are

---

[2] By psychologist James W. Pennebaker, PhD and his colleagues.

[3] Pennebaker, J.W. (1997). *Opening Up: The Healing Power of Expressing Emotion*. New York: Guilford Press. Pennebaker, J. W., Kiecolt-Glaser, J. K., & Glaser, R. (1988). Disclosure of traumas and immune function: Health implications for psychotherapy. *Journal of Consulting and Clinical Psychology*, Vol. 56, pp. 239-245.

expected to "get over it" and "move on." They are not supposed to dwell on their sadness for too long, and certainly not publicly.

The problem is that these mothers can't shut off the feeling of attachment to the babies. When considering the "psychological effects of baby loss on women and families, it is crucial to consider the gestalt of the experience and how broader systems influence individual outcomes. For example, mothers experiencing stillbirth are recognized as disenfranchised…For socially validated deaths, there is often community outpouring of sympathy and recognition of the deceased. However, individuals suffering from disenfranchised grief often do so in silence and may feel ashamed of their experiences, adding to the psychological complexity of their losses."[4]

These women and their husbands feel isolated and so alone. They feel empty. They feel like they are carrying around their own personal raincloud all the time. Many also report feeling intense guilt and believe that the loss was somehow their fault. They have a hard time hearing the message: It's incredibly painful, but it's not your fault. You did nothing to cause this.

How does grief manifest itself? It's common to feel tired all the time or never, to feel restless and have the inability to concentrate, to lose one's appetite or start eating more, or even have headaches or otherwise unexplained abdominal complaints. Emotionally, in addition to the isolation and feeling as if no one else in the world can possibly understand even a small part of what you're going through, it's common to see depression, denial, anger, guilt and a sense of failure. Some people also withdraw from social settings and others throw themselves into lots of activities, volunteering and work in order to stay busy, as a means of trying to disassociate themselves from the tremendous pain they are in.

The same dichotomy often plays out in the spiritual sphere. Families may become overly focused on the nuances of *halachot* surrounding *taharat hamishpachah*, *mikvah*, or any other mitzvah where they perceive their actions to have been substandard (as if, if they were following these *halachot* perfectly, the loss would not have occurred). They long for connection and a way to understand their pain. Other couples go completely the opposite way and start questioning their core beliefs. They start to distance themselves from G-d, learning and *halacha*. They are often angry at G-d but afraid to express this anger, as He will then punish them for their feelings. The *mitzvot*, both personal and communal, become unbearable. "Why?" and "Why me?" are constant refrains in their head. It is important to reach out to your Rebbetzin, *mashpia*, or mentor for *hashkafic* support as well.

---

[4] Psychological Effects of Stillbirth. Seminars in Fetal and Neonatal Medicine. 2012.

The Dream That Was: Understanding Pregnancy Loss

Another aspect of this loss that is unique is the fact that this is happening to the husband and wife simultaneously but in very different ways. For the woman, there is the medical aspect of getting the baby out by D&C or D&E, or a delivery vaginally or by cesarean. They have the same postpartum effects, just without a baby. Milk comes in (usually after losses in the second trimester and beyond), along with the usual bleeding, cramping, and hormonal shifts. They have also been the one carrying the baby, and therefore often have a stronger level of attachment. The males don't experience any physical changes but can have the same strong emotions of grief, sadness, and isolation.

Some people want to crawl into bed and not leave for months, and others want to resume "normal" life as soon as possible. Some want to talk about what happened to everyone and others want to keep it quiet (which is only possible with an early loss). These distinctions don't necessarily fall in line with gender stereotypes, and it's important to remember that grief is very individual. These differences in practical day-to-day living after a loss can sometimes become unbearable when one person desperately wants to share and the other demands privacy. It's important to respect each other's needs, desires, and methods of grieving. Sometimes this is best done with the help of a therapist or *rav* if the couple is clashing over how to handle the issue. This extra tension in a marriage is particularly hard, and it can drive people apart if not addressed right away.

The goal of the grief process is not to forget about your baby or the fact that this tragedy happened in your life. The ideal is to be able to think about your baby and feel a sense of sadness, but not the overwhelming, all-encompassing grief that tends to hover over the first few days and weeks. You won't ever "get over it" or forget about your baby, but you will be able to work through the pain and adjust to your "new normal." Grief is like an ocean. The waves keep coming and coming, but over time, they are further and further apart, and never as tall as the first waves you experienced during your loss.

What can friends, families, or communities do to support couples who have gone through baby loss?

DO:

- Reach out if you think something is going on, but don't pry. Be genuine and caring; they will share if/when they are ready.
- Allow for feelings to be shared without expressing judgment. Lend a warm, supportive listening ear. That's all they need.

- If they have given the baby a name and they have shared it with you, feel free to use it yourself. Using the name in conversation reminds the family that you care about their situation and remember the name of their child. It's incredibly special.

- Include them in Shabbat/holiday meals, family get-togethers, and parties, but understand if they decide not to attend or leave early. Withholding an invitation makes them feel even more alone and isolated. Give them the choice instead of making it for them.

- Continue to reach out in the days, weeks, and months ahead. A simple text saying "I'm thinking about you" is always appreciated and makes people feel loved. Due dates and/or the times of the year when a loss occurred also might be difficult for the couple. Reach out and tell them that you remember and that you care.

- Communities can provide meals or help with childcare if these are wanted. Some families don't want to be viewed as the subject of pity, and so they decline these offers. Respect their wishes.

- Find out if the family prefers visitors or if they want to be left alone. And also remember that this answer may change with time. During early weeks they might give a different answer than in later weeks.

- It's very common for the couple to take a long time to answer texts and phone calls. They also need a break from dealing with their emotions.

- Remember that this is a loss that affects the men, too. Don't forget about him and make sure that he's also thought of when considering meals, outings, and so forth. In addition, the grandparents are also grieving the loss of their grandchild while simultaneously trying to take care of the couple. They may be in a difficult spot. Reach out to them and give them the space and time to share their thoughts about the baby, as well.

- Helpful things to say:
    - "I've been thinking about you."
    - "Wow, that is really awful!"
    - "You've really been through so much."
    - "Would it be helpful if I came over with wine or chocolate?"
    - "I'm here if you want to cry."
    - "I'm so sorry that you've been through so much."

The Dream That Was: Understanding Pregnancy Loss

- "I'm at the supermarket now. What can I bring you?"
- "What can I do to support you today?"

DON'T:

- Stare pointedly at someone's stomach and ask how many children they have, or ask when they are finally going to be giving the family a grandchild, etc.
- Avoid the couple because you are afraid of saying the wrong thing.
- Tell them to just…try this doctor, use this medicine, relax, go on vacation, try adoption, etc.
- Change the subject if they are finally sharing what has been going on.
- Compare their situation to someone else's.
- Say any of these things:
  - "At least you didn't know your baby."
  - "At least you know that you can get pregnant."
  - "At least you have other children." (If they do)
  - "You can just get pregnant again and have another baby."
  - "I know how you feel." (even if you have been through the same situation)
  - "You should be over it by now."
  - "You'll see the baby when Mashiach comes."
  - "It's a test from G-d, and G-d only tests people He loves."

Often these kinds of losses occur in families where there are other children. Many have the predisposition to keep the loss a secret and not share the bad news, especially if it's an early loss. I always encourage parents to be as open and honest with their children as possible, according to their developmental age, because kids can often sense when something is wrong and when "Mommy has been so sad all the time." In addition, if the loss is public, the likelihood that someone will inadvertently spill the beans is very high, and you want to be the one to control the information. You don't want them to hear about it on the playground or the bus. There are also many times that the loss might affect their school performance or play activities with friends, and it will be important to advise the child's teachers and/or other parents as to what has happened.

One of the reasons why infertility and pregnancy loss take such a toll on those suffering is because of the communal norms and expectations about having a large family. When one's life doesn't exactly look like everyone else's, this disparity is striking. It's especially painful when coming into contact with people who don't know your story. The pointed looks at your stomach and constant remarks like "How many children do you have?" are like daggers in the heart each time they are uttered from someone's lips.

My suggestion? Don't ever ask.

What can you say when you run into an old friend at a wedding or other event?

"Tell me about your family."

This statement is very general and allows for a number of acceptable responses from different individuals.

- Someone going through primary or secondary infertility can talk about her husband, extended family, or children she does have.
- Someone who just had a loss can decide on what she wants to focus on and does not have to mention the loss if it makes her feel uncomfortable.
- Singles can talk about their parents and siblings; divorcees, widows or widowers can speak about others who are alive.

It immediately puts people at ease, instead of making them feel uncomfortable. And we all have the obligation to not embarrass people who already feel marginalized or disapproved of because of their experience.

Pregnancy loss has happened or is happening to you, someone in your family, your friends, neighbors, and coworkers. With the emphasis on children in our community and the *pru u'rvu* mandate, these kinds of losses are ubiquitous. Every community is affected. Every sect is affected. Every family is affected. We each have the responsibility to make sure that couples suffering such loss don't feel isolated and alone.

The days, weeks, months, and years after losing a baby can be some of the most isolating and demoralizing times that anyone can experience. The important thing to remember is that you do not have to go through it alone, as there are many different individuals and organizations that can assist you. Please reach out and get the support you need.

Aimee Baron MD, FAAP, is the founder and executive director of I Was Supposed to Have a Baby, a nonprofit organization that utilizes social media to support Jewish individuals and families as they are struggling to have a child. It provides a warm and nurturing space for those going through infertility, pregnancy loss, infant loss, surrogacy, or adoption, in addition to connecting those families to resources in the Jewish community at large. Dr. Baron was formerly the Director of Innovation and Growth at NechamaComfort and has also worked as an Attending Pediatrician in the Newborn Nursery and Neonatal Intensive Care Unit at St. Luke's-Roosevelt Hospital before taking a leave of absence after her third miscarriage. She lives in the New York area with her husband and five children.

Helpful Resources:

www.iwassupposedtohaveababy.org

www.NechamaComfort.org

www.mothersofcrownheights.com/pregnancy-loss

ATime Hug Program 718.686.8912#113

Knafayim 917.627.5528

Menuchas Hanefesh (Canada) 647-562-8147

Pamela Klein, LCSW, AASECT

Understanding Sexual Dysfunction:

AN OVERVIEW

The following essay is presented to help couples who are experiencing difficulty with sexual intimacy. If you are reading this out of curiosity or just to gain additional information, bear in mind that while sexual dysfunction does occur and can be redressed, by no means should you anticipate such challenges as part and parcel of your initiation into this aspect of life. It is best to approach intimacy with an open heart and mind, and trust that your natural desire and functions – created by Hashem – will lead you in the right direction.

Once you are married and begin to embark on the journey to build your intimate relationship, a range of emotions are evoked. There is a tremendous amount of excitement and joy and at the same time there can be worry, fear, and confusion. Creating physical intimacy requires an investment of both your physical and emotional self and the satisfaction often comes from the work that is put into it. The purpose of the physical relationship is to create a level of closeness that you have never experienced in other areas of your life. Over time, as the intimate relationship grows, your emotional connection will deepen.

A crucial part of a strong marriage is healthy sexual functioning: being able to experience sexual pleasure and satisfaction when the couple desires it. In recent years, scientists understand the intricacies of how we function sexually better than ever before. We are now aware that a combination of biological, psychological, and social factors are essential in producing a satisfying sexual experience. For us to understand how to intervene when these processes are not working, we need to first appreciate default sexual function.

To simplify things, the sexual response cycle includes four stages which can be referred to as desire, arousal, orgasm, and resolution. It is important to know that no two bodies are alike and everyone will experience these differently; there is no one "normal." The stages of the cycle can vary based on many different factors and will continuously evolve.

Desire and arousal are often brought on by physical and emotional interaction and stimuli such as the exchange of loving words, kissing, hugging, caressing, and other forms of foreplay. Especially for a woman, the physical and mental "setting" will make all of the difference in her being able to let go and be in the "zone." Physiologically, during this phase, there is an increase in heart rate and blood pressure, and breathing becomes heavier.

The buildup of sexual arousal and stimulation can lead to the pleasurable release of sexual tension known as orgasm. During an orgasm, muscle contractions occur in the genitals and often throughout the body. In men, these muscle contractions result in ejaculation or the release of sperm and semen. During an orgasm, the brain produces several hormones that are released in the body. One hormone produced is dopamine, which is responsible for feelings of pleasure and desire. The other hormone released is oxytocin, often referred to as the "love hormone." Oxytocin contributes to the connection we feel toward our spouse, as well as the satisfaction that accompanies the orgasm.

Following orgasm, in the resolution state, the body returns to its resting state. Men generally require a period of anywhere from a few minutes to a few hours before another orgasm is possible. Women can experience multiple orgasms within a short period of time if stimulating activities continue.

We now understand that many factors contribute to our sexual response cycle. While some people may experience the linear progression described above, many do not.

Because this is a private and sacred part of our marital lives, we do not know what others are experiencing and if our struggles are within the average range or not. Additionally, defining what is sexually healthy is difficult as there is a wide range of what is considered "normal" in sexuality. It is important to learn what the "average" person is experiencing so you know whether you are running into a problem. The best way to really know this is based on your own instincts and the level of distress you may be experiencing when things are not going as planned.

Understanding Sexual Dysfunction: An Overview

It is profoundly important to communicate with your spouse concerning what you are feeling. This essay is presented to help you figure out what you might be experiencing and to provide terminology you can use to articulate your experience. Most importantly, it allows you to understand that what you are feeling is a recognized struggle and that it can be successfully addressed with the right kind of assistance.

Sexual dysfunction refers to a problem – "a glitch in the system" – that occurs at any point in the sexual response cycle that prevents the person or couple from having a satisfying sexual experience. It can occur at any time; men and women of all ages can experience sexual dysfunction. Many factors can lead to sexual problems. However, these factors can be broken down into two simple categories: biological and psychological.

There are many biological/physical causes of sexual dysfunction. Common medical conditions such as diabetes, heart and vascular diseases, neurological disorders, hormonal imbalances, and other chronic diseases can negatively affect the normal physiological sexual response. Furthermore, the side effects of medications, such as antidepressants or blood pressure medications, can greatly impact sexual functioning.

The impact of psychological factors must be acknowledged as equally significant. Stress, anxiety, and depression can produce several sexual complications in men and women. Trouble can stem from concerns regarding sexual performance, relationship problems, feelings of guilt about sexual desires or activities, self-esteem or body image issues, and the effects of past trauma.

It is essential to assess which factors are causing the problem, and it is often the case that there are multiple contributory components. Identifying the underlying cause can help in treating the sexual issue. However, while many sexual problems can be traced back to a physical problem or an emotional issue, some lack an identifiable predisposing factor. Even in these cases, various medical and psychological interventions can still help the sexual problem.

Sexual dysfunction can be classified into four categories:

- Desire disorders – lack of sexual desire or interest in sex.
- Arousal disorders – inability to become physically aroused during sexual activity.
- Orgasm disorders – delay or absence of orgasm.
- Pain disorders – pain at some point in the sexual encounter.

Desire Disorders

> Ahuva is working full time, and Chaim is in yeshiva. She is hardly ever interested in sexual relations and Chaim is often the one that initiates it. She enjoys cuddling and being close but lacks desire for sexual engagement. She has experienced times where she started the process of intimacy and then became more interested in continuing, but when he initiates she usually says no as she is not in the mood. She would just rather go to sleep. She feels there must be something wrong with her that she could go for weeks without having sex and would be okay with it. They end up having sex about once a week but he is frustrated by the lack of intimacy or enthusiasm on her part.

Sometimes we desire sexual intimacy, and sometimes we don't – this is what the average person will experience. However, these oscillatory feelings develop into a problem when someone has ongoing low sexual desire and is bothered by this lack of interest. Sexual desire disorder can arise for both men and women and it is marked by a low level of sexual interest, causing a failure to initiate or respond to sexual intimacy. If this is distressing to an individual or their spouse, then it is something that should be addressed.

Very often the distress is exacerbated by one's reaction to their sexual dysfunction and the meaning that they deduce from their emotions. It can start with noticing that you don't have a desire for sex, which subsequently leads to thoughts such as, "There is something wrong with me" or "My husband will be frustrated with me for not being interested." Once those distracting thoughts exist, they further reduce sexual desire and start a vicious cycle. Individuals with these thought patterns begin to continually evaluate themselves in their sexual relationships and develop an internal anxious and self-conscious dialogue. This inner conflict removes a person from the sexual experience and will only diminish their desire to engage.

There is a powerful connection between our minds and bodies. When we have distracting thoughts, we fail to be in the moment, and consequently, we will/can not immerse ourselves in our feelings and sensations. When we participate in a sexual experience in a distracted state of mind, the interest in doing so will immediately diminish. Very often we have to ask if such sexual intimacy is worth desiring. If we notice something impeding our ability to desire intimacy, we should address the issue with the goal of living more in the moment and not concentrating on these thoughts.

Research has revealed that becoming more engaged in our feelings and sensations can limit our distractions. Investing one's complete attention in the moment, also known as "mindfulness," can be helpful for those experiencing lower desire. Imagine yourself riding a roller coaster. Upon ascending to the top and during the subsequent abrupt descent, are you thinking about whether you like this roller coaster or not? Are you occupied with thoughts about work or the pile of dishes waiting to be cleaned? Probably not. One would be too immersed in the moment of going downhill to think about anything else. In daily life, and especially during sexual relations, having thoughts about other things aside from what you are doing is very common. In mindfulness, one works towards noticing those thoughts and learning how to bring oneself back to the present moment. The more we practice becoming mindful in life, the easier it is to be present when participating in a sexual experience.

There are many other issues, aside from what is happening in that sexual encounter, that can distract either party. Two common concerns that can consume an individual are insecure body image and unresolved relationship problems:

Body image problems – It is quite challenging to enjoy one's sexual experience when he or she views their body negatively. This can create a lot of anxiety around being seen and touched and can interfere in multiple components of the sexual cycle. Not only is it unlikely that one will initiate sexual contact when experiencing this emotion, but it will likely interfere with their ability to get aroused and have an orgasm. Unfortunately, it is difficult to discard these thoughts; nevertheless, we should become more aware of them and the toll they take. By being aware that these negative thoughts are present, we can begin to address them.

Relationship problems – Our emotional relationship with our spouse strongly influences our sexual connection. Being intimate requires us to be vulnerable on both an emotional and physical level, making the feeling of emotional safety vital. It is challenging to feel interested in intimacy with your spouse when you are feeling disconnected due to a relationship problem. Stereotypically, women have a harder time being intimate after an argument, but it can apply for both genders. If we are insecure with our spouse, we will not be interested in becoming physical with them and immersing ourselves sexually.

There are many other biological and psychological factors that can contribute to low desire. Throughout the life cycle, the levels of desire will change based on the situation at hand. When a couple is trying to conceive, possibly facing infertility, hopeful of getting pregnant, and then raising children, they will experience fluctuations in their levels of desire. **Especially for women, who experience hormonal changes in addition to the emotional changes, pregnancy and lactation can bring variation.** It is important to note that if they can try to look at the broader picture and not get stuck in the downs, then their level of sexual desire will hopefully return to their personal baseline. Once we invest meaning into the dip in desire, we tend to become more stuck in it, and this can create a vicious cycle in our minds.

In addition, very often women do not experience spontaneous desire wherein they are overcome with a strong wave of desire for intimacy. In fact, many will only experience that desire once they get started, and becoming somewhat aroused will create desire for more. That pleasurable physical sensation will trigger a desire to continue being intimate. This means that sometimes getting started, even when you are feeling more neutral about it, will lead you to the place that you want to be although you initially were not feeling too excited about intimacy.

Desire Discrepancy

Desire discrepancy is when two spouses desire different levels, frequency, or kinds of sexual activity. The typical presentation of desire discrepancy is when one individual possesses more desire and wants sexual intimacy more often in the marriage. The spouse with higher desire is stereotypically the man, and the spouse with lower desire is the woman. However, this is not always the case and there are many times when it is the opposite.

In all relationships, there will be one individual who has "higher desire" and one who has "lower desire," utilizing these terms comparatively. This relative relationship is not an issue in itself. But often, because of the way a couple approaches it, it can develop into a problem. Making room for both spouses to accept the tension of being different from one another and consequently finding ways to collaborate is vital. It can be difficult for many couples to bear this discrepancy as they tend to start to interpret the inconsistency in their relationship negatively. The one with lower desire is perceived as inadequate and can hold feelings of guilt, which can prompt them to engage in sexual intimacy at times when they lack passion. This can consequently lead to feelings of resentment and avoidance over time. The one with stronger desire is often regarded as too pushy and will feel rejected by the other. They can interpret the rejection to mean that they are not desirable, and anger will often be the result.

Couples must remember that there is no "right amount" of sex to be desired. Whether couples enjoy having sexual intercourse often or not, this is not an indication of a problem with the relationship. Just as we differ in other areas of our lives, such as what type of food we prefer, so too there will be a difference in our levels of desire. It is important to take this as an opportunity to value our differences and work towards navigating these disparities together.

Understanding Sexual Dysfunction: An Overview

Finally, sometimes the discrepancy in desire is rooted in *hashkafic* concerns or preconceived notions. In this case, in conjunction with therapy, the couple can benefit from consulting with a *rav* who can guide them on the issue.

Arousal Disorders

> Moshe was a healthy man when he was a *bochur* and was very excited to start his married life with Sarah. Like many other boys, he was looking forward to the wedding night but also felt concerned about it at the same time. He was not sure what to expect and was worried about hurting his new wife. He was told to be sensitive and also to be encouraging so as to complete the act of intercourse, but he was confused about the mechanics of intercourse. He ended up struggling considerably to keep an erection that night. This created a psychological block where he felt that his body was betraying him and he experienced himself as a failure. This went on for months after marriage. He was told over and over again not to think about it. However, he felt that diverting his thoughts was impossible as he felt so much pressure to perform.

For some individuals, the desire to have sex may be present, yet their body or mind do not respond accordingly. Typically when a person becomes aroused, their body will react with physical changes in addition to mental excitement. For someone struggling in this area, their arousal response does not proceed as expected.

When women are struggling with arousal, the physical feelings of swelling, tingling or throbbing in the genital area and vaginal wetness will not be present. They often describe their genitals as being "dead." Similar to low desire, either physical or psychological factors can provoke this response. Very often, for younger women, the issue will stem from something psychological that is blocking her. One common explanation is a mere lack of knowledge about how one's body works, and her not realizing that her body needs foreplay to become aroused. She may then need guidance in what type of foreplay might bring her pleasure and how to explore this with her husband so as to figure that out. Another difficulty can be in allowing herself to let go due to ambivalence or negative feelings about sexuality. Many women have difficulty letting go sexually as they are uncomfortable with this new role. It is important to try to identify what is going on for the woman emotionally so that the problem can be addressed.

In men, an arousal problem would show up as Erectile Dysfunction. This can present itself as an inability to get an erection during sexual activity or to maintain an erection for an elongated period. Most men will occasionally have some difficulty in getting or staying firm, but this would only be recognized as a problem if it were a continuous issue. These difficulties can place a lot of stress on the man, lowering his self-esteem and causing relationship problems.

Erectile dysfunction can be attributed to either physical or psychological factors. It is imperative to check for any medical reason that could be causing or worsening erectile dysfunction. At times there could be a minor physical issue that causes a temporary problem with staying firm, but it subsequently transforms into a psychological problem. The male will start to worry about getting or maintaining an erection, and this anxiety often will lead to or worsen erectile dysfunction. Once this occurs, the anxiety will impede their sexual experience as the couple will have trouble staying in the moment.

Many relatively non-invasive medical treatment options exist for erectile dysfunction. One of the most common treatment methods is oral medication, such as Viagra, Levitra, and Cialis. The mechanism of action of these medications improves a man's erection by increasing blood flow to the genitals. They do not work without sexual stimulation as they are not "magic pills," but they have a high success rate of 65-70%. Other types of treatments exist as well, and a competent urologist should be consulted to explore those options.

Another way that an erectile issue would manifest itself would be in cases where a man feels that he is ejaculating too quickly or before penetration, also known as premature ejaculation. Most commonly, this occurs early in relationships and is rarely due to a medical condition. In most cases, premature ejaculation is due to psychological causes, making the outcome of treatment very successful. However, for men experiencing this problem, it can be quite difficult as it often leads to feelings of embarrassment, anxiety and distress in relationships. It can also be complicated by feelings of worry about *hotzaat zera levatalah*. The man must speak to his *rav* or *mashpia* about this very common scenario so his anxiety can be lessened.

There are several treatment methods for premature ejaculation. The most common are exercises that a man can try at home to "train" the timing of his ejaculation. A *halachic* authority should be consulted before utilizing these methods. In addition, men often have been prescribed antidepressants for a short period to help delay ejaculation and gain more control over their timing. There are also Kegel exercises that a man can perform, which strengthen the muscles that control ejaculation.

Orgasm Disorders

> When Chana was a kallah, her kallah teacher had briefly mentioned orgasm. She did not give her too much detail and told her she did not have to think about it just yet. Chana paid little attention to the fact that she didn't have an orgasm until about a year into marriage. She started to wonder at this point whether she was experiencing all of the pleasure possible in physical intimacy. She began to research ways to try and get to orgasm and tried all of the tips that were suggested. After a few months, she became increasingly frustrated as she felt she didn't get anywhere. In fact, the sexual relationship now focused exclusively on this goal and it was affecting her desire to be intimate.

Orgasmic dysfunction is when someone experiences difficulty achieving an orgasm. Individuals can become sexually aroused, but for no identifiable reason, the arousal fails to reach the level of orgasm. Men and women can experience this, but it is more common in women. Orgasm problems could be primary, which means that the person never had an orgasm, or they can be secondary, meaning they had orgasms in the past but cannot achieve one now.

Orgasms vary in intensity, frequency, and amount of time and stimulation it takes to attain an orgasm. The average woman will need clitoral stimulation to reach an orgasm and will usually not achieve it through penetration alone. Very often women or their husbands will be bothered by her difficulty in reaching orgasm. Having sex without experiencing orgasm can often be frustrating and may result in resentment when the woman watches her husband enjoying the sexual encounter. The husband might feel that there is something that he is doing wrong and feel like a failure for not being able to get his wife to that point.

Women need to be aware that the inability to attain an orgasm does not indicate that something is wrong with her or the relationship; the husband needs to know that it's not an indicator of his not giving his wife enough pleasure. Having an orgasm commences in a woman's mind, and if one's thoughts are not in the proper place, then orgasm will not be achieved despite the husband's efforts or the strength of the relationship. Often there could be fears of letting go, being vulnerable, or not being in control that can hinder a woman's ability to reach the point of orgasm.

It is important to note that a woman does not need to have an orgasm to enjoy sex. There are many feelings, sensations, and pleasurable thoughts that can arise from the sexual experience, even if there is no orgasm at its conclusion. Understanding this is key to relieving some of the pressure to always achieve an orgasm during every act of sexual intercourse. Some women who have orgasms still report that they don't enjoy sex, and the reverse holds as well. Therefore, it's important to not heavily focus on the need to have an orgasm as once it becomes a goal in itself, it often is even harder for the woman to attain one. While it is vital to keep the aforementioned in mind, therapy can be beneficial in understanding what might be impeding a woman's ability to attain orgasm, and she may subsequently be able to resolve these matters.

When a man has trouble having an orgasm, it is called delayed ejaculation. Delayed ejaculation is defined as difficulty or inability to reach an orgasm and failure to release semen altogether. Often the cause of this would be psychological; however, it can have a physical component as well. Some common psychological factors that could arise would be the following: an unwillingness to enjoy pleasure, negative religious beliefs about pleasure, fear of pregnancy, or a history of abuse.

Delayed ejaculation can be quite distressing for both the husband and wife. It often leaves the husband feeling like a failure and with a sense of inadequacy. Difficulties with ejaculation may be exacerbated when the couple cannot conceive due to the problem, which puts even more pressure on the husband to be able to ejaculate. Fortunately, men can achieve much success when they turn to therapy for this. Treatment does take time as the psychological blockages can be deeply rooted. However, in recent years, there has been much progress in the development of therapeutic methods to assist men with this challenge.

Pain Disorders

> Rivka had experienced sexual pain at the start of her marriage but at first thought, it was normal and would go away. She became pregnant a few months after marriage and told her OB/GYN that she always has some discomfort with intercourse. Her doctor explained to her that sex is something that should not be painful and worked with her to try to figure out what was causing the pain. She had noticed that she often became nervous before getting into bed as she anticipated intimacy being painful and that this was taking away much of her enjoyment.

Having sexual pain can feel very isolating as women do not talk about this amongst themselves, but it is a fairly common problem. Although precise statistics are unknown, it is estimated that about 15 percent of women experience sexual pain. Some common physical causes are infections, lack of lubrication, scarring from childbirth, breastfeeding, and pelvic floor dysfunction. Very often, even if the pain originated from a physical issue, it will progress to a psychological problem. This fear is exacerbated as the woman begins to anticipate the pain, which subsequently causes tightening of the vaginal muscles, a response that worsens the condition. A vicious cycle develops that needs to be resolved over time. All these factors can cause the woman to have diminished sexual desire and sometimes can lead to an avoidance of any genital touch.

One can experience sexual pain at the time of penetration or at any point during or after intercourse. The pain can occur in any part of the genital area and it can manifest itself in a variety of ways. The severity of the pain can range from not being able to endure penetration at all to being able to experience penetration in one situation but not another. For example, a woman may be able to do a *bedika* on her own but not be able to have intercourse with her husband.

One common way that sexual pain can present itself is in the form of vaginismus. Vaginismus commonly presents itself in *kallot* who are experiencing an involuntary tightening of their vaginal muscles, leading to pain when trying to penetrate. Vaginismus is psychological and regularly manifests itself at the start of the marriage when the couple is trying to consummate the marriage. Often, couples enduring these challenges feel very alone and grow frustrated due to their inability to resolve these issues. The underlying problem is often driven by anxiety and fears about having intercourse, which encourages the tightening of the muscles.

Some women will be able to consummate their marriage but will experience sexual pain at some later point in the relationship. A possible reason for this might be vulvodynia, chronic pain, or discomfort (burning or irritation) around the opening of the vagina (vulva), for which there is no identifiable cause. Other conditions cause discomfort or pain during the sexual cycle. A physical therapist specializing in pelvic dysfunction is a great resource for a proper evaluation/assessment and formulating a treatment plan.

Typically, there are physical and psychological factors that can contribute to sexual pain, and the treatment for it would involve addressing both sides. From an emotional perspective, therapy can address the anxiety that arises from the situation and assist the woman in gaining control of her body and mastering relaxation techniques. Therapy can also help the couple work through sexual pain and attain better communication about each of their needs.

To properly address the physical side, a qualified gynecologist who understands sexual pain is needed, as well as an experienced pelvic floor physical therapist. There are numerous treatments that women commonly use that can help to ease the pain and make it more manageable.

Although sexual pain is more associated with women, men can experience it as well. There can be a number of physical causes, including infection, an issue with the foreskin, or a deformity in the genitals. Although many men find it embarrassing to discuss, if a man is experiencing sexual pain it is important that he be seen by a doctor.

Sex Therapy

Reaching out for help when there is a sexual problem can be very difficult for many couples. There is most often an underlying discomfort in seeking sex therapy as most people are unaware of what is involved in such treatment.

Sex therapy is a specialized form of psychotherapy. General therapists can address sexual problems, but a sex therapist is specifically trained in sexual therapeutic methods. It is comparable to going to a dermatologist if you are experiencing a skin problem rather than going to your internist. Sex therapy involves talking; there is no physical contact at any time. It is generally short-term therapy and is very goal-oriented.

A sex therapist would start with a thorough assessment to understand a person's history and what sexual problem is presenting itself. Sexual problems can be complex, and it is, therefore, necessary to ascertain all of the contributing factors. Once there is more clarity on the issue, your therapist would explain what to expect from the therapy process and the plan to resolve the issue. Talking about a person's sexual relationship can be uncomfortable and awkward, but sex therapists are trained to help reduce that discomfort.

Sex therapy can be very successful in treating all of the aforementioned sexual problems, but it is vital to find a qualified sex therapist. It is also important to find a therapist that is a good fit for you as that will help in feeling more comfortable in opening up. If you are seeing someone whom you do not feel you can trust or communicate with, then you should discuss your concerns with them and ensure that you are compatible with one another. It is also important to find a sex therapist that has experience in couples therapy as the two issues are often intertwined.

One of the guaranteed outcomes of sex therapy is that it will lay groundwork for couples to be able to openly discuss their concerns. It is imperative that couples talk about what they prefer sexually and what is not working sexually; this can be challenging for many individuals. Being able to express what you are enjoying sexually can be equally as difficult as communicating your negative thoughts. With the help of a therapist, couples tend to become more comfortable about openly expressing their concerns. They will often notice the benefit to their sexual relationship as well as experience increased emotional connection and intimacy.

It is important that both the couple and the therapist speak on a consistent basis with a *rav* throughout the therapy process. The *rav* will serve as the *halachic* authority, and also tends to be the person to sanction the start and progress of the treatment. I have found that when a *rav* is involved in the work, the couple tends to develop a more positive attitude towards the therapy and will feel much more comfortable with it.

The nature of a sexual relationship is one of ups and downs, and it requires constant effort to build a mutually satisfying relationship. Sexual intimacy will take on a different role and form in various stages of your life (newlywed, mid-life, and growing older together) but it is always an essential part of marriage. Sexual intimacy is Hashem's gift to us, a unique and precious way to create closeness and connection between a husband and wife.

Pamela Klein is a licensed clinical social worker and a AASECT certified sex therapist. She specializes in helping individuals and couples with all kinds of relationship problems. Couples come to see her at various stages of their relationship and they come in with a wide variety of issues.

Pamela's specialization in sex therapy differentiates her practice from others. She helps people with sexual dysfunction, low desire, sexual pain and other sexual problems. Her treatment is tailored to the needs of each client and she utilizes practical methods to help make changes in a short period of time.

Pamela Klein has received her certification in sex therapy at the NYU Program for Human Sexuality. She has also been trained in Mindfulness, Somatic Intervention, and Emotionally Focused Therapy. She has a private practice in the Five Towns and now is working remotely with clients from all over New York. She can be reached at pamelakleinlcsw@gmail.com.

Lisa G Twerski, LCSW

I'm So Confused, Am I Being Abused?

GUIDANCE FOR THE ORTHODOX JEWISH SPOUSE AND THOSE WHO ARE TRYING TO HELP

Why is this Such a Difficult Question to Answer?

Perhaps you've been feeling that things aren't quite right in your marriage. In fact, much of it is not at all how you imagined it would be. On the other hand, you were told somewhere along the line that a good marriage takes a lot of hard work, so perhaps that's why things seem so difficult. But you've reached a point when you've been much more miserable than seems normal. You've started to wonder whether this is more than the expected "hard work" that marriage requires. You're just not sure.

> Sarah sought help because she was feeling very "down," and someone told her she was probably experiencing postpartum depression after the birth of her third child. She reported feeling overwhelmed and despondent, certain that she would never be able to manage, and didn't see the point in even trying.
>
> In exploring these feelings, it emerged that Sarah had been feeling overwhelmed and incapable for quite some time – years, in fact. These feelings were not due to postpartum depression, though her depressive feelings had increased during this most recent pregnancy. What took a long time to discover was where these feelings were coming from in the first place.
>
> Sarah talked a lot about how her feelings of despondency over her incompetence were based in reality. She explained that she never got the housework done sufficiently because she was so disorganized. The children were always missing something: enough clean clothing to last the week, healthy food for their lunches, and so on.

> But as Sarah continued to explore her feelings, it soon became clear that in her personal opinion, she really was doing okay. Her husband, on the other hand, was very certain that she was not measuring up. He would berate her constantly, make her come back and repeat tasks if they were not done to his liking, and compare her to his sisters, who he felt were the perfect wives and mothers.
>
> Sarah kept vacillating between feeling that she should have some say in the household and feel comfortable with her own approach, and defending her husband's right to "have needs," be particular and ask for things to be a certain way.
>
> At the end of the day, she knew she wasn't happy. But why? Was she causing the problem – or was it something else?

Though you may be unhappy – even very, very unhappy – it is not unusual to be somewhat confused and ambivalent about what is happening in your marriage. You can't quite define what's wrong, though you sense something is off. Even if you have toyed with the idea that something is drastically wrong, it can be difficult to define the problem.

To some extent, this is because no one wants to be having "marriage problems." Even harder to face is the possibility that the problem is abuse. Complicating matters is the fact that "marriage problems" can mean many different things. How is it possible to know if it's actually abuse, or something else?

Answering that question is just one of many things that may get in the way when a woman tries to face the disheartening possibility that she is living with an abuser.

Differentiating Between Dysfunction, Disorders, and Domestic Abuse

For people who feel abused in their marriage, or who are trying to help someone who is having problems in his or her marriage, it can be very confusing to distinguish between a dysfunctional relationship that may have some abusive features, and domestic abuse. In fact, if in two different marriages there is name-calling, demands about how time and money are spent, and demands about housekeeping and childrearing – in one case, these inappropriate behaviors may be part of the larger context of a dysfunctional relationship or spouse (particularly if one's spouse has a personality disorder), while in the other, these behaviors may be part of the larger picture of domestic abuse.

To effectively examine what might be going wrong, it's best to begin by exploring what a marriage looks like when things are going right.

A healthy, caring and respectful marriage is multifaceted. Much can be said about the subject, but in order to understand the dynamics of a healthy marriage it is helpful to have a guiding principle. This principle may also help us understand what is at the root of what may be going wrong in a marriage, how to conceptualize a particular problem, and what the appropriate intervention might be.

A healthy relationship is one in which *each* spouse feels responsible, and sees it as his or *tafkid,* her mission in life, to enjoy, consider and take care of the other – emotionally, spiritually, physically and psychologically. When this dynamic is present between spouses, it is at the heart of the most fulfilling and healthy marriages. This is not to say that everyone always gets what he or she wants, or that there are not some areas that are deferred to the husband or to the wife, even exclusively. What it does mean is that in a healthy marriage each spouse acts in consideration of the needs, feelings, opinions and perspectives of the other. In this way, both are getting their needs met, but from a position of giving. When this dynamic is present, we can refer to this as a functional marriage, because both partners are functioning in their intended roles, and the marriage works in the way it was intended.

In a dysfunctional marriage, one or both spouses is not abiding by this guiding principle. Even when one spouse is functioning in his or her proper role, if the other is not, the marriage can still be dysfunctional.

This may occur for a variety of reasons. There might be mental health issues that are getting in the way of the couple having a functional, healthy relationship. One of the spouses may have a serious mental illness, an addiction or an anxiety, mood or personality disorder. In some cases, that mental illness may get in the way of that person's ability to consider the needs of his or her spouse. That is because with a serious mental illness or disorder, or sometimes even a severe trauma, the person's emotional needs consume him or her and make it extremely difficult to be attentive to someone else, except to get his/her own needs met.

Sometimes, one or both spouses in the marriage may have the right ideas and are even trying to consider and care for the other spouse – he/she just doesn't know how. Sometimes a couple has poor or different communication styles, which leads to misunderstandings and discord. Sometimes the couple doesn't have a mechanism for healthy conflict management, acceptance or resolution. Sometimes one or both spouses will act out of misunderstood or inaccurate assumptions or expectations, leading to disappointment, anger and frustration. There are countless areas of misunderstanding which can – if a couple does not have the ability or mechanism to reconcile or manage their differences – lead to *shalom bayit* problems.

Another major cause of dysfunction in a marriage can be viewed as a basic lack of understanding of the role of a healthy, caring spouse. One or both spouses may be overly focused on him/herself and on what the spouse or the marriage, as a new chapter in life, can provide for him or her. That focus can permeate many, if not all, aspects of the marriage and cause tremendous tension and discord. This may be due to a lack of *chinuch,* education, regarding the proper role of a husband or wife.

In cases of domestic abuse, on the other hand, the abuser's focus on himself is not due to a mental illness, lack of proper *chinuch* regarding his role, or a lack of understanding of how to fulfill that role. An abusive spouse firmly believes that he is *entitled* to have his needs met by his wife and sees no place for the concept of considering hers. He expects to make all decisions he feels are important and to have the home and his spouse comply with exactly the way he wants things done. For the abuser, it's all about him. The abuser believes this so strongly that he is willing to instill fear by utilizing a variety of tactics to gain and maintain the control that will ensure that his needs, including the expectation of power over his spouse, are met.

In a dysfunctional relationship, although one or both parties are not making the spouse and his or her needs a priority, the spouse who is not being cared for, thought about or considered has a variety of options. This is because the neglect (or active exploitation) stems from some sort of deficiency in the ability, understanding, and emotional availability to care about the spouse. This is in contrast to the abusive spouse, who is convinced that this standard of being cared for without caring for his spouse is his entitlement in marriage.

What this means on a practical level is that someone who is married to a dysfunctional spouse may be hurt, disappointed or even intimidated by her spouse's disregard or demands. However, if she wished she could assert her needs, disagree or make decisions without fear of escalating repercussions.

Not that it would be easy. She would have to step out of the role of the caring, concerned spouse who puts her spouse's needs ahead of her own. This may be incredibly upsetting because the healthy spouse in a marriage has always wanted and expected to fulfill that role appropriately. Indeed, this intentional role change may be frightening, because the anger, or perhaps the fragility, that the unhealthy spouse displays seems difficult to challenge.

In fact, a challenge to the dysfunctional spouse's self-centeredness may at first make the marriage seem even more dysfunctional, because it increases discord, as both spouses are now "fighting" for their own needs. However, in a dysfunctional marriage it is possible to stop assuming the caretaking role and assert one's own needs. Often when this shift takes place, especially with professional help, that couple can experience profound change and improvement.

This is very different qualitatively from being married to an abusive spouse. The abusive spouse lives with the conviction that the marital relationship is all about him, and he will do whatever it takes to make sure that conviction is fulfilled. His spouse doesn't have the option of fighting to get her needs or her opinions considered, because if she did try to stand up for herself, she would have to contend with much more than just discord or unpleasantness. In an abusive relationship, the abuser will continue to escalate the consequences, making things increasingly unbearable or frightening for his spouse, until she feels she has no choice but to comply with his expectations. She is often too frightened to try to get help from an outside source because of the consequences the abuser is willing to impose in order to get his way and maintain his control.

In a dysfunctional marriage, there is a lot of pain, hurt and maybe even worry over a spouse's reactions. Ultimately, however, when the spouse of someone dysfunctional stands up to him or puts his or her foot down, there is a limit to how far the dysfunctional spouse will push for his way.

In an abusive marriage there is fear. This fear is based on the knowledge that the abuser will continue to escalate his tactics. It is a fear born of seeing that when things are not the way he insists, the consequences escalate until the abused spouse feels it is no longer worthwhile to assert her opinions or her needs. Alternatively, it may be fear for her own safety or wellbeing, or that of her children.

This is an extremely important distinction. For the dysfunctional couple, couple's counseling and other similar approaches may be the intervention of choice. But those same interventions, in the case of domestic abuse, could be anywhere from useless to unsafe.

What Does Abuse Look Like?

We tend to think of domestic abuse as manifested in violence, that only a woman who is being physically assaulted and injured seriously by her husband is the victim of abuse. If this is your definition of abuse and you are not being physically abused, you may be assuming that whatever it is you are going through does not constitute abuse.

The truth is that there are many women being abused and controlled by their spouses who have never been physically assaulted.

Domestic abuse has been defined as "a pattern of coercive control that one person exercises over another in order to dominate and get his way." Abuse is behaviors that physically harm *or* use other tactics to arouse fear so as to prevent a person from doing what she wants, or to coerce her to behave in ways she does not freely choose.[1]

Generating sufficient fear to gain control over one's spouse does not necessarily require physical violence. The abuser may use other tactics, or may include a combination of tactics along with physical violence, to achieve and maintain control. Sometimes his efforts have a sudden onset with an immediately obvious goal. Tactics aimed at control may also emerge gradually, almost imperceptibly, over a period of time.

Different Forms of Abuse

(There are many forms of abuse. We chose to elaborate on two forms followed by a summary and description of other types of abuse.)

Emotional Abuse

Emotional abuse is when your spouse attempts to control you by verbally attacking you, undermining your positive sense of self.[2] He attempts to make you question and doubt your worth or even your sanity. You become more dependent on him, and less likely to reach out to others, because of how worthless and hopeless you feel. This may include humiliating you, calling you names, putting you or your efforts down, or making you feel crazy so you begin to doubt your every thought and action. As an escalating tactic, emotional abuse is used to punish non-compliance, usually with a form of harassment that diminishes your self-esteem and fosters your dependence on him.

> Faigy said to me that at first her husband Yanky just seemed to be particular. He wanted his dinner ready when he got home. He wanted the towels in the linen closet folded and lined up in a particular manner. Faigy did not question these demands. In fact, Faigy worked very hard to satisfy them and to make her new husband happy. But whatever she did never seemed to be enough.

---

[1] Susan Schecter, Guideline for Mental Health Practitioners in Domestic Violence Cases, Washington, D.C. The National Coalition Against Domestic Violence, 1987, p.4.

[2] Definitions in this section are adapted from "Education Groups for Men who Batter: the Duluth Model," Ellen Pence and Michael Paymar.

> At first Yanky indicated his disapproval simply by muttering to himself, making some sarcastic remarks, and withdrawing from her. In time, however, he began to attack Faigy with barrages of outright insults.
>
> She told me that on one occasion he thought that she had said something "stupid" when they were visiting their neighbors for Shabbat lunch. He told her that they needed to "talk." When they got home, he told her to stand in front of him and explain to him why it was that she was so incompetent, why she didn't feel that it was important to please her husband, and why she couldn't correctly perform tasks that any "retard" could do. When he had finished berating her, he made her stand where she was and "think about" what she had done and what she would do differently in the future.
>
> These verbal assaults became longer and more vicious over time. They began to happen in front of their children. Yanky also started to include humiliating accusations of infidelity. He also called her stupid, ugly, and lazy.
>
> Finally, after one particularly bad incident, Faigy told a friend what was happening, who then encouraged her to seek help. As Faigy began to talk about all that went on, she realized how skewed her perspective had become. She used to be such a happy, confident person, perceived by others as capable and accomplished. And now she questioned everything she did. In fact, when she looked at the big picture, she could see that she accomplished the majority of what her husband asked of her. He would find the minor thing she had not, focus on that, and she would accept his assessment that she was incompetent. She had even started to rationalize his tirades in front of the children. She didn't understand what had happened to her.

There are a variety of ways an abusive husband can make you feel bad about yourself. The abuser may humiliate you by criticizing your physical appearance, your intellect, or your devotion to him or to your children. He may blame you for things that go wrong, regardless of your involvement in them. He may accuse you of various misdemeanors, ranging from inadequate care of the home to inadequate mothering.

He may ignore your comments in discussions, criticize your knowledge or logical reasoning in public, or tell others to "pay no attention to her." Usually, though, that only happens in front of people he doesn't care about. More commonly, even after severely damaging behavior, he will treat you well in public, perhaps even acting loving, caring or solicitous, in order to protect his reputation. His tactics will be reserved for the privacy of your home, demeaning you in private – or in front of the children.

He may insult you and call you names. He may pretend that the things you say make no sense. He may even imply that you are not completely in your right mind, or go to specific efforts to make you think you are crazy.

If you complain about his behavior or accuse him of being unkind or insensitive, he may claim that you are imagining things or that you are ungrateful. The possibility of evoking his anger will tend to make you afraid to speak up. You will be walking on eggshells all the time. He will focus intently on things you do not manage to do, even if the things you do get done are far greater and those you did not were unrealistic requests.

Women in this situation often find themselves endlessly second guessing all of their actions and decisions, fearful of how he will react. Often women also start to fear that others will "find them out" – in other words, see them as their husband does.

What makes this particularly confusing is that there is nothing wrong with trying to fulfill your husband's initial request. But when he isn't satisfied, you work harder, trying to make things better. That's when you lose sight of the line and when it gets crossed. It's not until something extremely egregious happens that you get shaken into realizing that your life is out of control – *your* control, anyway. At this stage, however, many women have already been isolated from potential support people, and so much has happened that it is hard to figure out how to reach out for help.

Sexual Abuse

Sexual abuse is one of the most difficult for women to talk about. It is frightening and demeaning. It's also a subject that in general *frum* women don't freely discuss, even in terms of a healthy sexual relationship.

Sexual abuse may include being forced into having sex when you don't want to, being forced to do things that you are uncomfortable with or cause you pain, or sometimes having affection withheld from you. An abuser may demand relations after a fight, he may be unfaithful, or he may compare you to other women, pointing out the various ways you don't measure up.

It can be very confusing for a *frum* woman with no previous experience or real understanding of healthy marital intimacy to know where the line is. Yes, there is an expectation in marriage of an intimate physical relationship. And yes, it is something that can be less comfortable or even a little painful at first. Even in a happy, healthy, respectful marriage, couples need to get used to each other and negotiate differences that may exist between them. However, there is a difference between sharing this experience with someone who is concerned for you and your pleasure, as is his *halachic* obligation, and someone who is demanding or forces you into things for his personal pleasure.

Sometimes women are confused about where the line is, and sometimes they are completely unaware.

> Rachel was a truly *frum* girl, with no awareness of the outside world. When she got engaged at 18 she had no inkling what went on between husband and wife "in the bedroom." Her kallah teacher taught her the practical halachot, and by way of education about relations between a husband and wife, told her, "your husband will know what to do."
>
> Years later, Rachel reflected that this might have been okay if her husband had been the *frum*, innocent *ben Torah* that she thought he was. Unfortunately, he was not. He seemed to be mainly concerned with his own gratification in general, and even more so in the bedroom.
>
> Rachel remembers being woken at all hours, being told all sorts of things that she was to do to him, and being kept locked in the bedroom doing them until her husband was ready to stop, which could take hours.
>
> Because she didn't know where the line was, Rachel told herself that this must be what happens in marriage. She wasn't happy, didn't enjoy any of it, and often was in pain, but figured that if this is what a wife is supposed to do, then she needed to deal with it. And she worked very hard to convince herself of this.
>
> When Rachel started sinking into a depression, she convinced herself that she was the issue. Looking back, Rachel realized that she was having a reaction to being treated like this. Unfortunately, it wasn't until six months later, when her kallah teacher called to check in and asked how things were going intimately, that she actually got the education she needed to recognize how far over the line her husband had gone.

As painful and abusive as situations like that are, one of the most painful forms of sexual abuse is when it comes in a form that compromises your religious standards, leaving you feeling undeserving in much the same way Rachel did. An abusive husband may demand that his wife engage in sexual behaviors that she considers inappropriate. He may browbeat her into engaging in a sexually intimate act that she has understood to be *assur*. She gives in, either because he physically forces her to do so, or because she hopes that by acceding to his demands, things will get better. But by giving in, the victim feels complicit, guilty, and not worthy of better treatment.

An abusive husband may also coerce his wife into sexual intimacy when she is a *nidah*. In this case, even if the woman was forced to have sex, she feels tainted by the enormity of the *aveira*, and she may be unable to differentiate his responsibility from her own. Even though she had no control over what happened, she feels as if she has been involved in behaviors that are terribly wrong. This leaves her feeling guilty, emotionally depleted, and unworthy. It contributes to the feeling that she deserves to be abused, and makes it almost impossible for her to reach out and tell anyone what is going on – she is just too embarrassed. She feels caught up with her abusive spouse, feeling bound to him by his tactics, rather than viewing what he has done as his responsibility.

Summary of Tactics of Control

Below are listed the most common tactics of control to which abused women are subjected. Depending on the particular relationship, over time the abusing partner may use any or all of these tactics in combination or separately. Generally, the tactics will escalate with time. If you have been a victim of domestic abuse, you have likely identified with a number of the cases that I have presented. However, just to avoid any ambiguity, take a look at this list of indicators of domestic abuse.

Examples of emotional abuse:
- Does your spouse put you down, or call you names?
- Does he blame you for everything that goes wrong, including when he abuses you?
- Does he destroy things that you care about in order to punish you?
- Does he try to make you think you're crazy, accusing you of things you know you did not do, mistreat you and then act as if everything should be normal between the two of you, making you doubt your sense of reality?
- Does he tell you that everything that is going wrong is because of something you did or did not do?
- Does he accuse you of everything that he himself does wrong?
- Do you feel that you never know what will make him angry – in fact, something that once made him happy can make him furious another time? Does it feel like you are walking on eggshells?

I'm So Confused, Am I Being Abused?

Examples of isolation:

- Does your husband (try to) prevent you from spending time with friends or family, by either aggressively getting in your way or punishing you for seeing them; or by subtly making it difficult (picking a fight, acting miserable when everyone gets together, embarrassing you so you don't feel it's worth it, coming up with other things you need to do when it's time to spend time with your family)?
- Does your husband try to intimidate you into isolation by accusing you of infidelity?
- Does your husband try to get you to give up certain friends, family members, or activities by putting them down, telling you how bad they are, and that you are negatively influenced by them?
- Does your husband tell you that if you pursue a relationship with someone he doesn't approve of, he won't be able to feel close to you?
- When you do go out with friends he doesn't approve of, does he call you an excessive number of times?
- Does your husband scrutinize every moment of your day, questioning where you've gone and what you've done?
- Does your husband check up on who you call, listen in when you're on the phone, check the cell phone bill, and so on?

Examples of intimidation:

- Does your husband scare you by punching walls?
- Does your husband drive recklessly with you in the car, though he knows it scares you?
- Does your husband get very loud, screaming in your face, scaring you to the point where you're not sure what else he might do?
- Is there a look that he gives you that lets you know you're in for it?
- Does your husband physically get in your way so you can't get out of the room or get away?
- Does your husband give you the angry silent treatment, so you never know when something might happen?

Examples of threats and coercion:

- Does your husband threaten to harm you, your children, your family?
- Does your husband threaten suicide as a consequence of making him unhappy?
- Does he threaten to cut you off financially?

Examples of using the children as a tactic of control:

- Does your husband threaten to take the children away or turn them against you if you talk to anyone or try to leave?
- Does your husband tell the children things that are untrue about you?
- Does your husband blame his behavior on your inability to control the children?
- Does your husband undermine your authority with the children?
- Have you noticed that if your husband gets upset with you he mistreats the children to get back at you?
- Does your husband withhold money for things the children need in order to punish you or get you to do what he wants?

Examples of using male privilege:

- Does your husband use *halacha* to justify his mistreatment of you? Have you explored whether this is a true interpretation of the *halacha* with a *halachic* authority (not your husband)?
- When you *do* have a differing opinion and he agrees to go to a *rav*, do you take an active part and speak to the *rav* yourself? Or does he ask the *rav* by himself and tell you what the *rav* said? Does the *rav's* supposed response usually follow your husband's opinion?
- If you want to speak to a *rav* yourself, does your husband refuse to let you or discourage you from doing this? Does he warn you that it will make one or both of you "look bad"?
- If you are part of the process of asking the *rav* a question, are you able to give all the details that are relevant, or are you intimidated by what your husband might do?
- Does your husband lie to the *rav* in order to get an answer he likes?

Examples of economic abuse:

- Are you on a strict budget while your spouse is not?
- Does your spouse harass you over every expenditure, questioning you endlessly?
- Does your husband tell you that you can't be trusted with the finances, that you are incompetent and spend too much on everything, as an excuse for limiting your access to the family funds?
- Do you have to hand over any money you make, but don't have access to money, except for what your husband decides to give you?
- Does your husband sabotage your ability to keep a job?
- Does he discourage you from getting the education you would need to get a job?
- Does he cut off funds as a punishment?
- Does he tell you there is no money and limit your spending, yet there's always money for the big purchases he feels are important?
- Do you find yourself lying about or hiding money because you're worried that you might not have any when you need it?

Examples of minimization:

- He dismisses what he has done with statements such as, "I didn't really do anything", "you just scare easily", "you're overacting", "you do get hysterical sometimes" or "I think you're just depressed, no matter what I do it's no good."
- He won't discuss something he has done that has upset you – he feels it wasn't a big deal and therefore you shouldn't be upset.
- Once a fight is over and *he* is over it, he expects you to be too.

Examples of denial:

- He denies that he has done anything. "I didn't do what you're saying I did. You lie all the time."
- When commenting on non-violent abuse, he makes statements such as, "You don't mind when I joke around like that" or "I didn't do anything. You're misunderstanding, or misinterpreting, or lying."

Examples of blame:

- He says things like, "You pushed my buttons", "you should stop when you know it's going to push me too far", "I was drunk" or "you know that upsets me but you did it anyway, what did you expect?"

- He tells you if you keep insisting on doing things that upset him he's going to kill himself and it will be your fault.

- He tells you that obviously, his behavior is your fault because everyone else thinks he's a great guy; no one else makes him this angry.

- He tells you that if you were a better mother, a better wife, more attractive to him, less busy with so many other things, things would be good between the two of you.

Examples of physical abuse:

- Punching
- Pushing
- Shoving
- Choking
- Slapping
- Burning
- Kicking
- Biting
- Using a weapon
- Pinching

Examples of false apologies:

- Does your husband apologize for his abuse when he sees that you are on the verge of doing something about it? Is this successful in weakening your resolve? Does it undermine your decision to reach out for help?

- Does your husband write apologetic notes, cry about what he's done, send flowers after a fight, or buy you a present as an apology, but you get the feeling it is another way of telling you, "Stop talking about it, it's over"?

- Does he expect that you will be "over it" because he is?

- Does he proceed to do the same things all over again?

What you might be feeling:

- Afraid of your spouse much of the time
- Avoiding certain topics for fear of arousing his anger
- Feeling that no matter what you do, it will not satisfy or please him
- Catching yourself thinking that you have done something that you deserve to be punished for
- Wondering if you are going out of your mind
- Realizing that you have become emotionally numb, that is, you have stopped experiencing spontaneous feelings.

If you have found yourself in this chapter you are probably feeling relieved about being understood, overwhelmed with all of the feelings that it has produced, and frightened about what it all means. Know that all it means is that you are understood. And understanding yourself usually is a great comfort.

All this sounds frightening and if in fact YOU are the one experiencing these behaviors in your marriage, often these questions come up.

You can't/don't want to imagine that *this* could be *you*.

When she thinks about her upcoming marriage, a *kallah's* focus is on how she is going to build her happy home. She is certain that her husband is the right person for her, that they share the same goals and have the same expectations and hopes for a healthy, fulfilled married life. This is true of *kallahs* who are young, and those who are a bit older, having waited for some time to find the right person. This is true of *kallahs* who are *re*marrying, hoping that, "*This* time, things will be good." This is true of *kallahs* who had a wonderful first marriage that ended due to a premature death, and would never dream that a second marriage would be any different. They are all happy at their weddings, convinced that they will be happy with their new husbands. And even if a *kallah* has some misgivings or concerns that she has pushed aside, she certainly did not think her concerns equaled abuse!

How and when things start to get difficult differs from situation to situation. Perhaps during the *sheva brachot,* or maybe a few weeks or months later, things begin to happen that make you uncomfortable. Perhaps the concern for you that he had shown previously has disappeared. Perhaps he ceases to show any interest in your well being or your opinions. He may become more demanding – perhaps unreasonably demanding. Your husband expects more and more from you, and he is not satisfied with your efforts. Perhaps he begins to complain about your inability to satisfy his wishes. Perhaps he begins to yell at you or to insult you. All of this comes as a shock to a new wife, and the possibility that your dreams of a happy home are falling apart is very hard to accept.

Under these circumstances, many new wives minimize the problem, make excuses for the behavior, choose to believe that what's going on is only temporary, didn't really happen the way they thought, or was just a misunderstanding. When I speak to women about the earliest instances of abuse, they often report that their initial reaction was, "That couldn't have really happened," or "He didn't mean for that to happen."

> Chaya had been married for twelve years when she came in for help. She started describing an abusive marriage, focusing primarily on what had been happening in recent years. Then she abruptly stopped. "You know," she admitted, "I knew during *sheva brachot* that things were not headed in a good direction."
>
> During one of the days of *sheva brachot*, Chaya's husband had gone out while she was in the bedroom getting dressed for the day, without telling her that he was leaving. Five hours later, without calling her once during that time, he walked back in as if what he had done was perfectly normal. Chaya told herself that he was planning a surprise for her, and even though his behavior was a bit unorthodox, that would make it okay. But when it became clear that he had disappeared without any reasonable excuse, Chaya told her new husband how she felt: "I feel hurt that you just disappeared for hours without telling me anything. I was so worried." The hurt inside was strong enough that she actually started crying.
>
> Her husband's response? "You're such a baby." Then he went to take a nap.
>
> This was Chaya's second marriage. At 24 years old, Chaya had already gone through a brief marriage that ended in divorce when her husband had a psychiatric break. Her immediate thought was, "Uh oh, what kind of man have I married?" But she immediately quashed that response with her second thought: "This can't be happening to me again!" Chaya refused to think about the implications of his behavior – it was too much for her to handle. So she shoved her thoughts aside and rationalized this incident.
>
> As time went by, more and more incidents occurred, moving from the inconsiderate to the overtly abusive. Because Chaya couldn't bear to think about being in another bad marriage, it wasn't until years later, when she just couldn't take it anymore, that she finally sought help.

I'm So Confused, Am I Being Abused?

Marriage is hard work. So you assume you just have to work a little harder.

Women who are abused often don't perceive it as abuse because they have so many messages about having to just "work a little harder" on their marriage. They spend so much time doing just that that they don't catch their breath, step back, and see the big picture: that the effort is completely one-sided, with her spouse expecting *her* to put all the effort into making the marriage work. He may also be exceptionally good at making her believe that *his* effort and hard work is putting up with her deficiencies.

> Yocheved knew that marriage is hard work. She heard this at different times both from her mother and her kallah teacher. So the fact that Heshy was very particular and became frustrated easily didn't concern her at first.
>
> Heshy couldn't handle it if the food didn't taste a certain way, or if she spilled something, or if the children were not kept neat on Shabbat. It bothered him to the extent that if any of those (or many other things) were to happen, he would not only berate her about them at that moment, but he would also bring it up countless times. He often punished her for being incompetent by denying her money, or privileges such as going out with a friend or agreeing to go to her parents for Shabbat. Yocheved kept reminding herself that "marriage is hard work," and she would just work really hard to keep Heshy happy.
>
> One Shabbat they went to a neighbor's house for lunch, and two things happened. Everyone started eating the *cholent* and it was clear that it had too much salt. The host started laughing, kidding with his wife about how she really did like to "spice things up." Then, a little later, the hostess knocked over a water glass. Her husband calmly got a towel to help clean things up, joking that she had done that because "you are such a *tzaddeket*, you wanted to make sure that if anyone else spilled, they wouldn't feel bad about it."
>
> That got Yocheved thinking. Yes, it's true that marriage is hard work. But maybe there was a deeper problem if it was this hard. Plus, she wondered, "Why do I have to do all the hard work in this relationship? Where's his hard work?"

When we prepare for marriage we learn how to have good *shalom bayit*. Some of these concepts include putting in effort, caring for the other person and considering his needs, making allowances for the differences between husband and wife while figuring out how to reconcile them, and so on.

The first reaction to the concern that something is not right, therefore, may be going to a lecture on *shalom bayit*, or reading books and listening to recordings/podcasts on this subject – all of which emphasize the need to work on our marriages.

It's no surprise that the natural tendency is to assume that *we* should take responsibility for making things work. And if things don't seem right, our first inclination is to work harder to make them right.

For certain types of marital difficulties, books and lectures of this kind can be quite helpful. Sometimes, however, the spouse who is healthy and functional tries to fulfill her role, losing sight of the fact that her spouse is not fulfilling his. So when demands are made, the initial response is usually an effort to satisfy the demands. And if those first efforts are unsuccessful, the next response is to redouble these efforts. It is easy to fall into a pattern of behavior where a woman spends so much time and energy trying to satisfy her husband's demands and to make things better that she loses sight of whether these demands are reasonable or fair ... whether it's really possible to make *shalom,* if the other person is making *milchama.*

> **He has such good qualities – he can't be an *abuser*!**
>
> Ahuva often really enjoyed Shimon's company. He was funny and so helpful at times, and they could have so much fun together. They had gone on a trip just recently and had a great time.
>
> But when they weren't having those fun times, he was on top of her about everything. He didn't like her friends, he thought her relationship with her family was childish, he told her she was careless with money and restricted her access to it. But he was also so popular with everybody as the *shul* youth group leader. It was so confusing.
>
> There was another really confusing aspect to Shimon's behavior. It wasn't just that he could be so horrible and so great, it was the juxtaposition of these two extremes that could make Ahuva doubt her sanity. Sometimes, right after being horrible to her, Shimon would tell Ahuva that he had made plans for them to go to a great new restaurant. Or after a horrible night, he would get up and cheerfully wish her luck on the test she was having in one of her classes. His complete switch into the normal or even caring mode could sometimes make Ahuva doubt her sense of reality. She would find herself wondering, "Did that really happen? He's acting so normal. Maybe I misinterpreted or overreacted earlier."

It can be *very* confusing for a woman to be mistreated by her husband and yet respect or enjoy him for his accomplishments, for how he treats others, or for the good times she does have with him. The degree to which there are positive aspects to your husband and your relationship may vary, but in almost every situation that I have seen, women who are grappling with whether this or not this is abuse will say, "But he's not all bad. He can be good!" Yes, that's true – that's what keeps you confused about what is going on, and uncertain about what to do about it. It is *also* true that his ability to be good, or your ability to have good times with him, does not diminish or make his bad behavior a figment of your imagination.

Women want to believe that the good times are the "real" him, and if you could just figure out what to do to keep *that* guy around, things would be great. The reality is that it's all him. The him that mistreats you is confusing because it is interspersed with good experiences, but it is still who he is. It does not eliminate the possibility that he is an abuser.

This ability to switch from abusive to caring – oblivious of any wrongdoing or bad feelings on your part – is commonly reported by women in these situations. It does not diminish what you know has happened. It's hard to know if this switch is itself a tactic, designed to make you doubt reality and sometimes even go so far as to make you feel crazy. Alternatively, perhaps for the abuser, once he's done putting you in your place, he's done. He can just move on. Deliberate or not, either way leaves most women feeling very disturbed and confused.

The people you've talked to say such different things – you don't know what to think!

Maybe you *have* talked to people about what's going on. But most people don't understand the nuances of abuse. Their reactions usually fall into one of two very rigid categories and mostly don't hit the mark in terms of making you feel understood.

Chances are you've run into those who tell you he doesn't mean it, or it will get better with time and effort, or he's a good/smart person and you should just talk to him. You've probably already tried all that. You know it doesn't help, but this person doesn't seem to get that. He or she just thinks you must not have explained yourself well enough, or really listened to him well enough. The problem is, this perspective just doesn't fit the picture you have of what's been going on.

Conversely, you may talk to someone who makes a quick pronouncement and starts pushing you to take steps you don't want to take. This category of person may say that he is just plain terrible, even evil, and you need to get away, no questions asked. This doesn't work for you either, and doesn't quite answer your questions about what's going wrong. Ultimately, you're left feeling confused and alone.

The good news is that this subject is much better understood today and there are resources available to help you. Do not remain in an abusive relationship, suffering quietly and hoping it does not get worse. Get help immediately.

This essay was excerpted from the book, I'm So Confused, Am I Being Abused?: Guidance for the Orthodox Jewish Spouse and Those Who Are Trying to Help, by Lisa G Twersky, LCSW.

Lisa Twerski, LCSW has advanced certification in pre-marital counseling and education. Mrs. Twerski, author of *I'm So Confused, Am I Being Abused?* is on the Board of Nefesh, The International Network of Orthodox Mental Health Professionals, maintains a private practice in Brooklyn, lectures nationally and is the host of the Creating Kesher podcast.

Helpful Resources:

Shalomtaskforce.org, 1-888-883-2323.

Zlata Gitlin

Everything Sheitel Untangled

Q. What can I do to make my wigs appear more natural?

A. When purchasing a new wig, many people might be hesitant to tamper with the product by cutting it because it is such an expensive purchase. However, wigs that are raw and uncut are bound to appear less natural. A good cut changes that especially if you ask your stylist to include a cutting method called texturizing.

Texturizing is done with a razor attached to a handle, and it cuts a *sheitel* in a way that gives it more movement. With this method, when you move your head, the hair will flow more naturally.

A *sheitel* can also look unnatural when it has a perfectly round or severe hairline. This can be solved by asking your stylist to add baby hairs. Although this is a tedious process it makes a tremendous difference in the look of the hairline and I usually include it in the price when someone purchases a new wig.

There is an option of adding a delicate lace front to the *sheitel*'s hairline. The lace is custom traced and mirrors the natural hairline exactly. Although this will give a flawless look, it does entail a lot of maintenance and can be very easily damaged, so it's not very practical for a *sheitel* one wears every day.

The above advice deals with the front of the *sheitel*. For an overall more natural look, I suggest you experiment with color by adding highlights, lowlights, and rooting. These can add dimension and a more natural look.

Q. Which wig choice is best for a sensitive scalp?

A. Some women with sensitive scalps find that wearing a wig cap (a thin stocking-like covering) between the *sheitel* and the scalp helps them a lot. Not only does it keep your own hair tucked in tightly, but it alleviates the sensitivity and makes the *sheitel* more comfortable to wear.

Purchasing lightweight *sheitels*, ones that are not too full, helps women with sensitive scalps to feel more comfortable.

Q. How should I care for my wig?

A. If you wear it every day, it should be washed at least once every two months.

You can add rollers to your *sheitel* at the end of each day to ensure a fresh look. However, because this is time-consuming and difficult to get right, many women today look for a "wash-and-wear" option when purchasing a *sheitel*.

Many stores, including my own, now carry these wash-and-wear wigs which have a natural wave and beautiful texture and body. You wash these *sheitels* at home by yourself with no blow-drying necessary.

I find that the older and younger generations all love these wigs because they look great and because of their easy maintenance which fits with today's busy lifestyle. It is especially helpful if you only have one wig and can't drop it off to be washed and set.

If you want to take care of a wash-and-wear *sheitel* at home, I recommend shampoo and conditioner (two separate bottles) by TRESemmé®. Lather in the shampoo once, rinse well, add in the conditioner, rinse well, gently brush out the wig, and hang it on a *sheitel* head to dry. In the morning, you can just put it on. A few days later or whenever it looks like it needs to be freshened up, brush it lightly and spray some water on it with a spray bottle.

With any *sheitel* that you own, it's really important to brush the back of it, at the nape of the neck, every day to avoid knots.

I recommend adding Moroccan Argan Oil once a month to add shine. Put a few drops in the palm of your hand; rub both hands together, then apply to your *sheitel*, starting from the bottom where it tends to be the driest and gently moving upwards.

Every six months or so, it is recommended that you deep-condition your *sheitel*. This is important especially during the winter months when hair can become dry and needs moisture.

Q. What are the different types of wig cap construction, and does it matter which I choose?

A. There are closed-net caps that are standard and very secure; hair does not get through the cap at all. It's thick but comfortable, strong and extremely durable. Most people will choose this net when purchasing a *sheitel*.

There are open-net caps which are very light, natural and airy. There is a big advantage here for people who get headaches from any weight on the head; however, hair does go through the net. I would recommend this type of net for special occasion use only because of this problem. They're simply not that durable (though very comfortable). Getting the hair out of the net is an expensive and time-consuming process, so these caps are not practical for everyday use.

Q. How do I figure out my wig size?

A. All wigs come in sizes S, M, L and XL. People have all different head sizes, and you might not find one that fits perfectly. If you choose the one that fits closest to perfect, your wig stylist can have it altered to ensure a perfect fit for you. First she will measure your head with a measuring tape very precisely, and then she will send the wig with measurements to a wig repair specialist to complete the process. This type of repair is very common, however, it should only be done for minor alterations. Major alterations may not be worth the time and money. If you try on a wig and find that there is an air pocket on top of your head, the repairs will be too extensive. You're better off finding a similar wig with a better fit.

Q. How should I go about choosing color?

A. If your hair is very dark, your wig stylist will show you a black or dark brown wig that corresponds to a color 2; it's usually an easy process. Once you move into the lighter browns, colors 4-6, it gets a drop more tricky and you might have to try on a number of options to find the perfect color. You want to wear a wig that matches your face, your skin type, and your eyebrows. The proper color wig will make your eyes shine and bring color to your cheeks. Your wig stylist will be happy to take the time to help you try on as many different shades of wigs as it takes for you to be comfortable with how you look. If you are blonde, colors 8-16/10, your stylist will usually add highlights or lowlights to get the most natural look for you. Some women buy a darker *sheitel* than needed because it'll invariably lighten over time, but I wouldn't recommend this because it could take a year or more for a *sheitel* to oxidize and change color. The goal is to walk out feeling beautiful today.

Q. What is the best way to make sure my *sheitel* stays put while also feeling comfortable? I don't like the look of a wig that's sliding down over the eyebrows but I also don't like the look of a wig that's falling back!

A. As mentioned before, focus on the fit. A *sheitel* that fits right is more likely to sit, and stay, in the right place. The *sheitel* should always start at your hairline, not on your forehead.

Then there's the question of how to anchor it firmly on your head. You should be able to walk outside on the windiest day, or hold the most energetic and curious baby, without worrying that it will move around at all.

People have different preferences for how to anchor a wig. One is to make a little braid on top of the forehead, in the center, right between the eyebrows, and then slide the *sheitel's* central comb into that braid. It should be immovable.

Another method is to use the clips installed by the ears in all wigs. Some people find these very uncomfortable, while for others it gives them a sense of security that the *sheitel* won't move.

The third method is to wear a wig grip made of velvet. It's soft and comfortable and you don't need to use any *sheitel* combs at all. Some say it makes them hot; other people love them. Many women will use this as a way to secure their *sheitel* because they find that the combs and side clips have a tendency to thin their hair over time. All of these methods are effective so it is a matter of personal preference.

Q. Can I curl or straighten my wig by myself?

A. The short answer is, yes. Styling your *sheitel* follows the same basic process as styling your own hair. So if you had a knack and the confidence to do your own hair before you were married, you can probably learn to curl or straighten your *sheitel*.

Just one note of caution: Unlike your own hair, most *sheitel*s cannot be repaired if damaged by a hot tool.

Quite a few clients have shown me their *sheitel*s that have had irreparable heat damage done to them by a neighbor or friend. You might not be able to tell right away that the *sheitel* is heat damaged, but over the span of a few months you will see split ends appear and feel the texture turning coarse.

So before you plug in the curling iron, keep in mind that there is some risk if you apply too much heat for too long.

Here are some tips for curling or straightening your *sheitel*:

Spray heat-protectant spray on the *sheitel* (my favorite drugstore brand is TRESemmé® heat protectant spray).

Wrap the hair around a curling iron or wand in the direction you want the hair to go.

Wait three seconds and release.

For a looser beach wave, run your fingers through the curl to separate the strands, then give it a light spray of hair spray to set it in place.

A little *sheitel* trivia. Back in the 1960s and 70s, women used curlers (rollers) on their wigs. They were slowly replaced, in the '80s, by electric (hot) rollers. These were later replaced by curling irons that came with a clamp; it was a little challenging to use that because you had to know exactly where and how to clamp it. Now there's a wand. It's much easier and you probably won't mess up. You just wrap the hair around the wand, hold for three seconds, and let go, for a beautiful curl.

If you have a straighter *sheitel* and want to give it a little lift, you can put two medium-sized dry rollers on the scalp of the wig overnight. You can also hang the *sheitel* upside down, which will give it a lot of volume, but to keep side bangs looking fresh, I prefer the rollers method.

Not sure you can do this? Practice on an old wig until you gain the confidence to work on your current one. If, after practicing, you still feel it's not your thing, you're in good company. Your *sheitel macher* (wig stylist) is only a phone call away.

Q. What is the best way to store my wig?

A. If you have a wig that you only wear occasionally, store it on a *sheitel* head with gift wrapping tissue paper on top. This will protect your *sheitel* from collecting dust when you aren't wearing it, and ensure that it keeps its shape for when you are ready to wear it. It is best to store the *sheitel* on a closet shelf to help prevent moisture or dirt from getting to it.

Storing your *sheitel* on your head-board pole or water bottle will stretch the netting and may give it a cone shape. It is not recommended.

Don't store it long-term in a bathroom, which becomes humid. A dry place is ideal.

Q. What's the best way to travel with my wig?

A. The ideal way of transporting a *sheitel* is in a firm-sided *sheitel* box, available in tall and short sizes to accommodate the length of your wig.

Before placing your *sheitel* in the box, be sure it is pinned tightly to the "head." To put the box through an airport X-ray baggage scanner, lay it down carefully, face up.

If you don't have a *sheitel* box, or you can't bring the extra piece of baggage, you can travel with the *sheitel* in your luggage and still have fine results. The key is to keep your *sheitel* away from clothes. With all the friction between clothes and hair, you'll have to re-wash and set the *sheitel* when you arrive at your destination. (This is especially frustrating if you're traveling to a *simchah* with little time to spare. Who wants to worry about rewashing an already set *sheitel* on arrival?)

There are two methods for transporting a sheitel in your suitcase, depending on the style of the sheitel:

For a straighter *sheitel*, stuff the inside of the cap with tissue paper and pack it until it is quite compact. Gently place your *sheitel* head up inside an adult-size shoe box. Close the shoe box lid, taking care not to squash the front bangs.

For a curly sheitel, turn the *sheitel* inside out, tucking all the curls inside, so that only the netting shows. Gently place it in a Ziploc bag, leaving some air in the bag so it is a little cushioned. When you arrive at your destination, unfurl the wig right away, give it a shake, spray some water on it and hang it up to dry.

If you don't take a *sheitel* box with you, bring along a collapsible sheitel head. These cost under $5, take up practically no room in a suitcase, and will ensure that your wig remains beautiful throughout your stay.

Q. My wig is thinning... should I repair it?

A. Sheitels inevitably thin over time, as there is no regrowth like regular hair. To minimize hair loss, proper brushing techniques are essential. With proper care, you should not see any thinning for at least the first year or two. If a substantial amount of hair does fall out, it is likely that the hair was not sewn properly to the cap. (Cap construction is a very important part of a quality wig!)

Adding hair can add life and longevity to your wig, but the value depends on the extent of the hair loss. If your wig still looks great, or if you're very attached to it and find it very comfortable, having your *sheitel macher* add some wefts (extensions) can make a big difference. If your wig is balding on the top, adding hair can be an expensive and time-consuming process. It may be worth putting that money toward a new wig.

Q. Do I need more than one wig?

A. From a styling and value perspective, having more than one *sheitel* will significantly extend the life of both, and add convenience to taking care of them. Additionally, it certainly makes it easier to fulfill the mitzvah of *kisui rosh* in the way the Rebbe promoted, with the wearing of a *sheitel*.

Q. What is the difference between processed and unprocessed hair?

A. Great question, and one that I am asked very frequently, so I am happy to respond in this forum!

First the similarities: Both processed and unprocessed wigs are crafted from human hair. The differences are in the natural quality, texture, and body of the hair:

"Unprocessed" refers to Virgin European Hair, the most natural, most luxurious, and highest quality human hair available. Because of its natural body and texture, it is desirable as is and is not treated with any chemicals. As a result, it is extremely easy to maintain on your own and can be washed and air dried easily. Though an unprocessed European wig can be very expensive, the benefits in look, feel, and care are great if it is within your budget.

"Processed" *sheitels* are made of human hair, usually from countries in the Far East. Manufacturers use a wide range of processes with this hair, from minimally invasive hair coloring to complete acidic baths to remove all natural characteristics so it can be dyed and permed as "new" hair. The more processed the wig, the more it affects the look, quality, maintenance ability, and longevity.

It is important to note that at first glance it is hard to tell how processed a wig is just by look and feel. (The differences in appearance between a minimally processed and highly processed wig are subtle and can be masked with conditioners and coatings. The difference in quality may only become apparent over time.)

These days you can purchase a very beautiful, minimally processed wig at a mid-level price. It's important to be comfortable with the person you are buying from to be sure she is selling a processed wig that has longevity and is priced fairly.

Q. How can I wash my *sheitel*?

Whether you're out of time or out of town, knowing how to wash your own wig is a great skill to have. Remember that it takes an average of 12-18 hours for a *sheitel* to dry properly, so give yourself a full day's time before you need to wear it again.

1. Hold your *sheitel* on four fingers, palm up, with your thumb holding your part in place. (You'll want to hold this position all wash long so you don't lose your preferred part line.)
2. Brush gently in downward motions. If your *sheitel* is especially knotty, lay it on a flat surface and gently brush back until it's smooth.
3. In a clean bathroom sink, run it under lukewarm water for about two minutes.
4. Put a small amount of salon-quality shampoo on your fingers (I recommend TRESemmé®) and run it through in gentle downward strokes. Concentrate on the hairs near your cheeks and neck, which attract the most oil. If you have bangs, shampoo them too. *But do not rub or scrub the scalp!*
5. Rinse under lukewarm water for five minutes, until the hairs feel squeaky clean.
6. Run a dime-sized drop of conditioner through the back of the *sheitel*, downward from about the ear line. Do not apply conditioner to the crown of the wig.
7. Rinse under lukewarm water for five minutes.*
8. Gather the hair like a pony and squeeze all excess water. Be sure not to wring, just squeeze!
9. Wrap in a clean towel and give another good squeeze to remove remaining water.
10. Brush gently in downward strokes, or if it's a curly *sheitel*, you can use some mousse on it.
11. Place on a *sheitel* head. If it has baby hairs, gently comb them back to dry nicely and naturally. For wavy *sheitels*, scrunch up the bottom a little to give it body.
12. Wait about 12 hours or 18 for very thick hair.

*If your hair is particularly dry, you can leave the conditioner in for up to half an hour, setting your wig carefully on a counter to keep your part line in place!

Q. What is so novel about "lace" wigs?

A. Conventional wigs are constructed by sewing wefts of hair into a fabric wig cap. Inevitably, this creates some bulk between your natural scalp and the *sheitel* hair.

Lace *sheitels* achieve a nearly seamless top by sewing each individual hair into a delicate lace cap. The result is the uniquely natural appearance of hair growing out of the scalp.

But a flatter—and more flattering—look is only the beginning.

As each hair is sewn individually, a lace *sheitel* replicates the free movement of natural hair. It also typically contains less hair—they are not multiplied in wefts—which means it weighs less, making it much easier to wear comfortably for an extended period of time. Finally, it is more versatile and easier to style, which is ideal if you like to wear your *sheitel* in a ponytail or bun sometimes.

Sometimes a woman's natural hair is visible through the lace cap. In such a case, ask your *sheitel macher* to line it for you so that it complies with *halacha*.

Q. What is the difference between a lace-front and lace-top?

A. The most natural-looking and most lightweight wig is a lace-top. This is when the entire scalp is made of lace. (As it is also extremely delicate, it is often lined with one or two layers of material to add durability and extend the lifespan of the wig.)

But what if you like the volume of a conventional wig?

A lace-front *sheitel* provides a natural-looking hairline with a small strip of lace in the very front, while the rest of the wig is structured with a regular cap. Seamless in the front, fullness all around.

Though it is possible to retrofit a lacefront to a conventional wig, this most often creates a noticeable bump or separation.

Q. Should I wear and care for my lace wig differently?

A. Yes. As lace wigs are extremely delicate, you'll want to handle yours with special care.

- **Putting it on:** Avoid touching the front. Hold the wig by its neck tags and flip it over to place it straight on your head. To adjust, grasp it by its sides and slowly pull it backwards.

- **Using a *sheitel* head:** Be sure to use a narrow stand or head. As lace stretches very easily, putting it on a head that is too wide will change the shape of your *sheitel*.

- **Tucking in hairs:** Although this may be a hard habit to break, never slide your fingers under the lace front to tuck in loose hairs. It will stretch the lace. Instead, try to prevent loose hairs by wetting the front of your hair and smoothing it back before putting on your wig.

- **Washing and styling:** I recommend having your wig washed and styled by an expert who has specific experience with lace. As every hair on a lace wig is individually sewn in, washing the scalp like a regular wig is likely to result in bald patches and stretched lace.

- **Fixing stretched lace:** If your lace does stretch, it can be tightened by your *sheitel macher*. At Zlata's we leave a little extra lace in the front when we first fit you so we can fix, tighten or repair frayed edges that happen over time.

With gentle handling and care, your lace wig will have a long and luscious lifespan.

An earlier version of this essay appeared in the N'shei Chabad Newletter.
Special thanks to Rishe Deitch, editor.

Zlata Gitlin, a NY-licensed cosmetologist, has been in the wig industry for 12 years. She is the owner of Zlata Wigs in the Crown Heights section of Brooklyn, and a respected authority in the wig and hair industry. Originally from Cleveland, Ohio, Zlata now lives in Crown Heights with her husband and their four daughters.

Esther Piekarski

Yakar Mikol Yakar:
THE MOST PRECIOUS TIME OF OUR LIVES

Engagement in Chabad practice and some thoughts on Shana Rishonah

Dear *kallah sht',*

Mazal tov! Welcome to the wonderful world of *kallot*.

How glorious it must feel to be past the decision-making process and doubts. You made it, *Baruch Hashem*! Enjoy every minute of your engagement. A new galaxy is now opening for you: the world of wedding plans, apartment hunting, shopping for clothes and household needs, and so much more.

Surely you just want to spend time relishing the excitement and enjoying this precious, rapturous, once-in-a-lifetime experience. The Rebbe referred[1] to this time as *yakar mikol yakar* – the dearest of all dearest – which it truly is.

The engagement period passes by quickly – you're busy, busy, busy. You're filled with an energy that seems to come down from heaven to help you with all the decisions, pressure, and details. Is this what you expected it would be like? There's so much emotion in the air. Where did it come from?

I like to compare this time to the world of *tohu*. *Tohu* literally means void. In Kabbalistic teachings, the term *tohu* refers to the world that preceded this world we inhabit which is termed *tikkun*. In *olam hatohu* each *sefira* was revealed in its fullest capacity, leaving no room for integration with the others; i.e. *chessed* presented as unlimited kindness, *gevurah* as severity that knew no bounds, *tiferet* as infinite compassion, etc. Each *sefira* was uncompromising. Each existed only for itself without any regard for intertwining or partnership with another.

So, if you suddenly feel all excited and then swing to a tense, anxious mode, welcome to the world of a *kallah*: welcome to the world of *tohu*! If you move from jumping with joy to falling into doubt, then you are in the world of *tohu*, my dear *kallah*. The wonder of *tohu* is that the energy is strong and pure. The downside of *tohu* is that it lacks "vessels" – the capacity to achieve balance– to contain and keep that energy from overflowing. The expression, *orot bli keilim* – light without containers – comes to mind.

You may go through your day thinking, "I wish my *chatan* would call," and then you think, "I need my space." At one moment you may think, "Maybe we shouldn't rush" and then shift to "I wish we could get married tomorrow!" You may decide, "I want to be involved with *all* the plans" … and then say, "I don't care as long as there's a wedding." If this sounds familiar you are in the world of *tohu* and in good company. Many – although not all – *kallot* and *chatanim* experience this type of vacillation. Understanding the conscious and unconscious factors that play a role at this time can help a *kallah* and *chatan* experience a more calm engagement period, grow spiritually, and set down cornerstones for their future home.

Some *chatanim* and *kallot* date for a long time and start becoming very familiar and comfortable with each other. After a while, they decide to set a date to get engaged. Then comes the "surprise" proposal. This is a romantic and fun option. A lot of planning goes into the dates and especially into the marriage proposal. Yet I'm afraid that a lot of tension and competition is also involved. I feel that a very private, emotional, and historic moment in a couple's life is being displaced by a frivolous plan meant to impress the outside world. As chassidim, the most important decision in our life is made by the Rebbe's *Ohel* with the seriousness and respect this momentous decision deserves.

Once engaged, we want this time to be a fun time. We want to have pleasant memories that will last forever. We want to get to know each other. We want to be with each other. We want to be married. We want to be sure. We want to be happy. We want to know we made the right decision!

But this is, after all, a very unique stage and should be understood and respected as such. While the *kallah* and *chatan* are strengthening their relationship, they must be careful not to become too emotionally enmeshed lest it lead to a strong urge for the physical closeness they cannot share at this time. Understanding this conundrum of *orot bli keilim*, strong feelings that lack proper outlet at this time, the Rebbe strongly advised that the *kallah* and *chatan* spend minimal time together;[2] just as much as necessary (see below for further elaboration on this point). Eliminating extra activities, dates, and expenses can alleviate possible tensions.

As a *kallah* teacher living in Israel where the custom is that many Lubavitcher *chatanim* travel after the *l'chaim* to 770[3] to learn and prepare for the wedding, I certainly see the difference in the *kallah* after the *chatan* leaves, she is calmer and more focused.

Why? you ask.

Because when the "lights" are fewer, it's perfectly fine that there are no "vessels." The *kallah* is still on a high, but she is concentrating her energies more fully on practical accomplishments. She feels a great deal of longing and happiness but is focused on the tasks at hand. The couple's connection is via long distance communication (thanks to technology) without being tested by the need for physical connection. Love is being developed step by step, at the right time, within the right " vessels."

To teach a child to walk before he stands is harmful; to put a large pot of soup into a small container is silly. For *chatan* and *kallah* to connect physically before their *chuppah* is forbidden, and indeed dangerous. They do not – they *cannot* – access the vessels. The *keilim* come down from the moment of *kiddushin* under the *chuppah* and no sooner – not a minute before the *chatan* says, – הרי את מקודשת לי בטבעת זו כדת משה וישראל, With this ring, you are consecrated to me according to the law of Moshe and Yisrael.

I remember once standing on the dance floor of a wedding *seudah* (celebratory meal) when the *chatan* and *kallah* were lifted onto a table by their friends. The *chatan* and *kallah* were holding hands. A woman nearby remarked to herself, "You can tell it's not the first time they are holding hands. That is a pity. It's so nice to see a new couple together when they are still bashful with each other." She felt that they had lost out on an important step in developing together as a married couple, and that this treasured step was forsaken. They had a precious *keili*, the sense of touch, and by partaking in it before its right time, they forfeited precious "lights".

You might say, "I'm not that gushing, overwhelmed, emotional *kallah*. I'm the mature *kallah*. I do not need these guidelines. I don't believe that if we are less careful with the *halachot* of 'negiah,' we will fail in other areas, nor do I believe that it will harm our marriage." I understand your point of view. You feel that you have control over

---

2 *Shaarei Halacha U'minhag, Even Ha'ezer,* p. 92.

3 770 is the affectionate shorthand for 770 Eastern Parkway, the address of Chabad-Lubavitch World Headquarters in Crown Heights, Brooklyn, NY.

your emotions. Perhaps you feel that these *hanhagot*, modes of conduct, are for the real *chassidish* folks and not as much for the mainstream people.

The Gemara states אין אפוטרופוס לעריות, There is no guarantee regarding promiscuous behavior.[4] Anyone can be tempted. Everyone, even great rabbis, are obligated to keep the laws of *yichud* because the attraction between men and women is so strong. And if it isn't strong, then we should ask why it isn't! To hear a *kallah* say she won't be tempted is scary, because she and her *chatan* should be attracted to each other, and that's why they must be careful. And if she says she doesn't feel that they have to keep the *halachot* of *yichud* because she's getting married anyway, she is cheating herself and her *chatan* out of *yakar mikol yakar*. A more measured reaction which puts long term gain over immediate gratification allows us a better vantage point.

Each *kallah* has her own personality and way of dealing with things. That's because every *kallah* is different, as every couple is unique. Some couples can speak for hours with each other. Others have shorter conversations, which is wonderful too since it suits their personalities. Some don't like to talk on the phone much and prefer to save conversation for when they meet, instead of constant texting. Often however, when they meet, they feel that all has already been said via Whatsapp and they are at a loss for conversation starters. Incidentally, even when you are married, texting should be kept to a minimum so you don't forget the sound of each other's voices! Start practicing now! Are text messages and Whatsapp real communication? Or are they just a way to convey information and messages? Nothing can compare to person-to-person-communication. We should start to develop this as *chatan* and *kallah*. Each *kallah* and *chatan* should discuss with their respective *mashpia* as to how often they should meet and speak. The Rebbe's advice was to speak and meet once a week[5] and he clearly counseled that *kallah* and *chatan* not remain in the same city during the engagement[6] nor travel long distances together before their marriage.[7] Creating parameters to begin with makes it easier to go forward in strength. If necessary, the original parameters can always be re-evaluated and adjusted. The meetings between *kallah* and *chatan* should take place in accordance with the laws of *yichud* and with extra care. Inappropriate conduct can lead to closeness that will cause distance after their wedding. It is a great

---

4 *Kesubos* 13b.

5 *Shaarei Nissuin*, p. 245.

6 See *Toras Menachem*, vol. 39, p. 11, fn. 24. *Me'Otzar Hamelech*, vol. 2, p. 167. *Mikdash Melech*, vol. 1, p. 48.

7 *Shaarei Nissuin*, p. 245.

pity to lose out on the tremendous *brachot* promised to the *kallah* and *chatan* for their future life together through upholding modest conduct during their engagement.[8]

Of Rivkah *Imeinu*, it is written that when she saw Yitzchak for the first time, she took her scarf and covered her face.[9] The Radak explains this conduct: "The Torah is teaching us the ways of *tzniut*. An engaged woman should be shy (bashful) with her *chatan* and shouldn't show her face until she is married to him."[10] Of course, this might sound extreme in today's era. However, it gives us a perspective on the beautiful way engaged girls felt when in the presence of their *chatanim* in days of old. A modicum of reserve is the hallmark of respect and refinement. It is a quality that should never be abandoned and should, to a certain extent, continue into married life.

The Midrash[11] tells of a matron who remarked to Rav Yossi, "I was to marry my uncle, but we grew up in the same house and I became ugly in his eyes. He married a woman who is not as pretty as I am." Becoming overly familiar with each other should be saved for after the wedding. What might sound and even feel exciting can be detrimental[12] to the future bond they hope for.

Halachically, the connection and expressions between *chatan* and *kallah* can be only verbal. Even that is limited, because they are not married yet. There is only so much that is *halachically* appropriate to express to the other before you are married. Treasure that. Invest in that emotional feeling of looking forward to meeting and speaking to each other. If you run out of topics to speak about, it's okay. Being silent in another person's silent company should be a pleasant experience too. It's much better than speaking about topics that should be left for after the wedding.

This is what I mean by *orot bli keilim*: The lights are on. The excitement exists but you have no vessels available for it. The navigation of this stage of life is delicate and

---

[8] *Shulchan Ha'ezer*, vol. 2, p. 131b.

[9] *Bereishis* 24:65.

[10] *Radak* to *Bereishis* 24:64.

[11] *Bereishis Rabbah* 17:8.

[12] In a letter to a *kallah* who wanted to travel to Israel, to visit with her *chatan*, the Rebbe writes: "I understand your feelings about wanting to go, but on the other hand, if you look into the idea you would admit that it is not fitting for a Jewish and *chassidishe* person to do so. Even when *chatan* and *kallah* live in the same city or nearby cities, they refrain from meeting before the wedding. So how can you make a special trip, with all the publicity it entails, not to mention to spend money, time and energy, all to do something that *lechatchilah*, from the outset, isn't right? Please don't take it to heart. Just realize that you and your *chatan* are building a *binyan adei ad* for many tens of years, with happiness and harmony, the *chassidishe* way." From this letter we can see just how much the Rebbe felt that spending a limited amount of time rather than elongated time together was to the couple's benefit. The Rebbe was so careful with the *kallah's* feelings and at the same time wanted the best for her regarding her future happiness and harmony. It's so calming to see how the Rebbe writes that they will *iy"h* be building a home for many years to come with happiness and harmony. The separation during engagement, as hard as it is (we all know that), is a small price to pay. Keep busy – it helps!

crucial. It is a balancing act. And we must never forget that it is *yakar mikol yakar*, the dearest, most foundational time in our life.

What can/should we do to maximize the engagement period?

The Rebbe teaches us that this special time is so unique that it influences the rest of our lives[13] it should ideally be used as a time to reflect on and grow in our spirituality.[14]

There is the story told about the *chatan* who went into the Rebbe for *yechidut* after his engagement and the Rebbe inquired how the preparations were going. The *chatan* described to the Rebbe the apartment, furniture, and so forth and what he still had left to buy. The Rebbe said to him, "I meant your spiritual preparations. How are they going?" At about the same time, another *chatan* went into *yechidut* and, when asked the same question, he told the Rebbe everything he had learned and which *maamorim* (chassidic treatises) he had prepared for sharing during the *sheva brachot*. The Rebbe answered him, "I meant your physical preparations. How are they going? Have you bought a *kapote,* (a long black coat worn by Chassidic men on Shabbat and holidays) yet, etc.?"[15]

One of the key skills of marriage is balance. We start practicing this skill from the day we get engaged. Yes, we should have wonderful memories of this time. Yes, we should be shopping, working, learning, and preparing. Yes, it is a pressure filled period in our lifetime. Add to this the way the excitement can affect your hormonal balance, all the "stuff" of everyday life, plus gown fittings and *sheitel* appointments. What is best at this time, is to follow the Rebbe's guidance which he gave throughout the years to *chatanim* and *kallot*. These instructions help to enrich this beautiful time capsule.

The Rebbe's guidance is not a set of restrictions. On the contrary, every single piece of advice opens our eyes as to how to behave as a married couple. If the Rebbe tells us that it's best not to meet too often as *chatan* and *kallah*, we learn that a married couple should be close. If we are counseled to speak once a week or so, it teaches us the value of communication.

This is because *orot bli keilim*, light without vessels, can cause the *keilim* to burst. Too many stories are told, and there are many letters from the Rebbe addressing this exact issue to *chatanim* and *kallot* on the verge of breaking their engagement. The

---

13   *Igros Kodesh*, vol. 14, p. 82.

14   *Igros Kodesh*, vol. 14, p. 80. Ibid., vol. 16, p. 40.

15   *Hiskashrus*, issue 70, p. 14.

Rebbe's message was: "They were too close, too much involved with each other, spoke too much, met too much and now have run out of energy"[16] – *orot bli keilim*.

When the Rebbe Rashab, Reb Sholom Dovber, and his brother, the Raza, were young boys they would often visit their grandfather, the Rebbe the Tzemach Tzedek. Once, the Raza couldn't find the hat he customarily wore when entering his grandfather's study, so he told his younger brother to go in without him. The Tzemach Tzedek gave his young grandson a kiss and a coin. When the Raza heard about this, he grabbed the coin from his brother. The young Sholom Dovber cried, but then calmed himself and said, "*Nu*. You [take the] money, [and] I [will keep the] kiss." The Raza realized he was wrong and offered to return the coin. Again, his younger brother insisted, "You [take] the money, [and] I [will keep] the kiss." Their mother, Rebbetzin Rivka, related this story and added that from a young age her son already had his priorities straight.[17]

A kiss is a beautiful act of love. In Chassidus we learn the different levels of expressions of love. A hug, a kiss, looking into each other's eyes, all reflect different levels of connection.[18] To scoffingly say, "What is the value of a kiss?" or to misuse it at an inappropriate time is to underestimate its beauty. This is the equivalent of the child's fixation with a coin.

• • • • •

The Torah relates the stories regarding the *shidduchim* of our *Imahot* and *Avot* at great length underscoring important themes:

For instance, where was Yitzchak while Eliezer was traveling to Charan and then returning with Rivkah as his bride? The *mefarshim* explain that Yitzchak spent the time before his wedding in Gan Eden.[19] Yitzchak knew that his father would prepare all the physical and material elements for a home, wedding, and so forth, so he went to prepare himself in the most spiritual way.[20]

Rivkah also made her preparations. As the Torah tells us, she was familiar with the *mitzvos* of *challah*, Shabbat candles and *taharat hamishpachah*. She had learned about them so well prior to her marriage, that the Torah tells us that she returned to Avraham's home, the joy and blessings that departed when Sarah died. Due to Rivkah's

---

[16] *Igros Kodesh*, vol. 9, pp. 209-210. Ibid., vol. 14, p. 21. Ibid., vol. 28, p. 103.

[17] *Divrei Yemei HaRabbonis Rivkah*, p. 44. *Oros Ba'afeilah* (Avtzon), pp. 121-122. *Reshimos Sippurim* (Mishulovin), vol. 1, p. 57.

[18] See *Likkutei Dibburim*, vol. 1, pp. 4-6.

[19] *Riva Al Hatorah* to Bereishis 24:64 and 25:27.

[20] See *Likkutei Sichos*, vol. 1, p. 52.

investments of time and effort, the couple's dwelling place merited the blessings of the *challah*, the candles that stayed lit from week to week and, when they wed, a cloud that hovered over their home, a sign of *shalom bayit* and *taharat hamishpachah*.[21]

The Rebbe's father, Reb Levik, expounds[22] on the dialogue between Eliezer and Rivkah's family before Rivkah joined him to travel to Avraham and Yitzchak:

The family wanted Rivkah to stay at home longer to prepare for her wedding (preparations mostly involving gifts and jewelry). They suggested, תשב הנערה אתנו ימים או עשור, she should stay with us for days or ten months.[23] Rashi says "days" mean a year. (This might be the basis for the *minhag* of some different groups of chassidim to have a year-long engagement.)

Reb Levik explains that this dialogue alludes to the *Yamim Nora'im;* teaching us how to prepare for our wedding.

Yamim - Days, allude to the two days of Rosh Hashanah.

Asor - Ten, is Yom Kippur, the tenth of Tishrei.

The climax of Tishrei is Sukkot, the most joyous and festive of all holidays.

The seven days of Sukkot symbolize the wedding day and the festivities of *sheva brachot*.

To achieve the true happiness of Sukkot and Simchat Torah, we must first go through Rosh Hashanah and Yom Kippur.

For a marriage to be truly happy, the preparation beforehand should be worthy of Rosh Hashanah and Yom Kippur. Rosh Hashanah is the day we crown Hashem as our king without any doubts. So, too, we express that type of unconditional commitment in marriage. Yom Kippur[24] is the day we repent on the past and prepare ourselves for the future. So, too, the days and months prior to the wedding should be spent in retrospective thinking and positive resolutions regarding the future.

Further in the Torah, we learn about Yaakov marrying his wives. After Yaakov left his parents' home on a quest to find his wife, he first stopped in the *yeshivah* of Shem and Ever to study Torah, only then did he proceed. Yaakov wanted to marry Rachel. He worked for her for seven years: seven years spent working and learning.

---

21   See *Chizkuni, Gur Aryeh, Bartenura,* and *Be'er Mayim Chaim* to Bereishis 24:67.

22   *Likkutei Levi Yitzchak, Likkutim al Pesukei Tanach,* pp. 21ff.

23   Bereishis 24:55.

24   The Rebbe discusses the *inyan* of a *kallah* and *chatan* fasting and being forgiven for all of their sins on the day of their marriage which is akin to Yom Kippur (*Likkutei Sichos,* vol. 30, pp. 161ff.).

As Yaakov took over Rachel's task as shepherdess, she was free to study and prepare herself to become a befitting wife to Yaakov. We are told that Yaakov taught her the *halachot* a woman should know for a Jewish home. When Rachel realized that Yaakov would be marrying Leah, she subsequently taught her sister Leah everything she herself was taught.[25]

Yaakov married Leah, and then one week later he married Rachel. Leah's primary mode of preparation for her marriage was prayer. Leah prayed she would marry Yaakov and she thus changed her destiny. Rachel, on the other hand, prepared through self sacrifice, by giving her would-be husband to her sister, a sign of deep and unconditional love.

Our holy *Imahot* and *Avot* recognized the importance of using the time before marriage for Torah, prayer, and love for another. Immersing ourselves in these acts propel us forward in moving from the "me" to the "us" of marriage and family.

This is the time to build a good, solid foundation for the new home. It is the time for a couple to discuss important topics like who they will choose as their *rav* and *mashpia*, and continue their discussion of topics presumably discussed while they were dating such as the *chassidishe* behaviors they will uphold in and out of the home, the children's education, and their *hiskashrus* (connection) to the Rebbe.

From the Rebbe's guidance to parents of engaged couples we clearly understand that most of the wedding plans and details should be left up to the parents.[26] The idea is to give the couple as much time as possible to study and prepare themselves in the spiritual aspects and *halacha*. The Rebbe once said that "If on regular days we need to strengthen ourselves and hold onto Torah— that it is our source channel for bringing down blessing and success— how much more so during the time of preparation for the wedding."[27] Of course, a certain amount of shopping and decision-making is inevitable for any *kallah* and *chatan*. When they are busy shopping for new clothes, items for their new home, etc., it should all be done in a most calm way, avoiding confrontation and arguments. It is written that the *Satan* tries to cause tension and argument before a *chuppah*.[28] We don't need to help him.

There is a story told that once during a *Kinus Torah*, a plenary convened for the purpose of teaching Torah, the Rebbe saw a future father-in-law talking to his future

---

25   See *Daat Zekeinim* to *Bereishis* 29:25.

26   See *Toras Menachem*, vol. 12, pp. 153-155.

27   *Igros Kodesh*, vol. 5, p. 53.

28   See Shabbat 130a. *Igros Kodesh*, vol. 6, p. 171.

son-in-law. They excused themselves that they were talking about the wedding. The Rebbe reacted by saying, "In the middle of the *Kinus Torah*?! In the middle of the Kinus Torah?! For wedding preparations, use the time of sleep and not the time of learning Torah!"[29] The Rebbe's message was that they should be busy with the *ikar,* the truly important thing, and not the *tofel,* the insignificant.

During the year 2020 due to the Coronavirus and the protocols it engendered, we witnessed many restricted-participation weddings due to health concerns. They were extremely beautiful and meaningful. Quite a few of those *kallot* expressed their happiness with having a smaller group of guests, a simpler venue, and so forth. Many people realized how much time, energy and money were too often spent on things that were unimportant. Even so, we do wish for every *kallah* to have her expectations for her wedding day met to their fullest. A wedding should be the most joyous and wonderful *simchah.*

Studying Torah

Both the *kallah* and *chatan* should study the laws of *taharat hamishpachah* with veteran teachers with whom they feel comfortable so they can continue their relationship after the wedding. I suggest that the *kallah* take classes soon after the engagement so she can calmly learn these new topics.

As the *akeret habayit*, it is a good idea for the *kallah* to refresh her knowledge of the laws of *kashrut* and Shabbat. It is good for *kallot* to start being more careful with lighting candles on time (18 minutes before *shekiah*) as the wife is the one who brings the Shabbat into the home.

The wife's *tzniut* is her responsibility to her family. She sets the tone for her whole family. She should be knowledgeable about all the *halachot* of *yichud*, and *tzniut* in behavior and dress. Experience has shown that the young men do not really know the *halachot* of *tzniut*, and they rely on their wives to be well-versed in these laws. I've heard girls say, "My husband likes me in ..." or "My husband never said I should be careful with that..." Much of the time it's because he doesn't know the pertinent *halacha*. It is the woman's privilege to set the tone and she can best do this when she is familiar with the relevant *halacha* and *hashkafah*.

---

29   *Hiskashrus,* issue 573, p. 16.

Tefillah

Time should be set aside for extra *Tehillim* and prayer. The *chatan* and *kallah* should involve themselves in true *teshuvah*, the forgiveness of others, and prayer that the wedding should be *b'shaah tovah u'mutzlachat* and that they should build a *binyan adei ad*.

Tzedakah

Increased amounts of *tzedakah* – beyond what would be given at any other time in life – should be distributed during this time.[30] Keep an eye out for a nice *tzedakah* box for the kitchen in your new home.[31] *Tzedakah* is based on the concept that everything belongs to Hashem, a concept we want to feel palpably in our new home. The Rebbe wrote: **A tzedakah box is gifted [to the new couple] to serve as a reminder that this is a home built on Torah and** mitzvos**.**[32]

I also like to think that *tzedakah* finetunes the concept of sharing with someone else. This is the time to start making room in our mind and heart for our other half, transforming "me" into "we."

Gifts

In Chabad there are very few customs regarding the gifts given to *chatan* and *kallah*. I personally feel that this relieves a lot of pressure from the parents as well as from the *chatan* and *kallah*.

It is customary for the *chatan's* family to buy the *kallah* candlesticks and for the *kallah's* family to buy the *chatan* a *tallit* and *kittel*.[33] The rest is very individual.

The Rebbe suggested concentrating on giving gifts of holy books that would increase the holiness at home.[34] It is customary for the *chatan* to receive a *Shas* and Chassidic *sefarim* from the *kallah* and her family.[35] Generations ago, a *kallah* would

---

30 *Hisvaaduyos* 5751. vol 2, p. 53. In addition, the Rebbe spoke on a few occasions about the *kallah* and *chatan* setting aside a large sum of money to distribute for *tzedakah* on their wedding day. See *Hisvaaduyos* 5744. vol. 2, p. 899.

31 See at length *Toras Menachem* 5748. vol. 4, pp. 342-347.

32 *Sichos Kodesh* 5739. vol.1, p. 364.

33 *Tallit* and *kittel* as presents are mentioned in the *nusach* of the *tenai'm*.

34 *Sefer Hasichos* 5748. vol. 1, p. 191.

35 *Toras Menachem* 5745. vol. 2, p. 1181.

be gifted with a Siddur Korban Mincha. Today, this is replaced with *halacha sefarim* pertaining to running a home, as well as other *sefarim*.[36] In this regard, the Rebbe wrote:

> **"Presently, since women study much Torah, are knowledgeable, and so on, they do not need a simplistic Yiddish translation. In fact, receiving such a gift may even cause them embarrassment. Instead they should receive books of Jewish law that relate to conducting one's home in the proper Jewish way. The more books the better."**[37]

There is one near-universal gift about which the Rebbe adamantly expressed himself: **"In my opinion, it is advisable, for obvious reasons, that a ring not be among the gifts that are given to the *kallah*** [during the engagement period]."[38] At a farbrengen[39] the Rebbe addressed this topic in greater detail and explained that this seemingly benign, widely held practice can have serious *halachic* ramifications. A *chatan* gifting his *kallah* a ring might be considered *kiddushin (safek kedushin)*, since the act is so similar to the iconic act of *kiddushin* effected with a ring under the *chuppah*. Preempting those who claim that the engagement ring is not for the purpose of *kiddushin*, the Rebbe countered that it is most certainly evocative of *kiddushin* as the gift is conceptually about formalizing their union. The problem, the Rebbe continued, is especially acute if the *chatan* puts the ring on his *kallah*'s finger which involves an additional *halachic* issue, that of *kirvah shel chiba,* an overture denoting closeness that comes as a result of love. Such physical manifestation of closeness is not permitted until after the couple is married.

The Rebbe rhetorically asked: Why involve oneself in a potentially *halachically* problematic– if not dangerous –situation, when many other gifts can be given, such as other types of jewelry etc. The Chabad custom is therefore for the *chatan* to give his *kallah* the diamond ring after the *chuppah*, whether in the *yichud* room or at some point after that.

---

36   See *Sefer Hasichos* 5748, vol. 1, p. 191.

37   *Sefer Hasichos* 5748, vol. 1, p. 191.

38   *Likkutei Sichos*, vol. 19, p. 510.

39   *Sichos Kodesh* 5741, vol. 2, p. 512.

Kallah Jitters

Find me a *kallah* who doesn't experience pre-wedding jitters at some level!

There is the garden variety of jitters, that includes second guessing oneself. It's understandable for a girl to ask herself. "How did I make a lifelong decision on my own?! Do I really know him?!" Add to that the hormones that play an important role at this time and can contribute to emotional disequilibrium.

Then there are levels of anxiety that can be cause for concern. A *kallah* should not ignore her feelings if she has serious doubts. Her parents, *kallah* teacher or rabbi can be a source of help. Sometimes a therapist needs to be involved to assess the broader situation.

Week Before the Wedding

It's customary that *chatan* and *kallah* don't see each other or speak during the week leading up to the wedding.[40]

It is also customary for the *chatan* and *kallah* to have accompaniment for a few days before the wedding in the form of a *shomer/shomeret*.[41] Just as Yitzchak Avinu was in Gan Eden before his wedding, *chatan* and *kallah* should try to be in a Gan Eden-like environment before their wedding.[42] They should be surrounded with pure things, people and thoughts. The person who accompanies them (*shomer*) should make sure that the atmosphere surrounding the *kallah* and *chatan* is saturated with positive energy and *kedushah*. The Gemara[43] teaches "Three things have to be guarded: a sick person, a woman after childbirth, and a *chatan* and *kallah*." We guard what is holy, precious, and fragile.

The customary *shemirah* (accompaniment) after the wedding is for the purpose of providing the young couple with an "honor guard", as *chatan* and *kallah* during the week of their *sheva brachot* are likened to a king and queen.[44]

---

[40] See *Sefer Haminhagim*, p. 75.

[41] *Likkutei Sichos*, vol. 1, p. 52.

[42] See *Likkutei Sichos*, vol. 1, p. 53.

[43] *Brachot* 54b.

[44] See *Sefer Haminhagim*, p. 76. *Likkutei Sichos*, vol. 1, p. 52.

Aliyah to the Torah

It is customary that the *chatan* receives an *aliyah* to the Torah on the Shabbat before the wedding.[45] The reason for this is to receive extra strength from the Torah which is the basis of their new home.[46] It is also customary to throw candies upon the *chatan*, blessing him with sweetness and goodness.[47] A *kiddush* is prepared,[48] usually followed by a *chassidishe farbrengen*. The Rebbe's instructions regarding imbibing alcohol in moderation[49] should be adhered to so that the *aliyah* leads to elevation on the part of all present.

Shabbat Kallah

The *kallah* celebrates this Shabbat with a gathering of friends who come to bless and wish her *mazal tov*. *Divrei Torah* are offered with words of wisdom for the *kallah* on her upcoming wedding.

I find it beautiful that the Shabbat before the wedding and the Shabbat after the wedding are both times *kallah* and *chatan* spend with family. It illustrates our priorities: we understand that we are contributing a new link to the existing family chain. Rather than travel on our honeymoon[50] we spend the week after the wedding with *sheva brachot*, strengthening our familial connections.

The First Year

If the engagement period is a time of *tohu*, the first year of marriage is a period of transition from *tohu* to *tikkun*.

We learn the importance of this year from a letter written to the Rebbe, after his wedding, by his father, Harav Levi Yitzchak Schneerson. In the letter[51] Reb Levik writes that in the world of *tohu* a person is alone. In the world of *tikkun* he makes room for another.

---

45   *Magen Avraham, Orach Chaim* 282:18.

46   See *Sefer Hamaamorim Kuntreisim*, vol. 1, p. 38. *Toras Menachem*, vol. 1, p. 125.

47   Based on *Brachot* 50b (*Shulchan Ha'ezer*, vol. 2, 14a).

48   *Piskei Dinim Leha Tzemach Tzedek* 192:6. *Shulchan Ha'ezer*, vol. 2, 14a. See also *Pirkei D'rabbi Eliezer*, end of ch. 17.

49   See *Toras Menachem*, vol. 36, pp. 351-354.

50   See *Toras Menachem*, vol. 15, p. 323. Ibid., vol. 52, p. 153.

51   *Likkutei Levi Yitzchak, Igros Kodesh*, pp. 315-321.

Tohu is a plane of distinctiveness while *tikkun* is about interinclusion. We model our married life on the world of *tikkun* which is about *hiskallelut and achdut*, inclusion and unity. Only in this way do we get closer to achieving true harmony and love. One of the first steps in this process is understanding the ways in which each spouse complements and completes the other. *Tohu* was about me and *tikkun* is about us.

Reb Levik continues in this beautiful Kabbalistic letter by describing the eternal impact the work of the "builders," the *kallah* and *chatan*, has on their descendants for all time. The level of refinement they achieve in this first year, accomplished together, with love and harmony on the basis of the Torah, will not only prepare them to take on the challenges of life, but will also refine their children.

The Mitzvah of Shana Rishonah

The Torah forbids enlisting a newlywed, even for the important purpose of waging war.[52] In contemporary application, this more broadly includes leaving home for purposes of business, or for a Yom Tov and other occasions.[53] There are of course exceptions, and a *rav* should be consulted. In cases where it is permitted, it is predicated on the wife's permission.

The *Sefer Hachinuch* explains this mitzvah referred to as *shana rishonah* (the first year), in the following way:

> על כן גזר עלינו העם אשר בחר להיות נקרא על שמו, שנשב עם האשה המיוחדת לנו להקים זרע שנה שלמה, מעת שנשא אותה, כדי להרגיל הטבע עמה ולהדביק הרצון אצלה ולהכניס ציורה וכל פעולה בלב

> …This is why Hashem instructed His nation, the ones He chose to carry His name, to spend a complete year together with the woman with whom they will establish progeny. During this year, her husband will become familiar with her. His desire for her will grow ever closer. Her appearance and all her actions will enter his heart.[54]

This mitzvah is a statement on the primacy of Jewish family in Jewish life and provides deep psychological insight into human nature. The *Sefer Hachinuch* teaches

---

52   *Devarim* 24:5.

53   *Kitzur Shulchan Aruch* 149:13. See also *Likkutei Sichos*, vol. 24, p. 468.

54   *Sefer Hachinuch*, mitzvah 582.

that as a rule, people gravitate to what is familiar. Familiarity brings comfort, security, and faithfulness.

The Torah teaches us that a groom must stay close to home for the first year of marriage nourishing and nurturing the fledgling relationship and thus establishing the "familiarity" that is a basis for so much else. We come to learn our spouse's characteristics, and try to adopt them as our "second nature."

Emotional intimacy is the soul and predictor of physical intimacy. Emotional intimacy is a sense of security; a feeling of belonging and togetherness. The Torah recognizes that it takes (at least) a year to solidify a close relationship. We learn this from Hashem, who stayed with *Bnei Yisrael* in the camp of *Har Sinai* for a full year after *Matan Torah*.[55]

Hashem desires a stable, moral and decent world; a world filled with children born to parents who conceived them with love and joy. In order for that to happen, Hashem gave us the mitzvah of *shana rishonah*, a year to study and concentrate on each other exclusively. This is a year with a learning curve; a year used to build strong foundations for an eternal home.

There is a beautiful letter from the Frierdiker Rebbe, the Previous Lubavitcher Rebbe, that has much to teach us about marriage in general and the first year in particular.[56]

I call this letter "The Ten Steps to a Healthy Marriage":

29 Nissan, 5700 (1940)
Lakewood, NY

To Mrs.......shetichyeh,

Blessings and greetings!

Before I left Riga, I tried several times to call you, but you were not home and then I was very busy, and it was simply impossible for me to spend the time needed to talk to you about what I wanted to tell you. In short words, I tell you that family life demands from the man, and even more so from the woman, relating sincerely to one another with dedication and gentleness, which must take a lot of time and energy.

---

55   *Rabbeinu Bechaye* to *Devarim* 24:5.

56   *Igros Kodesh* of the Frierdiker Rebbe, vol. 5, pp. 57-59.

According to our holy Torah, and according to healthy intelligence, there is nothing in human life more important than the beautiful and pure way of Torah, where we are taught that even the mitzvah of honoring one's father and mother gives way to a certain extent in favor of the mitzvah of family life.

A true family life according to the Torah requires understanding, effort, devotion, patience, kindness, purity/cleanliness, calmness, orderly appearance, a happy mood and a welcoming face, and a friendly disposition.

This is how they should both behave, the husband and the wife; however for the most part it depends on the woman, as it is written,[57] חכמות נשים בנתה ביתה, the wisdom of women built her home – the home, a wife builds.

The word "home" does not refer to a building or a place of residence, but refers to a place where a person lives in general, as it is written,[58] כתפארת אדם לשבת בית, as the glory of man to dwell in a home. That is to say, this refers not only to the physical apartment, but also the spiritual and moral level of the home. And of this home it is said, "The wisdom of women built her home."

Of course, it is imperative that each and every one take part in communal religious life, and the more the person Baruch Hashem is in a good situation, the more he must devote himself to this. But first of all, she "builds her home" – she builds the private home.

I have to say something that is very painful for me to say: I had great grief and for the time being, I have not felt better about it, and do not be angry at me for my direct expression – over the carelessness with which you value family life.

You are still young and not too experienced, and you certainly lack the necessary Torah knowledge and the necessary explanations to know the tremendous everlasting effect family has on human behavior for many generations.

---

57 *Mishlei* 14:1.

58 *Yeshayahu* 44:13.

Everything, without exception – Torah and mitzvos, health, children, livelihood, giving nachas to parents and good friends, and being loved, as in the saying[59] כל שרוח הבריות נוחה הימנו רוח המקום נוחה הימנו, Anyone who is favored by man is favored by Hashem – everything in life is dependent on the proper family life.

I bless you that Hashem will enlighten you and awaken your heart, to understand everything I have spoken to you. All this will penetrate your mind and your heart well, in order that you will fulfill it successfully. Hashem, blessed be He, will strengthen your health and the health of my dear friend your husband, and will delight their hearts with zara chaya v'kayama, living, healthy children, and will give you livelihood in abundance, materially and spiritually.

With blessing,

The Frierdiker Rebbe's signature

I find this letter fascinating, firstly because of its date. It was written shortly after the Frierdiker Rebbe miraculously escaped Europe, during World War II. A month after he arrived in New York, after a tumultuous journey and amidst great world wide chaos he sat down to write a letter to a young woman left behind in Riga. He wrote her a detailed, fatherly letter about the importance of investing time and effort in marriage.

The Rebbe mentions ten attributes necessary for building a happy marriage:

Understanding

Effort

Devotion

Patience

Goodness and kindness

Purity/cleanliness

Calmness/easygoing behavior

Orderly appearance

---

[59] *Pirkei Avot* 3:10.

A happy mood and happy facial expression

A friendly demeanor

Each above point can be elaborated upon at length. I would like to suggest one thought on each point.

Understanding: Women were blessed with a deeper understanding, an intuition concerning human nature. Use that understanding wisely.

Effort: Marriage is an investment. Marriage needs to be cultivated, nurtured, and protected.

Devotion: Put your heart into your marriage. It's your true life and love.

Patience: Take your time. Don't rush to conclusions quickly. Be patient.

Kindness: Giving is receiving. *Ahavat Yisrael* starts at home.

Purity and cleanliness: A pleasant home is a clean home and pure atmosphere. The tone of the home is usually set by the woman of the house.

Calmness and easygoing behavior: Tension and stress drain us of our energy. Life has challenges. Try to meet them calmly and with balanced proportions.

Orderly appearance: Structure and order are basic human necessities. An orderly appearance in and out of the house helps the person feel better about themselves.

A happy mood and facial expression: This is a very fundamental point. Spouses should always greet each other happily and try to be in a happy mood. *Simchah* is an *avodah,* as the Chassidic saying goes, *Tracht gut, vet zein gut,* think positively and it will bring about good results.

A friendly demeanor and behavior: Be a good and faithful friend. Friends trust each other, respect each other and protect one another. Be there for him and he will be there for you.

It is instructive that in his letter, the Previous Rebbe doesn't write about love. If we follow the steps he mentions above, love will naturally flourish in the home.

I once met with a young couple who came for advice after they celebrated their first wedding anniversary. Unbeknownst to them, I had met the day before with another couple who had recently celebrated their first wedding anniversary, too. I couldn't help but compare the two couples (in my mind, of course). They were both dealing with similar issues.

Couple Number One was a young couple who came to get advice on how to make their marriage better. They wanted reading material, asked what they should do to change and improve, and so on.

Both members of Couple Number Two were a bit older than the first couple. They each had been living on their own for a while before marriage. Their opening sentence was, "We tried marriage for a year, and it isn't working for us."

The difference between the two couples was very obvious. The first got married and spent the first year learning about marriage and how it works. The second couple "tried marriage to see if it works." Couple Number One was investing, while Couple Number Two was testing and experimenting.

Hashem married us, the Jewish people, and we said *Naaseh v'nishma,* we will do and then we will understand. We weren't just going to give it a try, like a "why not?" type of agreement. We went into our bond with Hashem with complete devotion.

This is the attitude we each need to embrace, and in the above mentioned words of the Previous Rebbe, "with patience, tenderness, time and energy." The first year is not a "test drive," it is a precious period in time meant to help the new couple develop their couplehood from a place of sincere commitment.

In the words of our Rebbe: May you and your *chatan* merit to build a: בית נאמן בישראל בנין עדי עד על יסודי התורה והמצוה כפי שהם מוארים במאור שבתורה זוהי תורת החסידות, an everlasting Jewish home based on the foundations of the Torah and *mitzvos,* as they are illuminated with the inner light of the Torah, that is the Teachings of Chassidus.

Mrs. Esther Piekarski and her husband are *Shluchim* to North Tel Aviv, Israel. She has taught *Bayis Yehudi* for the past two decades in seminaries throughout Israel and is a premarital counselor for the Ministry of Religious Affairs, preparing brides and grooms to marry "according to the law of Moses and Israel." Mrs. Piekarski was cited by the Israeli daily Ma'ariv, as one of the "Top Ten Speakers in Israel" and has lectured around the world on the topics of marriage and *Taharat Hamishpachah -* Family Purity.

Sara Morozow

The Holiness of the Wedding Day

CHABAD MINHAGIM FOR THE YOM HACHATUNA

Your wedding is a day to remember! A tremendous investment of time, effort, thought and money goes into preparing for this grand occasion. Given the world we live in, with *gashmiyut*, materialism, front and center, it is easy to overlook the spiritual power of this day. If we want to harness the *ruchniyus'dike, spiritual,* energy of the wedding experience, it requires focus and preparation.

In this respect, preparing for the wedding is similar to bringing Shabbat into our homes. The *ruchniyus'dike* beauty of Shabbat is reflected in the *gashmiyut*—in the way we prepare our home and in the special foods and clothing we set aside to enjoy on this day. The same is true of the wedding day. As much as we want every detail to be perfect *b'gashmiyut*, we must ensure that this does not overshadow the *ikar* (essence)*;* the physical beauty should reflect–not muffle–the holiness of the day. The awareness that we are preparing to establish our lives on the foundation of holiness and purity should pervade our preparations. In the words of the Mitteler Rebbe:[1]

---

1   *Maamorei Admor Ha'emtzai. Drushei Chatunah* vol. 2. p. 728 (printed as a *hosafah* to *Likkutei Sichos Parshas Yisro* 5748).

> הטעם שמעמידים החתן תחת החופה ביום חתונתו, כי החופה היא בחינת מקיף
> וכל מה שיעסוק בעבודת השם עד ימי חייו נמשך לו ממקיף בעת הזאת ולכן צריך
> לקשר מחשבתו בה'.....

Why is the chatan made to stand beneath a chuppah on his wedding day? The chuppah represents a transcendent level of divine energy known as makif. During these moments, the makif influences whatever you will do to serve Hashem your entire life. To release the energy of the makif, you must focus your mind on Hashem at this time...

The spiritual power of a *chatunah* is so unique that when a *chatan* and *kallah* get married, the *simchah* is not solely for themselves, their family, and their friends. It is shared by the entire community and all of *Klal Yisroel*. For example, for the whole week of *sheva brachot*, *tachanun* is not recited in shul if a *chatan* is present. And it is a mitzvah to participate in the *simchah* of a wedding and to dance and rejoice with the *chatan* and *kallah*. Why is this so? Indeed, why can't the *chatan* and *kallah* solidify their union in private? Why the necessity for a big public display?

The Mitteler Rebbe[2] compared a wedding to two close friends who, after being separated for a long time, are reunited. The joy of reunion depends on how close the friends were, how long they were separated, and the reason for their separation. If one was in peril – such as in captivity or seriously ill – the intensity of the joy upon reunion will naturally be greater.

The *chatan* and *kallah* are not just close friends but one *neshamah* that descends into two separate bodies. They have been separated for a long time. Furthermore, they have been sent down into *olam hazeh*, a world filled with the danger of ubiquitous *kelipah* and *sitra achara*, which pose a profound risk to what their *neshamot* are meant to accomplish. For all these reasons, the joy at a Jewish wedding is especially great. And since all *neshamot* are essentially one,[3] the joy of one *neshamah* is shared by all.

When the two halves of this particular *neshamah* finally reunite, they do not merely revert back to their previous oneness. The *chatan* and *kallah*, together, create something new. Together, they embark on building a new Jewish family. We've all done the science experiment whereby you form a volcano by mixing baking soda and vinegar. When two substances come together to form a new compound, energy is

---

2   *Maamorei Admor Ha'emtzai, Vayikra* vol. 2, pp. 696-698.

3   Tanya ch. 32.

The Holiness of the Wedding Day

released. At a wedding,[4] the union of the two halves of this *neshamah* releases an *or makif* a transcendent, encompassing light and energy[5] that impacts the entire *seder hishtalshelut,* the whole chain-like evolution of spiritual worlds from the highest heavens down to our physical realm. Every detail of a Jewish wedding must therefore reflect the unprecedented *kedushah* released at this moment.

During the engagement, the *kallah* has a lot on her mind. She needs to shop for – everything! – in addition to finding and furnishing an apartment. Most likely, she is working, taking *kallah* classes, and worrying about her future. It is, therefore, impractical to leave all of the *ruchniyus'dike* preparations for the engagement period. Ideally, as soon as we reach marriageable age, we should begin exploring the spiritual and *halachic* underpinnings of a *chatunah* and married life in general. Many *sefarim*, in both Hebrew and English, explain in detail every aspect of the wedding day and marriage in general. You can highlight what inspires you and revisit it during your engagement period and then closer to the wedding day itself.

We all want to feel the *kedushah* of the wedding. But in reality, the wedding day often goes by in a blur. Especially for the *kallah*, there is hair, makeup, pictures, and more pictures. When, during this hectic day, does she get an opportunity to focus her thoughts on what really matters? Like everything important in life, this requires planning.

Four Themes of the Wedding Day

As we learn about the wedding day and the significance of the wedding *minhagim*, four themes emerge:

Rosh Hashanah: The wedding day is a personal Rosh Hashanah for the *chatan* and *kallah*. Just as Rosh Hashanah draws *chayut,* vivifying force, into this world that lasts for the duration of the entire year, so do the *kallah* and *chatan* draw down *brachot* for their entire lifetime. We are taught that the way we utilize the day of Rosh Hashanah affects our whole year, so too (and more so) the way the *kallah* and *chatan* utilize this singular day impacts the trajectory of their marriage and beyond. Rosh Hashanah was also the first wedding day in history—the wedding of Adam and Chava. Indeed, many details of a Jewish wedding reflect what happened at that first wedding. For example, the custom that a married couple accompany the *chatan* and *kallah* to the *chuppah*

---

[4] For the above, see The Jewish Home by SIE.

[5] *Likkutei Torah, Shir Hashirim* 48c.

reminds us of how Hashem had the angels Michael and Gavriel attend to the first couple when they married in Gan Eden.[6]

Yom Kippur: The wedding is a personal *Yom Kippur* for the *kallah* and *chatan*, which explains the strong *minhag* to fast on this day (health permitting, and if it is not *Rosh Chodesh* or some other calendrical date that precludes fasting).[7] The *chatan* also wears a *kittel* under the *chuppah*. Additionally, the couple's sins are forgiven on this day, just as on Yom Kippur, when an *or makif*, an all-encompassing light, empowered to override the sins of Bnei Yisroel, flows down into the world. The *chatan* and *kallah* say *vidui* at *Minchah* on their wedding day. They should focus on what this day means for them and be filled with a sincere feeling of *teshuvah*.[8]

Matan Torah: The giving of the Torah is likened to the wedding between Hashem and *Knesset Yisroel*. When we stand under the *chuppah*, we recreate the moment of *Matan Torah*. The candles used in escorting the *kallah* and *chatan* to the *chuppah* remind us – among other things – of the lightning and fire at Har Sinai.[9]

Yemot Hamoshiach: Finally, the marriage between the Jews and Hashem was not finalized at *Matan Torah* because we went into *galut* afterwards. It will only reach full actualization in the future, when Mashiach comes. The *kallah*'s seven rotations around the *chatan* under the *chuppah* is an allusion to – as well as a taste of– the prophetic words of Yirmiyahu Hanavi who described the times of Mashiach as a time when: *Nekeivah tesovev gever*,[10] the feminine [energy] will not only encircle but prevail over the masculine.[11]

Minhagim of the Wedding Day

On Yud Daled Kislev, 5714, at a *farbrengen* marking the Rebbe and the Rebbetzin Chaya Mushka's wedding anniversary, the Rebbe spoke about the importance of the *minhagim* of the *nessi'ei* (the Rebbes of) Chabad, in general,[12] and more specifically

---

6 *Bereishis Rabbah* 18:13. *Mateh Moshe, Hachnasas Kallah* 1:2.

7 Check with your *rav* if you should fast on another day instead.

8 See *Likkutei Sichos*, vol. 30, pp. 161ff.

9 *Mateh Moshe, Hachnasas Kallah* 1:2.

10 *Yirmiyahu* 31:21.

11 See *Toras Chaim, Vayeishev* 70c-71a.

12 In that same *sichah* (*Toras Menachem*, vol. 10, p. 197), regarding the general importance and power of *minhagim*, even seemingly "small matters" the Rebbe quoted the *maamar Chazal* (see *Shir Hashirim Rabbah* 5:2), "Open for Me an opening the size of the eye of a needle, and I will open for you an opening the size of a hall." We offer Hashem a small overture, "the eye of a needle" and He reciprocates with immense *brachah*, "An opening the size of a great hall."

The Holiness of the Wedding Day

about the *minhagim* related to the wedding day. The Rebbe explained that marriage necessitates the revelation of an infinite power – the power of generation, of a *dor yesharim yevorach,* upright and blessed generations or progeny. Because, the Rebbe added, this power comes via the agency of the *nassi hador*, it is important to abide by the *minhagei chatuna* of our *nessi'im*.[13] Careful observance of the wedding *minhagim* opens up a channel for remarkable *brachot* that last the couple's entire life.

Among other *minhagei chatuna*, the Rebbe discussed the text of the wedding invitation. Nowadays, this may strike us as especially minor as so many use paperless invites. The *minhag Chabad*, however, is to use the precise wording (and timing) that the Frierdiker Rebbe used in the invitation to the wedding of the Rebbe and Rebbetzin.[14] It is known that the invitation entails four paragraphs, and, together, the first letter of each paragraph spells out the word *ahavah*, love. The Rebbe said that the Frierdiker Rebbe didn't want this to be made conspicuous. One should, therefore, not design the invitation with these letters in large type. Another *minhag* the Rebbe mentioned is that the *taba'at kiddushin*, the ring given under the *chuppah*, be made of gold specifically (rather than silver), and that the ring be round and smooth.[15]

In the 1980s, the Rebbe underscored the importance of the *kallah* and *chatan* giving *tzedakah* on the wedding day; including family and friends doing the same in the *zechut* of the *chatan* and *kallah*.[16] Coins and *pushkas* should be prepared at home as well as in the wedding hall for this purpose. Besides placing a *pushka* on the head tables of both the *chatan* and the *kallah*, as the Rebbe suggested,[17] it is wise to arrange for a *pushka* on each table along with some coins so that the guests can easily give *tzedakah* in the *zechut* of the *kallah* and *chatan*. The *chatan* and *kallah* themselves should be reminded to put coins in the *pushka* throughout the day of the wedding. Chassidus explains the great advantage in giving small sums at frequent intervals, versus giving one large sum at one time.[18] Furthermore, the Rebbe underscored the global impact of the *kallah* and *chatan* giving *tzedakah* on their wedding day:

---

[13] *Toras Menachem*, vol. 10, p. 198.

[14] Including insertion of the phrase, *bshaa hachamishis*, at 5 o'clock, even when the wedding is called for a different hour.

[15] *Toras Menachem*, vol. 10, pp. 198-200. See there for additional *minhagim* discussed in that *sichah*.

[16] *Toras Menachem* 5744, vol. 4, p. 2242. Ibid. 5746, vol. 2, p. 488. Ibid. vol. 4, p. 84.

[17] *Toras Menachem* 5749, vol. 1, p. 286.

[18] *Iggeres Hakodesh*, siman 21.

In light of the saying of our Sages, "Great is tzedakah, for it hastens the Redemption,"[19] there is a special quality to the tzedakah given by chatan and kallah – "king and queen" – to hasten and bring about the imminent true and complete Redemption[20].

Another wedding day *minhag* is for the *kallah* (and *chatan*[21]) to say the entire *sefer Tehillim*. This is traced to the Frierdiker Rebbe's request that his daughter, Rebbetzin Chaya Mushka, recite specific *perakim* of *Tehillim* on her wedding day. Since we don't know which chapters he enumerated, the *minhag* to say them all was adopted.[22] Depending on how fast the *kallah* reads, completing the *Tehillim* can take two, or even three hours, or more. With everything going on throughout the wedding day, the *kallah* may find it difficult to focus on her *ruchniyus'dike* preparations. It may be a good idea, therefore, for the *shomeret* to take the *kallah* to a private place where she can *daven* and say *Tehillim*. If the *kallah* will not manage to complete the whole *Tehillim*, some arrange to divide the remaining *perakim* for recitation by family members and friends.

For chassidim and all those aspiring to live a spiritually attuned life, a most important *minhag* is the visit to the Rebbe's *Ohel*.[23] The *minhag Yisroel* to visit *kivrei tzaddikim*, the gravesite of *tzaddikim*, on one's wedding day has always been a custom cherished in the Chabad community. Since the Rebbe's passing, however, visiting the *Ohel* of the Rebbe has taken on a new dimension for chassidim, akin to the *yechidut* that *kallahs* and *chatanim* would merit in honor of their wedding. Therefore, even many who live a great geographical distance from the *Ohel* make this trip a priority, and preferably as close to the wedding as possible. This important visit to the *Ohel* is not something to rush; the *kallah* and *chatan* (each one separately if this on the day of the wedding or within the week preceding) should take their time and think deeply about what they will request in their *pa"n* (*pidyon nefesh*, the note that is customarily written with requests), and write the *pa"n* out slowly and with care. For this reason, some choose to go to the *Ohel* a bit earlier than the actual wedding day (consult a *mashpia* beforehand). The engaged couple should speak to parents and *mashpi'im* beforehand to get *hadrachah*, proper guidance, in how to write the *pa"n* and what to include.[24] The

---

19   *Bava Basra* 10a.

20   *Toras Menachem* 5744, vol. 4, p. 243.

21   See *Shaarei Nissuin*, pp. 261-262.

22   *Sefer Haminhagim*, p. 75.

23   See *Mekadesh Yisroel*, pp. 175 and 293.

24   Suggestions for what to include in this *pa"n* include: Asking specifically for the *brachah* with which the Rebbe blessed *chatanim* and *kallahs* within

The Holiness of the Wedding Day

day of the wedding is an *eit ratzon,* an auspicious time, for the *chatan* and *kallah,* and it is important to properly tap into the spiritual bounty of this singular energy.

Standing Under the Chuppah

The Rebbe once offered the following piece of advice:[25]

הנה מבואר בספרים הקדושים, שבעת החופה עת רצון הוא, והחתן וכלה יש להם חשיבות מיוחדה, וכדאי שהוא יבקשם להתפלל למילוי משאלות לבבו לטובה, בעת עמדם בחופתם.

It is explained in Sefarim, that the time of the chuppah is an auspicious moment, and the chatan and kallah carry special significance. Therefore, ask them to daven on your behalf when they stand beneath their chuppah.

The Mitteler Rebbe explains that the *chuppah* is *bechinat makif* – a level of *kedushah* that transcends the world and cannot be accessed through human overtures. (This transcendent dynamic finds concrete expression in the way the *chuppah* hovers above the couple.) This unique level of divine revelation pours down upon the *chatan* and *kallah* as they stand under the *chuppah,* and it is this energy that they draw upon to build their lives together and to bring a *dor yesharim yevorach,* a blessed and upright generation, into this world. Thus, at this moment, the couple needs to connect their thoughts to Hashem, to make themselves into appropriate vessels to draw this holiness into their lives in a revealed manner. As noted, standing under the *chuppah* parallels standing at *Matan Torah*. The *chatan* and *kallah,* therefore, strive to fill themselves with a sense of *bittul,* self abnegation, and a tremendous desire – even if it will entail *mesirat nefesh,* self sacrifice – to fulfill Hashem's will.[26] The *kedushah* of a *chuppah* creates an *eit ratzon* so powerful that the *tefillot* of all of the guests – not only that of the *kallah* and *chatan* – take on additional potency.[27]

---

the letter he sent on the occasion of the wedding (the letter customarily read under the *chuppah*), asking for the all encompassing *brachot* of בני חיי ומזוני רויחי. abundant (*nachas* from) children, health, and *parnassah*. asking for specific *brachot* for oneself, one's (almost) spouse and your impending marriage, requesting *brachot* for family members and friends who are in need, and a general request for *bias Moshiach*. Generally speaking. Chassidim include a *hachlatah tovah,* a good resolution, undertaken in order to provide a vessel and conduit for blessing.

25   *Igros Kodesh*, vol. 20, p. 274.

26   *Maamorei Admor Ha'emtzai, Drushei Chatuna* vol. 2, p. 728 (printed as a *hosafah* to *Likkutei Sichos Parshas Yisro* 5748).

27   See *Toras Menachem*, vol. 9, p. 154.

Since a *kallah* and *chatan* are vested with such extraordinary powers on their wedding day and their *tefillot* are accepted more readily, many people ask *kallahs* and *chatanim* to *daven* for them on their special day. A *kallah* and *chatan* should absolutely keep all of these individuals in mind. They should remember, however, to concentrate most fully on their personal *tefillot* for their future together as, in fact, this is the day that impacts their union eternally.

Wedding Pictures

We all want beautiful memories and gorgeous pictures of our special day. At the same time, we do not want the photographers to intrude on – or assert control over– the atmosphere of the wedding itself. When you hire a photographer, you are the boss, and he wants to please you. Think about what you want your wedding to be like. Communicate to the photographer, so he knows his place at the wedding. How much time does he really need before your *chuppah* to catch a considerable amount of poses? You may want to limit the amount of pictures taken before and after the *chuppah*. The *kallah* may choose not to be present while all of the family pictures are taken and use that time to complete her *Tehillim* and *Minchah* privately. Alternatively, the schedule of pictures can be planned to minimize the time the *kallah* and *chatan* must be involved.

When the *chatan* and *kallah* stand under the *chuppah*, they are joined by the souls of three generations of ancestors.[28] In some cases the *chatan* and *kallah* are blessed, and all three generations are present in person. Their parents, grandparents and great-grandparents *tzum lange yohren* may all stand under the *chuppah*. You may want to remind the photographer to treat the grandparents and great grandparents with respect and, certainly, not to shove the elders in their effort to capture the best shot!

Chatan and *kallah* should be mindful of this as they pose for pictures that will be shared publicly. They may stand next to each other and their clothing may touch (if the *kallah* is *tehorah*), but they should not take any suggestive poses[29].

The Dancing

Dancing at a wedding is not just an enjoyable way to express our happiness for the new couple; it is a mitzvah of profound spiritual significance. Remember that a wedding is a reunion of two halves of one *neshamah*. At this moment, the elevation

---

28 *Sefer Hamaamorim Kuntreisim*, vol. 1, p. 76א.

29 See chapter 2 for a full discussion on public displays of affection.

of the *neshamah* is so palpable that it lifts the body off the ground. When we feel this *kedushah*, our dancing is different.

According to Kabbalah, the *chatan* and *kallah* represent two opposite forces. The *chatan* is the *mashpia*, and the *kallah* is the *mekabel*. In this vein, the *chatan* represents water, which flows downward, and the *kallah* represents fire, which draws upward. How do these two opposite forces unite? עושה שלום במרומיו, Hashem makes peace in heaven. All forces in the world unite when subjugated, in humility, to serve Hashem. (An important lesson and source of empowerment to remember and draw upon throughout marriage.) The lifting up of the *chatan* or *kallah* during dancing represents the couple's elevated access to this higher holiness, a holiness that allows them to fuse their opposite modalities and become one.[30]

Clearly, the wedding dance is imbued with an otherworldly *kedushah* we hope will suffuse our marriages. But that's only possible when we facilitate and safeguard the presence of this spiritually-sensitive energy. Speak with the band and tell them exactly what type of music you want them to play to ensure that your *simchah* will reflect the true holiness of the event. Find a musician/DJ who will work with you to create a beautiful, lively, and specifically Jewish atmosphere at the wedding.

With proper planning, we can enjoy a wedding that is both materially and spiritually beautiful. We can tap into the tremendous *brachot* Hashem is waiting to bestow upon us. May we merit to dance straight into *Yemot Hamoshiach* with the wedding of *Knesset Yisroel* and the *Shechinah*, speedily in our days!

I understand the importance and spiritual significance of the music and dancing at a wedding, and of course, we are planning to have separate dancing, but what about family?

Early on in his leadership, the Rebbe campaigned, fought to reinstate two very important observances that had fallen by the wayside in the larger Orthodox community. One was for married women to cover their hair completely, optimally with a *sheitel* (See Chapter 8, Hide and Seek: The Mitzvah of Kisui Rosh for complete treatment of this subject). The other was to ensure the placement of kosher *mechitzahs* in shuls and at weddings. There was a time in America when mixed seating even at "very *frum*" weddings was the norm. During the dancing, even if men and women danced in separate circles, the absence of a *mechitzah* allowed them to see each other.

---

30 *Likkutei Torah, Shir Hashirim* 48d.

Al pi halacha, it is forbidden for a man to watch women dancing.[31] Chassidim – and all those aiming to chart a spiritual path – therefore plan the wedding with an eye towards upholding the *halachot* of *mechitzah* in optimal fashion.[32]

Regarding mixed or "social" dancing at weddings, the Rebbe explained:[33]

> **Kiddushin and marriage consist of "You are consecrated unto me" – that the husband and wife are coupled only to each other. When the assembled express their joy and blessings to the couple, it is to be in a similar manner – at least, not in a conflicting manner.**
>
> **The theme of mixed dancing is the following: Someone who is married to one individual dances with another, or an unmarried young man dances with an unmarried young lady – thereby indicating that the institution of marriage is entirely superfluous. And all this is done publicly and with a clamor!!**
>
> **Hashem's reaction is in line with our behavior below. When someone indicates that the joy of marriage leads to such behavior of illicit closeness, then, Heaven forfend what can result from such behavior!**

There are exceptions to the rule of women and men dancing together. A woman may dance with her father and grandfather, and a man with his mother or grandmother (as long as the women dancing are not visible to other men). Brothers and sisters should not dance together in public.[34]

There are many Chassidic communities that observe the *minhag* of a mitzvah *tantz*[35]. The *kallah* typically comes to the men's side of the hall and holds a *gartel*, prayer sash, as her father and other male relatives and distinguished guests hold the other end of the *gartel* and dance. In some cases, she wears a veil; she might also dance with the *chatan* holding hands.

---

31   See *Shulchan Aruch, Even Ha'ezer* 21:1.

32   This includes the manner in which the *chatan* and *kallah* enter the ballroom, up until the conclusion of the wedding.

33   *Likkutei Sichos*, vol. 14, p. 305.

34   See *Nitei Gavriel, Nisuin*, 45:3.

35   Many Chassidic *sefarim* explain that the *mitzvah tantz* carries great spiritual importance (see *Derech Pikudecha*, mitzvah 35, os 14; *Nitei Gavriel, Nisuin*, 45:1 and fn. 1).

The Holiness of the Wedding Day

A *rav*[36] once asked the Rebbe why it is not *minhag Chabad* to have a *mitzvah tantz*. The Rebbe's reply to him consisted of four points. 1) We can try to understand the reasoning behind it and why there are exceptions, but that does not change the fact that dancing together is not our *minhag*. 2) Just by looking around we can see that this practice (dancing with the parents) has evolved at many weddings [into something completely inappropriate]; whoever has actually seen this can understand why we avoid it. 3) In the times of the *Avot*, they used to build *bamos* (private *mizbachos*, altars) for *korbonot* and this was acceptable. After the Mishkan was built, it became completely a*ssur* to build a *bamah*.[37] Some things that are completely fine in one generation are inappropriate in a different time. 4) Ask the *rav* of your community [about dancing with family members of the opposite gender at the wedding].

This final point underscores the Rebbe's all encompassing vision. On the one hand, the Rebbe wanted to obviate behaviors that contravene *halacha* that might evolve from a *mitzvah tantz*. On the other hand, he did not close the door on the possibility that there might be a time and place for a *kallah* to dance with her father or grandfather or a *chatan* with his mother or grandmother.[38]

Halacha states that in the case of a wedding where men can see women dancing, or any other form of dancing occurs not *al pi halacha*, the specific words שהשמחה במעונו (there is happiness in Hashem's abode), which are traditionally added to the *zimun* before *sheva brachot*, may not be recited.[39] The Rebbe explains [40] that when a proper *mechitzah* is upheld throughout the wedding, Hashem's name is mentioned in connection with the *simchah*, and He bestows *simchah* to the world at large—first and foremost to the *chatan* and *kallah*. This causes the *chatan* and *kallah* to be "*tzufriden*" (content) throughout their lifetime. When there is dancing against *halacha* – this represents a breach of the boundaries of *tzniut* or worse – we cannot then include שהשמחה במעונו – which means Hashem's happiness is removed from the wedding, in effect removing Hashem's blessings of happiness to the couple. Why would anyone want to tamper with or jeopardize their future happiness?

When the youngest child in a family gets married, many households enjoy a poignant "tradition" called the *mezinke* (youngest child) *tantz*. In the dance, the

---

36 Rav Gavriel Tzinner, see *Nitei Gavriel, Nisuin*, ch. 45, fn. 4. *Likkutei Sichos*, vol. 34, p. 291.

37 See *Rashi* to *Devarim* 16:22.

38 Especially in cases where children are more observant than their parents and their parents have already "compromised" considerably in allowing what is absolutely *halachically* necessary.

39 *Beis Shmuel, Even Ha'ezer* 62:11.

40 *Igros Kodesh*, vol. 9, pp. 1-3.

parents of the bride or groom sit together, while family and friends form a circle and dance around them to the tune of an upbeat Klezmer melody, "*Di Mezinke Oysgegebn*, The Youngest Daughter/Son is Given Away." Typically, all of the children – the *kallah* and *chatan* as well as the *mezinke's* siblings – often with their spouses – and all of the grandchildren – often with their spouses – dance around the parents/grandparents. This practice has become so entrenched that people assume it must have a storied place in our history.[41] In truth, the *mezinke tantz* is actually not a *minhag Yisroel* and in point of fact can easily lead to behaviors that contravene *halacha*.

Marrying off the youngest child is indeed a huge *simchah*, and we should show our gratitude to Hashem for bringing us to this occasion. The way we celebrate, however, must appropriately reflect *halacha* and our holy *minhagim*.

Understanding the holiness of the *chatuna* day, learning the deep meaning of the *brachot* said under the *chuppah*, and exploring the significance of the *minhagim* helps us approach this day with awe, humility and deep gratitude for the remarkable blessings Hashem showers on the *kallah* and her *chatan* on this day.

An earlier version of this essay appeared in the N'shei Chabad Newletter.
Special thanks to Rishe Deitch, editor.

---

[41] Often a "crowning ceremony" takes place wherein the mother holds a broom and laurels are placed on the heads of both parents. How did this non Jewish custom become so prominent at Jewish weddings? According to Lubow Wolynetz, curator of the folk art collection at the Ukrainian Museum in New York: "*When the [Ukrainian] wedding celebrations (during the second half of the nineteenth century) were coming to the end (after a few days), wedding guests would put the parents of the bride or groom on a wagon and take them to the village inn (bar) for the so-called "selling of the parents," which meant the parents had to buy everyone a drink. If the parents married off their last child (son or daughter) then the guests would make wreaths and place them on the heads of the parents and thus take them to the village inn. In this frolicking way the wedding celebrations would come to the end.*"

In the 1800s, many village inns and taverns in the Ukraine were owned or operated by Jewish families. Wolynetz noted, therefore, every time the parents of the newlyweds came into the taverns wearing wreaths and treated everyone to a drink, the Jewish tavern owners saw this. It is very likely that this is how the custom came to be part of the Jewish wedding. Dr. Ruth R. Wisse, professor of Yiddish literature at Harvard, for her theory opines: "The spread of the *mizinke krensl* custom in America is due to the bands that perform at weddings. They organize [the *mizinke*] as part of their routines — without necessarily consulting the families (and occasionally to their great surprise). Cited from *Exploring One of the Most Puzzling Rituals at a Jewish Wedding By Rabbi Reuven Becker.*

Glossary

achat bashana. [Only] once a year.

adamah. Earth.

ahavat Yisrael. Love for a fellow Jew.

Aibershter. Literally translated from Yiddish as the one above, is an endearing term to refer to Hashem.

akeret habayit. Literally the anchor of the home. This phrase is used to describe the woman's role in her family.

Am Yisrael. The nation of Israel.

Arizal. Also known as Rabbi Yitzchak Luria, lived from 1534-1572 and is one of the most celebrated Kabbalists of all time.

aron kodesh. A closet where the Torah is housed in synagogues, most often referred to as the holy ark.

aseret hadibrot. The ten commandments.

Aspaklaria meira. Literally translated from Hebrew as a clear and illuminated lens. In Hebrew, this phrase refers to an exalted (and rare) form of prophecy.

Aspaklaria she'eina meira. Literally translated from Hebrew as a lens that is blurry and unclear, dark and unlit, this phrase refers to a secondary form of prophecy.

aveirah. Transgression.

avodah. Work, particularly spiritual work.

Avodat hakodesh. Holy work in Hebrew, this is a phrase used to keep the mitzvot and Hashem's will.

Azarah. Refers to the courtyard, the largest area in the Mishkan.

Bais Rivkah. The flagship girl's high school of the Lubavitch movement located in Crown Heights, Brooklyn, New York.

baal(at) teshuvah. Literally translated from Hebrew as a master of return, this term refers to a Jewish person who takes on the observance of Torah and mitzvot without necessarily having been raised and schooled in that lifestyle.

balabuste. Translated from Yiddish as owner (feminine) the term is most often used to describe a woman with superior domestic skills.

Baruch Hashem. Thank G-d.

bashert. Literally translated from Yiddish as meant to be or destined, the term most often refers to one's predestined soul mate.

bat melech. Literally translated from Hebrew as a daughter of a king, this a phrase used to refer to Jewish women and girls, who are G-d's daughters.

Batei Mikdash. The first and second Temples in Jerusalem. Plural for Beit Hamikdash.

bayit ne'eman b'yisrael. A faithful home among the Jewish people.

bechirah chofshit. Hebrew for free will.

bedeken. Literally translated from Yiddish as the covering, this term refers to the chatan veiling his kallah's face just before they are led to the chuppah.

bedika cloth. Check in Hebrew. This phrase refers to a white cloth that women use to check their nidah status in compliance with halacha. The cloth is sometimes referred to as ed, Hebrew for witness since it provides testimony regarding her status.

be'ilat mitzvah. Literally translated from Hebrew as the intercourse of mitzvah; this term refers to consummating the marriage. This is the final aspect of the nissuin, marriage.

beinoni. Literally translated from Hebrew as average, this term, as used in the Tanya refers to one who never sins yet continues to struggle with the evil inclination or animal soul.

Beit Hamikdash. The Jewish temple in Jerusalem.

bentching. Yiddish for grace after meals. In Hebrew, this is called birkat hamazon.

Glossary

betulah. Virgin.

biah. Literally translated from Hebrew as coming, this term is used to mean coming together in sexual relations.

binah yeteira. Translated from Hebrew as additional understanding. Colloquially, it refers to the extra measure of feminine wisdom and intuition.

binyan adei ad. Translated as an everlasting edifice, this refers to an eternal familial structure built up through children and their children's progeny.

bitachon. Faith.

bittul. Self effacement.

b'kedushah u'b'taharah. In sanctity and purity.

Bnei Yisrael. The children of Israel.

bodeket. (plural: bodkot) Translated from Hebrew as an examiner, the term refers to women with both medical background and halachic training who examine women to determine the facts surrounding gynecological issues that have a bearing on hilchot nidah.

bracha. Blessing.

brit milah. Circumcision.

b'simchah. In joy.

b'tzelem Elokim. In the image of the divine. This is how the Torah refers to human creation: that humans were created in the image of the divine.

b'yichud. Alone together.

Chabad Chassidut. A chassidic movement and very specific philosophy founded by Rabbi Schneur Zalman of Liadi in the latter part of the 18th century. Chabad emphasizes the concepts of studying and understanding G-d and His relationship with the world as well as ahavat yisrael, love for every Jew. The movement is also known as Lubavitch, the name of the town in White Russia that served as the center of the Chabad Chassidism for four generations.

chachamim. Sages.

chadar hamitot. The bedroom.

chagorot. Literally means girdles. In context, it refers to what Adam and Chava used to clothe their bodies.

chas v'shalom. G-d forbid.

chassid. Literally pious. (a) One who goes beyond the letter of the law (b) a member of the chassidic community. One who follows the ways of chassidism and studies its teachings.

chassidut. The movement was founded in 1734 by Rabbi Yisrael Baal Shem Tov. It aims to inspire Jews with the mystical concepts of the Kabbalah, teaching everyone at their level how to understand these concepts and use them to build a personal, loving relationship with G-d.

chatan. (plural: chatanim) Groom.

chatan teacher. Instructor for the laws of family purity for bridegrooms.

chatzot. A halachic term referring to midday or midnight.

chayot hakodesh. Literally translated from Hebrew as holy animals, this is a liturgical term that refers to celestial angels.

cheshbon hanefesh. Taking stock of your spiritual standing.

chet. Sin. When referred to as pre-chet or post-chet, this refers to Chava and Adam partaking of the Tree of Knowledge.

Chet Eitz HaDaat Tov v'Ra. The sin of the Tree of Knowledge of Good and Evil in Gan Eden.

chibbur. Connection.

chizuk. Literally translated from Hebrew as strength, the term is used to connote encouragement and bolstering.

chovah. Responsibility.

chuppah. Marital canopy.

chumra. Stringency.

daat. Knowledge or consciousness.

dam makkah. Blood due to injury. This term refers to vaginal bleeding as a result of a wound or naturally occurring injury to the cervix, vaginal walls, or labia, which does not cause a woman to become nidah.

dam nidah. Literally translated as blood of nidah, this term refers to uterine based bleeding which causes a woman to become a nidah.

dat Moshe. Translated as the law of Moshe, the term when used in primary Jewish texts refers to Biblical law.

Glossary

dat Yehudit. Translated as the law of the Jewish Woman, the term when used in primary Jewish texts refers to the laws of normative modesty accepted by Jewish women and codified in Jewish law.

daven. Pray.

dinei harchakah. Literally translated as the laws of distancing, it refers to the laws and customs that delineate a couple's physical relationship during her time of nidah.

dirah betachtonim. Literally translated as a dwelling in the lower realm, refers to the spiritual transformation of this world into an abode for the Divine presence.

dirah lo yitbarech. A dwelling place for the blessed G-d. See the above entry.

Dirah na'eh. A beautiful home.

d'orayta. From or of the Torah.

d'rabanan. From or of the Rabbinic teachings.

echad. One or oneness.

eidim. Legal witnesses acceptable to a beit din, a Jewish court.

Elokut. G-dliness.

emunah peshutah. Simple [pure] faith.

erusin. The betrothal phase. This is also referred to in halacha as kiddushin. In a halachic marriage, there are two phases, and betrothal is the first.

erva. Defined in halacha as nakedness or those parts of the body that are meant to be concealed.

Even Ha'ezer. One of the four books of the Shulchan Aruch that primarily deals with marriage and relations. For more, see Shulchan Aruch.

Farbrengen. A gathering of chassidim where honest discussion, Torah learning, and singing of niggunim, Chassidic melodies, takes place.

frum. Traditionally observant of Jewish law.

gashmiyut. Physical, material matter.

Gan Eden. The garden of Eden.

Gan Eden Mikedem. Literally Gan Eden of the east, this term refers to the pristine wholeness and wholesomeness that preceded the original sin.

Gehinom. The Jewish concept most akin to hell or purgatory.

Gemara. Also referred to as the Talmud, this is Jewish oral Torah, as codified in the Babylonian and Jerusalem Talmud.

Gematria. The numerical value of each letter in the Hebrew Alphabet, i.e. alef=1, bet=2, etc. In Jewish study, specifically in mysticism, the names of the letters, their shapes, and their numerical value are each laden with meaning.

Get. Religious divorce. The Get is the literal divorce document that a man gives to his wife as a means to formalize the divorce process. This is done through a Beit Din, a religious court.

geulah. Redemption.

gezeirah. Decree (usually of negative variety).

gilgulim. Literally translated as those who came back through the process of reincarnation, it is the term for the concept of reincarnation in Hebrew.

guf. (plural: gufim) Body.

Hakadosh Baruch Hu. The Holy One Blessed be He, a name for G-d.

halacha. Codified Jewish law. The term is etymologically rooted in the Hebrew word halichah, to walk. (plural: halachot; adjective: halachic)

hanhagah. (plural: hanhagot) Practice or practices.

Har Habayit. Temple Mount.

harchakot. Laws of distancing. This is the spoken vernacular for dinei harchaka.

Hashgachah Elyonah. literally translated as celestial oversight, a term used to refer to the concept of Divine providence.

Hashgachah pratit. literally translated as individualized oversight, a term used to refer to the concept of Divine providence.

hashkafah. Outlook, perspective. (adjective: hashkafic)

hatzlachah (Rabba). (Great) Success.

hefsek taharah. This term refers to the simple vaginal inspection a woman makes to ascertain the end of her period. At that point, she begins counting her sheva nekiyim, seven clean days, before immersing in the mikvah.

heter. Halachic dispensation.

hilchot yichud. The laws about members of the opposite gender (barring immediate family members) being secluded.

hirhur. Sexual thoughts or ideation.

Glossary

hishtadlut. Efforts.

hitkadshut. Elevating and consecrating each detail of our corporeal lives.

hitkashrut. Connection.

hotzaat zera levatalah. Literally translated as releasing seed/sperm in vain. This is a halachic concept that refers to ejaculation outside of a woman's vagina.

Imahot. Literally mothers, this Hebrew word most often refers to the Biblical mothers, Sarah, Rebecca, Rachel and Leah.

issur d'orayta. Biblical prohibition.

issur karet. A specific type of Biblical prohibition, whose consequence is being spiritually cut off from the Jewish people.

Kabbalah. Jewish mysticism.

Kabbalat Ol. Literally means accepting the yoke, This refers to accepting all of G-d's commandments and submitting to the Divine desire.

Kadosh. Holy.

kallah. (plural: kallot) Bride.

kallah teacher. A woman who instructs engaged women about the laws of taharat hamishpachah, and often imparts more general relationship advice as well.

Kashrut. The dietary laws as delineated in the Torah and halacha, may also be used to refer to the kosher status of a given food.

kav. Translated as a line, this is a Kabbalistic term for the vector of concentrated G-dly light that exists in the universe.

kavanah. Intention.

kavyochal. As it were.

kedushah. Holiness.

kedushat hazivug. Literally the holiness of the couple, this means consecration within sexual intimacy.

keilim. Vessels. In Kabbalistic and Chassidic teachings this often refers to a conduit or receptacle for spiritual energy or blessing.

kelipah. Literally translated as the outer shell, this term is used widely in mystical teaching to refer to unholy powers that both obscure and at the same time feed off of the sacred just as the shell of fruit receives its vivifying force from the fruit itself.

keruvim. The cherubs that were located atop the ark in the Batei Mikdash.

ketoret. Incense. This was burned daily in the Batei Mikdash.

ketubah. Marriage contract.

kiddush. Ritual prayer over wine on Shabbat and holidays.

Kiddush Hashem. Sanctifying G-d's name.

kiddushin. Literally translated as the consecration, this is the term most often used to refer to Jewish marriage.

kisui rosh. Literally covering of the head, the term used for the mitzvah of a married woman covering her hair.

Knesset Yisrael. Literally translated as the community of Israel, this endearing term for the Jewish people is used often when describing the relationship between the Jewish people and G-d.

kochot hanefesh. Literally translated as the strengths of the soul, this refers to the kabbalistic and chassidic teachings regarding the ten aspects of our psyche, which are subdivided into our cognitive abilities, chochmah, binah, and daat, and our seven emotive expressions, chessed, gevurah, tiferet etc.

Kodesh Hakodashim. The holy of holies in the Batei Mikdash.

Kohen Gadol. (plural: Kohanim Gedolim) High priest.

kolanit. The Gemara uses this term to describe a woman whose voice can be heard by others, specifically regarding matters involving sexual intimacy.

korbanot. Ritual sacrifices.

Kriat HaTorah. Reading of the Torah.

Kudsha Brich Hu. A mystical term that refers to the male aspect of the G-dhead.

levushim. Garments. In Chassidic teachings, this term often refers to "garments" of the soul.

Lubavitcher Rebbe. Rabbi Menachem Mendel Schneerson (1902-1994) was the seventh leader in the Chabad Lubavitch dynasty, and is considered to have been one of the most phenomenal Jewish personalities of modern times.

Luchot. The tablets that were brought down from Mount Sinai containing the ten commandments.

maasim tovim. Good deeds.

machshavah. Thought or contemplation.

malachim. Celestial angels.

Glossary

Mamlechet Kohanim V'goy Kadosh. Quoted from the verse in Vayikra, Leviticus, this term means a kingdom of priests and sacred nation and refers to the Jewish people.

Mashiach. Messiah.

mashpia. A mentor for spiritual matters and questions.

Matan Torah. The giving of the Torah.

mekabel. Receiver.

melicha. Salting meat and chicken to make it kosher.

menorah. The gold candelabrum lit by the Kohanim, in the Mishkan and Batei Mikdash each day.

menuchat hanefesh. Literally rest of the soul, this means calm and equanimity.

mesader kiddushin. The wedding officiant.

mesirat nefesh. Self-sacrifice.

mesorah. Tradition.

midbar. Desert.

mikdash me'at. Literally a small temple, this refers to how each home is ideally a microcosm of the Temple.

mikvah. Ritual bath.

minhag. (plural: minhagim) Custom.

minyan. A quorum of ten men, necessary for many formalized Jewish rituals.

mishna. Codified oral law.

mishkan. The Tabernacle in the desert.

Mitzrayim. Biblical Egypt.

mitzvah. (plural: mitzvot) Commandment or deed written in or based on the Torah.

mitzvot asei. Positive commandments or deeds.

mitzvot lo ta'aseh. Negative commandments or prohibitions.

mivtza'im. Literally campaigns, this term refers to the Rebbe's ten point Mitzvah campaign.

mizbeach hazahav. The golden altar in the Beit Hamikdash.

nachat. The singular happiness and pleasure derived from the accomplishments and achievements of loved ones, especially children and grandchildren.

Nefesh Eloki(t). Literally the G-dly soul, the term used in the Tanya to refer to the spiritual aspect or force within the person that is driven by the Divine alone.

nefesh habehamit. Literally the animal soul, the term used in the Tanya to refer to the vivifying force of the person that is driven by selfishness.

neshamah. (plural: neshamot) Soul.

nesiut. Leadership.

neviim. Prophets.

nevuah. Prophetic perception of the Divine or Divine visions.

nidah. Biblical term for a menstruant woman.

nigleh. Literally, the revealed, this term refers to the exoteric dimensions of the Torah.

niggun. (plural: niggunim) Wordless melody.

nissuin. A halachic term for marriage, specifically, the second aspect of marriage which is preceded by erusin, also referred to as kiddushin.

nisyonot. Trials and tribulations.

nitzotzot. Sparks.

Nitzut Eloki. G-dly spark

nitzutzei kedushah. Sparks of divinity.

Olam Haba. The world to come.

Olam Hazeh Hagashmi. This physical world.

onah. (plural: onot) Literally translated from Hebrew as season, this term, when used within Jewish law refers to the Biblical commandment for a man to provide his wife with sexual pleasure. When used within the system of family purity, this term also refers to particular increments in time.

Or Ein Sof. Literally, the endless light, this kabbalistic term refers to the infinity of G-d.

Or Eloki. A Divine light.

or makif. The kabbalistic concept meaning an encompassing celestial light or energy.

or pnimi. The kabbalistic concept meaning an internal celestial light or energy.

orot. Plural for lights. In Kabbalistic and Chassidic teachings this often refers to a celestial emanation or energy.

parnassah. Livelihood or income.

Glossary

parochet. Curtain.

passuk. (plural: pessukim) Biblical verse.

pru u'rvu. Translated as be fruitful and multiply, this is how the Torah phrases the mitzvah to have children.

psak. a Rabbinic ruling on Jewish law.

Ratzon Ha'Elyon. Celestial will.

ruchniyut. Spirituality.

sefer. Holy book.

sefirot. In Kabbalah, this refers to the ten aspects of the Divine, and the way this is mirrored in each individual's inner landscape.

segulah. A spiritually propitious action or conduit for blessing.

sh'aila. (plural: sh'ailot) Translated from Hebrew as question, the term refers to a question regarding Jewish law.

shalom bayit. Martial peace and domestic harmony.

shamayim. Heaven, the place of the Heavenly throne.

shana rishonah. The first year of marriage.

Shechinah. Divine presence.

Shechinta. The mystical term for the female aspect of the G-dhead.

sheitel. (plural: sheitlach) The Yiddish word for wig.

Shem Havaya. The name of G-d often referred to as the Tetragrammaton. It is synonymous with Divine thought and emotion.

shemitah. The Sabbatical year.

shemoneh esrei. Literally translated as eighteen, this term refers to the silent devotion, otherwise referred to as the amida, which is the central aspect of Jewish prayer.

sheva brachot. Seven blessings recited under the chuppa and for the week after the wedding, every time a quorum of ten men is present at a meal.

shidduch. Literally translated from Hebrew as a match, the term most often refers to the traditional way in which many observant Jews meet each other upon the suggestion of a third party.

Shir Hashirim. Translated as The Song of Songs, a Biblical text written by King Solomon that describes an intense love understood to refer to the relationship between G-d and the Jewish people.

shitot. Opinions.

shivah nekiyim. Literally translated from Hebrew as the seven clean ones, the term refers to the week preceding a woman's immersion in the mikvah. After a woman does her hefsek tahara, thus confirming that her period is over, she counts these seven clean days and then immerses in the mikvah.

shlichut. The concept of being sent as an emissary or proxy for someone.

shluchah. A female emissary of the Rebbe of Chabad. Her male counterpart is a shaliach.

shulchan. Table.

Shulchan Aruch. The Code of Jewish Law which is comprised of four sections: Orach Chaim, Way of Life, covers prayer, Shabbat and holidays, and other issues encountered in day to day life. Yoreh Dei'ah, He Shall Show Understanding, includes the intricate laws of kosher, usury, vows, and other areas in which a rabbi is generally consulted. Even Ha'ezer, Stone of Assistance, contains laws of marriage, divorce etc. Choshen Mishpat, Breastplate of Justice, is devoted to monetary laws, torts, and other issues relevant to a rabbinic court.

simchah. Happiness.

sitra achara. Literally translated as the other side, this Kabbalistic concept refers to the forces of evil.

tahara. Purity.

taharat hamishpachah. Literally defined as family purity, the term refers to the halachot surrounding marital intimacy.

talmidei chachamim. Scholars.

Tanach. An abbreviation for **T**orah (5 books of Moses), **N**eviim (Prophets), and **K**etuvim (Writings).

tashmish hamitah. Literally means using the bed, a halachic term for sexual relations.

tefillot. Prayers.

tehorah. Ritually pure.

teshuvah. Repentance.

tevilah. The act of immersion, bathing in a ritual pool.

Glossary

tichel. Kerchief.

tikkun. Rectification.

Torah Shebaal Peh. Oral Torah, comprised of the Mishna and the Gemara.

toveling. Bathing in a ritual pool.

tzaddik. Righteous individual.

tzemichah. Growth.

tzimtzum. Contraction.

tzniut. Modesty.

yahrzeit. Anniversary of death.

yechidut. A private audience with the Rebbe.

Yemot HaMashiach. The days of the Messianic era.

yeridah. Descent.

yetzer hara. Bad inclination.

yetzer tov. Good inclination.

yichud. Secluded privately.

Yiddishkeit. Judaism in Yiddish.

Yom Kippur. The day of atonement, the Holiest day of the Jewish year.

yovel. The Jubilee year.

zechut. Merit.

zivug. Coupling.

Zohar. The Zohar is the primary text of Jewish mysticism, Kabbalah. Written as a commentary to the Torah, the Zohar itself attributes its disclosure of the Torah's mysteries to R. Shimon bar Yochai (known by the acronym "Rashbi"), a second-century sage, and his disciples, including his son R. Elazar.

About the Authors

Sara Morozow

Sara Morozow is a Brooklyn based scholar, beloved *mashpia* and much sought after counselor. Morozow teaches and mentors at the Beth Rivkah Seminary in Crown Heights and is the program director at Mikvah.org. In that capacity she has created a host of online programming focusing on various aspects of family life. After teaching *kallah* classes for over two decades, Morozow created the curriculum for, and is the dean of Mikvah.org's Kallah Teachers Training program. She is also a consultant to Kallah teachers of all backgrounds from around the globe.

Rivkah Slonim

Rivkah Slonim is the Associate Director at the Rohr Chabad Center for Jewish Student Life at Binghamton University which she co-founded with her husband Rabbi Aaron Slonim in 1985. A self described Chassidic Feminist, Slonim is an internationally known lecturer, and activist. Slonim is the editor of Total Immersion: A Mikvah Anthology (Jason Aronson 1996, Urim 2006) and Bread and Fire; Jewish Women find G-d in the Everyday (Urim 2008). Slonim serves on the Editorial Board of the Rohr Jewish Learning Institute and is co-author of one of JLI's most popular courses, Fascinating Facts. She sits on the executive boards of Tamim Academy as well as the Institute of Jewish Spirituality and Society.

Made in the USA
Middletown, DE
13 March 2025